Mayo Clinic
GUIDE TO SELF-CARE
SEVENTH EDITION

Answers for everyday health problems

Cindy A. Kermott, M.D., M.P.H.
Medical Editor

Martha P. Millman, M.D., M.P.H.
Medical Editor

Seventh Edition

Mayo Clinic
Rochester, Minnesota
Jacksonville, Florida
Scottsdale/Phoenix, Arizona

Published by Mayo Clinic

© 2017 Mayo Foundation for Medical Education and Research

Mayo Clinic Guide to Self-Care provides reliable, practical, easy-to-understand information on issues relating to good health. Much of its information comes from physicians, nurses, dietitians, research scientists and other health care professionals at Mayo Clinic. This book is intended to supplement the advice of your personal physician, whom you should consult about your individual medical condition. *Mayo Clinic Guide to Self-Care* does not endorse any company or product.

For bulk sales to employers, member groups and health-related companies, write Mayo Clinic, 200 First St. SW, Rochester, MN 55905, call 800-430-9699, or email *SpecialSalesMayoBooks@Mayo.edu*.

Library of Congress Control Number: 2009938854

Seventh Edition

Printed in the USA

Introduction

Nearly two decades ago, Dr. Philip Hagen had a vision for developing a Mayo Clinic guide for consumers that would empower people to take charge of their health. He called on his colleagues to share their expertise on more than 150 topics. Today that number has grown to more than 300 topics — from how to handle medical emergencies to how to deal with common problems such as back pain.

It all started with a review of the top reasons adults and children visit a doctor, based on discussion with Mayo Clinic physicians, nurses and others. The team also consulted with health care providers, employers and managers of corporate health programs to learn what illnesses and injuries are common in the workplace.

The result is an invaluable resource that focuses on how to *prevent illness*, how to *detect illness* before it becomes a serious and costly problem, and how to *avoid unnecessary trips* to the clinic or emergency room.

New in this 7th edition

It is our pleasure to provide an upgraded, now the seventh, edition of the *Mayo Clinic Guide to Self-Care*. Following the tradition of collecting expert recommendations of our colleague physicians and other health professionals, we offer guidance on the care of over 300 health conditions. We continue to focus on ways to reduce illness risk and strategies for the evaluation and early treatment of common conditions.

We thank our Mayo Clinic colleagues who reviewed every page of this edition and added the latest guidelines, medical recommendations and self-care tips to help you take charge of your health. In this edition you will find:

- A completely revised CPR section, including easy-to learn hands-only CPR for adults
- New adult screening guidelines, as well as new adult and pediatric immunization guidelines
- The latest on smoking cessation and managing alcohol use
- Research and recommendations on popular integrative medicine therapies and approaches
- Healthy cooking tips, updated fitness recommendations — and much more

We hope you'll keep this book handy so you can learn what to do in an emergency, when to contact your doctor, and what steps you and your family can take to maintain the best of health. That's what self-care is all about.

Cindy A. Kermott, M.D., M.P.H.
Medical Editor

Martha P. Millman, M.D., M.P.H.
Medical Editor

Editorial staff

Medical Editors
Cindy A. Kermott, M.D., M.P.H.
Martha P. Millman, M.D., M.P.H.

Editorial Director
Paula M. Marlow-Limbeck

Senior Editor
Karen R. Wallevand

Managing Editor
Jennifer L. Jacobson

Product Manager
Christopher C. Frye

Illustration and Production
Kent McDaniel
Gunnar T. Soroos

Editorial Research
Abbie Y. Brown
Deirdre A. Herman
Erika A. Riggin
Katie J. Warner

Proofreading
Miranda M. Attlesey
Alison K. Baker
Julie M. Maas

Indexing
Steve Rath

Administrative Assistants
Katie S. Palbicki
Terri L. Zanto-Strausbauch

Contributors

Daniel A. Assad, D.D.S
Sophie J. Bakri, M.D.
Keith A. Bengtson, M.D.
Christopher L. Boswell, M.D.
Jeffrey S. Brault, D.O.
Sara W. Brevik, RDN, LD
Lisa K. Buss-Preszler,
   Pharm.D., R.Ph.
Petra M. Casey, M.D.
Tony Y. Chon, M.D.
Bart L. Clarke, M.D.
David W. Claypool, M.D.
Edward T. Creagan, M.D.
Diana S. Dean, M.D.
Martin G. Ellman, D.P.M.
Floranne C. Ernste, M.D.
Kevin C. Fleming, M.D.
Amy E. Foxx-Orenstein, D.O.

Matthew T. Gettman, M.D.
Karthik Ghosh, M.D.
Donald D. Hensrud, M.D.
Cynthia A. Hogan, Ph.D.
W. Michael Hooten, M.D.
Robert M. Jacobson, M.D.
Amer N. Kalaaji, M.D.
Mary J. Kasten, M.D.
Frank P. Kennedy, M.D.
Stephen L. Kopecky, M.D.
Lois E. Krahn, M.D.
Esther H. Krych, M.D.
Edward R. Laskowski, M.D.
Devyani Lal, M.D.
James T. Li, M.D., Ph.D.
Sharon E. Libi, M.D.
Timothy J. Milbrandt, M.S., C.T.T.S.
Robin G. Molella, M.D.

Brian A. Neff, M.D.
Eric J. Olson, M.D.
David E. Patterson, M.D.
Gregory A. Poland, M.D.
Stacey A. Rizza, M.D.
Carrie (Beth) E. Robertson, M.D.
Teresa A. Rummans, M.D.
Nicole P. Sandhu, M.D., Ph.D.
Priya Sampathkumar, M.D.
Terry D. Schneekloth, M.D.
James M. Steckelberg, M.D.
Sandra J. Taler, M.D.
Carmen M. Terzic, M.D., Ph.D.
Jacqueline N. Thielen, M.D.
Maria G. Valdes, M.D.
Andrew I. Vaughn, M.D.
Gerald W. Volcheck, M.D.
Debra A. Zillmer, M.D.

How to use this book

Mayo Clinic Guide to Self-Care, Seventh Edition, provides reliable, practical, easy-to-understand information on more than 300 common medical conditions and issues relating to your health.

No book can replace the advice of your doctor or other health care provider. Instead, our intent is to help you understand and safely manage some common health problems. In addition, you'll learn how to recognize serious problems so that you'll know when to contact your health care provider and when to call 911 or your local emergency number.

How this book is organized

Most chapters in *Mayo Clinic Guide to Self-Care* begin with a general discussion of the health topic, sometimes including signs and symptoms and a summary of the cause. Next, look for:

- Self-care and prevention suggestions highlighted in blue shading
- "Medical help" headings, which advise you when to see a doctor or other health care provider and what kind of treatment you might expect
- "Kids' care" headings when there's special information regarding children (however, the book is not meant to be a comprehensive resource of childhood illnesses)
- Information in gray boxes related to topics on a page

In the table of contents, you'll find eight major sections:

- Emergencies and urgent care
- General symptoms
- Common problems
- Specific conditions
- Mental health
- Staying healthy
- Your health and the workplace
- The healthy consumer

Browse the contents to get familiar with the topics and the format. Don't forget the index at the back. Scan the book so that you know where to look when specific health concerns arise.

What the blue symbol means

Many pages have words that are in blue and underlined. At the bottom of those pages, you'll see a blue symbol. This means that you can find more information on the underlined topic by going online. See the back cover of this book for information on the website.

Ready, Check, Go!

For a quick health check, before reading on, go to "Ready, Check, Go!" on page xiii. In just a few minutes, you'll be started on your personal self-care program. You'll find brief health tips that you can use right now!

About Mayo Clinic

Mayo Clinic evolved from the frontier practice of Dr. William Worrall Mayo and the partnership of his two sons, Drs. William J. and Charles H. Mayo, in the early 1900s. Pressed by the demands of their busy practice in Rochester, Minnesota, the Mayo brothers invited other doctors to join them, pioneering the private group practice of medicine. Today, with thousands of physicians and scientists at its three major locations in Rochester, Minnesota, Jacksonville, Florida, and Phoenix/Scottsdale, Arizona, and its regional community-based health care practices, Mayo Clinic is dedicated to providing comprehensive diagnoses, accurate answers and effective treatments.

   With this depth of knowledge, experience and expertise, Mayo Clinic occupies an unparalleled position as a health information resource. Since 1983, Mayo Clinic has published reliable health information for millions of consumers through a variety of award-winning newsletters, books and online services. Revenue from the publishing activities supports Mayo Clinic programs, including medical education and research.

Table of contents

READY, CHECK, GO!   xiii

EMERGENCIES AND
URGENT CARE   1
CPR   2
Choking   4
Heart attack   5
Stroke   7
Poisoning emergencies   9
Severe bleeding   10
Shock   11
Allergic reactions   12
   Food allergies   12
   Drug allergies   13
Bites and stings   14
   Animal bites   14
   Human bites   14
   Snakebites   15
   Insect bites and stings   15
   Spider bites   16
   Tick bites   16
Burns   17
   Chemical burns   18
   Sunburn   19
   Electrical burns   19
Cold-weather problems   20
   Frostbite   20
   Hypothermia   21
Cuts, scrapes and wounds   22
   Simple wounds   22
   Puncture wounds   23
Eye injuries   24
   Corneal abrasion (scratch)   24
   Chemical splash   24
   Foreign object in the eye   25
Foodborne illness   26

Heat-related problems   28
Poisonous plants   29
Tooth problems   30
   Toothache   30
   Tooth loss   30
Trauma: Bones and muscles   31
   Dislocations   31
   Fractures   31
   Sprains   32
Trauma: Head injuries   32

GENERAL SYMPTOMS   33
Dizziness and fainting   34
Fatigue   36
Fever   38
Pain   40
   Common forms of chronic pain   41
   Treatment for chronic pain   43
Sleep disorders   44
   Insomnia   44
   Other sleep disorders   45
Sweating and body odor   46
Unexpected weight changes   47
   Weight gain   47
   Unexplained weight loss   47

COMMON PROBLEMS   49
Back and neck   50
   Common back and neck problems   51
   Other back and neck problems   53
   Preventing back injuries in the
     workplace   53
   Preventing common backaches
     and neck pains   54
   Your daily back routine   55

Digestive system   **56**
    Abdominal pain and discomfort   56
    Colic   57
    Constipation   58
    Diarrhea   59
    Excessive gas and gas pains   60
    Gallstones   61
    Gastritis   61
    Hemorrhoids and rectal bleeding   62
    Hernias   63
    Indigestion and heartburn   64
    Irritable bowel syndrome   65
    Nausea and vomiting   66
    Peptic ulcers   67

Ears and hearing   **68**
    Airplane ear   68
    Foreign objects in the ear   69
    Ruptured eardrum   69
    Ear infections   70
    Ringing in your ear   72
    Swimmer's ear   72
    Wax blockage   73
    Noise-related hearing loss   74
    Age-related hearing loss   75

Eyes and vision   **76**
    Black eye   76
    Dry eyes   77
    Excessive watering   77
    Floaters   77
    Pink eye   78
    Sensitivity to glare   79
    Other eye problems   79
    Common eye diseases   80
    Problems related to glasses and
       contact lenses   81

Headache   **82**

Limbs, muscles, bones and joints   **85**
    Muscle strains: When you've
       overdone it   87
    Sprains: Damage to your ligaments   88
    Broken bones (fractures)   89
    Bursitis   90
    Tendinitis   90

    Fibromyalgia   91
    Gout   92
    Shoulder pain   92
    Elbow and forearm pain   93
    Wrist, hand and finger pain   95
    Hip pain   97
    Leg pain   98
    Knee pain   100
    Ankle and foot pain   102

Lungs, chest and breathing   **107**
    Coughing: A natural reflex   107
    Bronchitis   109
    Croup   109
    Wheezing   110
    Shortness of breath   110
    Chest pain   111
    Palpitations   111

Nose and sinuses   **112**
    Foreign objects in the nose   112
    Loss of sense of smell   112
    Nosebleeds   113
    Stuffy nose   114
    Runny nose   114
    Sinusitis   116

Skin, hair and nails   **117**
    Proper skin care   117
    Acne   118
    Boils   118
    Cellulitis   119
    MRSA infection   119
    Corns and calluses   120
    Dandruff   120
    Dryness   121
    Eczema (dermatitis)   121
    Fungal infections   122
    Hives   123
    Impetigo   123
    Itching and rashes   124
    Baby rashes   124
    Lice   126
    Scabies   126
    Psoriasis   127
    Moles   127

Shingles	128
Signs of skin cancer	129
Warts	130
Wrinkled skin	130
Hair loss	131
Nail fungal infections	132
Ingrown toenails	132
Throat and mouth	**133**
Sore throat	133
Bad breath	135
Hoarseness or loss of voice	135
Mouth sores	136
Other oral infections and disorders	138
Men's health	**140**
Testicular pain	140
Enlarged prostate	141
Prostatitis	142
Erectile dysfunction (ED)	142
Male birth control	143
Women's health	**144**
Lump in your breast	144
Breast cancer	145
Pain in your breast	146
Menstrual cramps	146
Irregular periods	147
Bleeding between periods	147
Premenstrual syndrome	147
Menopause	149
Urination problems	150
Vaginal discharge	150
Cancer screening	151
Other common medical conditions	152
Pregnancy	154
Common problems during pregnancy	155

SPECIFIC CONDITIONS	**157**
Respiratory allergies	**158**
Thyroid disorders	**160**
Arthritis	**161**
Exercise	161
Medications control discomfort	163

Other methods to relieve pain	163
Joint protection	164
Asthma	**165**
Cancer	**168**
Signs, symptoms and screening	168
Diabetes	**172**
Heart disease	**177**
Hepatitis	**180**
High blood pressure	**182**
Sexually transmitted infections	**184**

MENTAL HEALTH	**187**
Addictive behavior	**188**
Alcohol use disorders	188
Treating alcohol use disorders	189
Individualized treatment	190
Smoking and tobacco use	192
How to stop smoking	192
Nicotine replacement therapy	193
Coping with nicotine withdrawal	194
Teenage smoking: What can be done?	195
Drug use and dependency	196
Compulsive gambling	197
Anxiety disorders	**198**
Generalized anxiety disorder	198
Social anxiety disorder	198
Post-traumatic stress disorder (PTSD)	199
Panic attacks and panic disorder	199
Depression	**200**
Causes of depression	201
Treatment options	202
Domestic violence	**203**
Memory loss	**204**

STAYING HEALTHY	**205**
Weight: What's healthy for you?	**206**
Determining your body mass index	206
Tips on losing weight	208

Physical activity: The key to
    burning calories 209
Healthy eating **210**
    Mayo Clinic Healthy Weight Pyramid 211
    Healthy cooking 212
Lowering your cholesterol **213**
Physical activity and fitness **215**
    Aerobic vs. anaerobic activity 215
    Starting a fitness program 216
    Walk your way to fitness 217
    Stretching exercises for walkers 219
Keeping stress under control **221**
    Stress suppresses immune system 221
    Stress increases risk of heart and
      blood vessel disease 221
    Stress worsens other illnesses 222
    Signs and symptoms of stress 222
Screening and immunization **225**
    Adult screening tests and
      procedures 225
    Adult immunizations 226
    Well-child immunization schedule 227
Protecting yourself **229**
    Emergency preparedness 229
    Reduce your risk on the road 231
    Reduce your risk at home 231
    Preventing falls 232
    Lead exposure 232
    Carbon monoxide poisoning 233
    Indoor air pollution 233
    Hand washing 234
Aging and your health **235**
    How age can affect your health 235
    Maintaining your health as you age 236

**YOUR HEALTH AND
THE WORKPLACE** **237**
**Health, safety and injury
    prevention** **238**
    Protect your back 238
    Hand and wrist care 238
    Coping with arthritis at work 239

Exercises for office workers 239
Safety in the workplace 241
Sleeping tips for shift workers 241
Drugs, alcohol and work 242
Stress relievers **243**
    Burned out? Get a tuneup 243
    Co-worker conflict: 6 steps to
      make peace 243
    5 tips for managing time 244
    Get to know your boss:
      Build a healthy relationship 244
    Halt hostility: Talk it out 244
Coping with technology **245**
    Computer screens and eyestrain 245

THE HEALTHY CONSUMER **247**
You and your health care provider **248**
    Start with primary care 248
    How to find a doctor 248
    Specialists you may need 250
Home medical testing kits **253**
Your family medical tree **254**
Medications and you **255**
    Ordering medications on the internet 256
    Pain relievers: Matching the pill
      to the pain 257
    Cold remedies: What they can
      and can't do 259
    Home medical supplies 260
Dietary supplements **261**
    Whole foods are your best source 264
    Should you take supplements? 264
    Vitamins and minerals: How much
      do you need? 265
    Choosing and using supplements 266
Integrative medicine **268**
    Check out claims of treatment
      success 269
    Natural products 270
    Mind-body medicine 272
    Other approaches 276
    5 steps in considering any treatment 278

The healthy traveler   **280**

    Traveler's diarrhea   280

    Heat exhaustion   280

    Blisters   280

    Altitude sickness   280

    Motion sickness   281

    Traveling abroad   281

    Vaccines for international travel   282

    Air travel hazards   283

    Questions and answers   284

    Travel information sources   286

INDEX   **287**

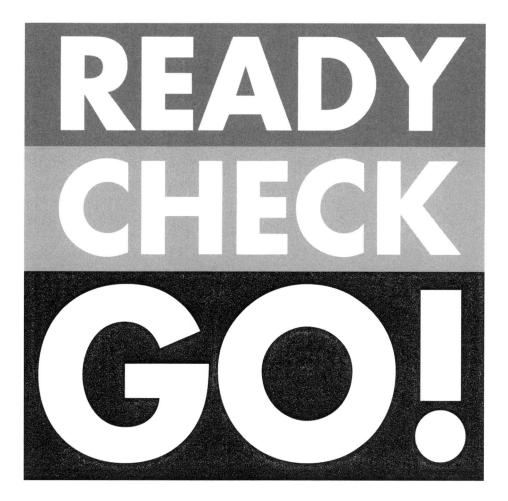

Put this book to work for you and your family today. Use "Ready, Check, Go!" to help you plan a healthier life.

Self-care is something you do every day. This book will help with many health problems — both routine and emergency — during the year. But these first pages have tips you can use *right now*. It takes just a few minutes to do the "Ready, Check, Go!" checklist. And what you learn may add years to your life.

What you'll need
- Pencil
- Bathroom scale
- Tape measure

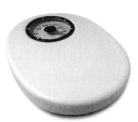

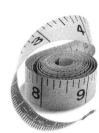

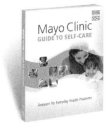

Get started

"Ready, Check, Go!" asks some basic questions about living a healthy life. If you breeze through them, you're probably already very healthy. If not, you'll have a good idea of what changes to make. First, make sure that you don't have a medical condition that might make it unsafe or unwise for you to make lifestyle changes.

Check all that apply

Do you have a significant medical condition for which you see a doctor regularly or take daily medication (examples include cancer, diabetes, heart disease, significant arthritis, asthma)?

Yes _____ → Go ahead and answer the "Ready, Check, Go!" questions, but before you follow the recommendations in this book, get your doctor's OK. In addition, look through "Specific Conditions" beginning on page 157 for more on your condition.

No _____ → Go to the next question.

For women: Are you pregnant?

Yes or not sure _____ → Talk with your doctor first. Read the pregnancy information, beginning on page 154.

No _____ → Go to the next question.

Do you have a condition for which you follow a special diet or that might be worsened by losing weight or exercising?

Yes _____ → Answer the questions, but before starting a weight-loss or exercise program, get your doctor's OK. Also look for information on your condition in "Common Problems," beginning on page 49.

No _____ → You're ready to go!

Step

Do you use tobacco?

Do you smoke or use smokeless tobacco (chew or snuff)?

Yes _____ → Tobacco use is a tough habit to break, but stopping could be the single most important health change you make. Smoking causes heart disease, strokes and cancer. It's never too late to stop. See pages 192-194 for how to stop smoking.

No _____ → Go to the next question.

Basic tobacco quit plan

1. List your top five reasons for quitting.
2. Identify your triggers and make plans to deal with them.
3. Set a quit date and get rid of all tobacco on that date.
4. Talk with your doctor about options such as nicotine replacement therapy or prescription medications.
5. Get support from family, friends and co-workers.

Tobacco facts: More than 480,000 Americans die of tobacco-related illness each year. Smoking can significantly increase your yearly health care costs. Figure out your yearly cost and see how much money you'd save if you stopped smoking.

How's your weight?

Find out your body mass index (BMI) and your waist size to see whether you're in the healthy weight zone and what your percentage of body fat is. To do this, you'll need a bathroom scale and a tape measure.

First, determine your BMI. To do this, use the handy BMI chart on page 207 and write your BMI here. _____

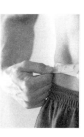

Or, for a more specific answer, use an online BMI calculator.

Next, measuring at the narrowest part of your abdomen, determine your waist circumference and write it here. _____

Generally:
If your BMI is less than 18.5, talk with your doctor — you may be underweight.
If your BMI is between 18.5 and 24.9, you're at a healthy weight.
If your BMI is 25 or greater, consider starting a weight-loss program (see page 208).

An ideal waist size is 40 inches or less for men and 35 inches or less for women.

Basic weight-loss plan
1. Set a weight-loss goal of 1 to 2 pounds a week.
2. Eat five or more servings of fruits and vegetables a day.
3. Increase your physical activity so you're doing at least 150 minutes a week.
4. Recruit a friend or family member for support.

Weight facts: More than two-thirds of all Americans are overweight. Being overweight increases the risk of diabetes, arthritis, heart disease and sleep disorders.

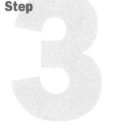

Step

Good nutrition

How many servings of:
Fruits do you eat each day? → _____
Vegetables do you eat each day? → +_____
=_____ *Total*

If your total is 5 or greater, go to the next step.
If not, see "Healthy eating," page 210, for tips on good nutrition.

Serving size

Vegetables	Calories	Visual cue
• 1 cup broccoli	25	1 baseball
• 2 cups raw, leafy greens	25	2 baseballs

Fruits	Calories	Visual cue
• ½ cup sliced fruit	60	Tennis ball
• 1 small apple or medium orange	60	

Carbohydrates	Calories	Visual cue
• ½ cup whole-grain pasta, brown rice or dried cereal	70	Hockey puck
• ½ whole-wheat bagel	70	
• 1 slice whole-grain bread	70	
• ½ medium baked potato	70	

Protein and dairy	Calories	Visual cue
• 3 ounces of fish	110	Deck of cards
• 2–2½ ounces of chicken or meat	110	½ deck of cards
• 2–2½ ounces of hard cheese	110	4 dice

Fats	Calories	Visual cue
• 1½ teaspoons peanut butter	45	2 dice
• 1 teaspoon butter or margarine	45	1 die

See the Mayo Clinic Healthy Weight Pyramid on page 211.

Basic healthy nutrition plan

1. Add one additional fruit or vegetable serving each week until you're getting five or more servings on most days.
2. Try at least one new healthy recipe each week.
3. Make sure you eat three healthy meals — including breakfast — every day.

Nutrition facts: Eating healthy foods can help prevent disease. For example, if you eat plenty of fruits and vegetables as part of a healthy diet, you may lower your risk of strokes, heart disease and certain types of cancer. Replacing butter, lard and other solid, saturated fats with healthier substitutes such as olive, canola and peanut oils can help lower your risk of heart disease.

Prevent disease or find it early

Here are suggested frequencies for having a preventive checkup with your doctor —
if you're in good health without symptoms or a chronic medical condition. However,
follow your doctor's recommendations.

Age	
20 to 29	At least twice in your 20s
30 to 39	At least three times in your 30s
40 to 49	At least four times in your 40s
50 to 59	At least five times in your 50s
60 and older	Yearly

Have you had a preventive checkup in the time frame for your age?

Yes _____ → Go to the next question.

No _____ → Make an appointment for a checkup.

Basic preventive care plan

1. Call your doctor to schedule a preventive checkup.
2. Use a birthday or anniversary to remind you to make your appointment.
3. Know your blood pressure, cholesterol and blood sugar numbers after your
   checkup, and keep track of those and other numbers that are important to
   your health.

Screening facts: Cancer is the leading cause of death among Americans age 45
to 64. Heart disease is the leading cause of death for Americans over age 65. Your
doctor can screen for breast, colon, cervical and prostate cancers. Cholesterol and
blood pressure screenings can help you detect and manage heart disease. (See
"Adult screening tests and procedures," page 225.)

How's your mood?

For at least the past two weeks, have you persistently felt down, depressed or hopeless?

Yes _____ → Talk with your doctor.

No _____ → Go to the next question.

For at least the past two weeks, have you had little interest or pleasure in doing things?

Yes _____ → Talk with your doctor. (See pages 200-202 for more on
depression.)

No _____ → Go to the next question.

Basic stress management plan

1. Do aerobic activity at a moderate level at least 150 minutes a week.
2. Try for an average of eight hours of sleep a day.
3. Stay connected with family and friends.

Mood facts: Stress and a depressed mood contribute to an increased risk of heart
disease and can intensify your physical symptoms.

6

Get moving and keep moving

How many minutes a week do you spend doing moderate or vigorous physical activities?
Check the time that comes closest.

(*Note:* For most people, examples of moderate or vigorous activities include brisk walking, dancing, biking, swimming and running.)

0 to 30 minutes   _____ → You're just getting started. If there are health reasons why you're not more active, ask your doctor about a physical activity plan that's right for you.

30 to 90 minutes   _____ → Good for you! You've got a good start. Make a goal to gradually increase the amount of time that you do moderate aerobic activity. If you're doing vigorous aerobic activity, you've reached a reasonable goal when you're doing 75 minutes or more a week.

90 to 120 minutes   _____ → You're well on your way to maintaining a good fitness program!

120 minutes or more _____ → You're an active person and probably at a good level of fitness. If your aerobic activity is moderate, you should be doing at least 150 minutes a week, with the goal of being active at least three days a week. If weight loss is part of your plan, you'll likely need at least 200 minutes a week of moderate physical activity.

See "Physical activity and fitness," page 215, for more on getting and staying fit.

Basic activity plan

1. Try to be physically active most days of the week. That includes any simple movement that burns calories, from gardening to walking up stairs.
2. Set a goal of a specific number of minutes or steps a week.
3. Keep a log to help remind you and track your progress.
4. Recruit a friend or family member to keep you company.
5. Build up slowly, but steadily. If you're having difficulty or not feeling well while doing physical activities, see your doctor.

Fitness facts: Only one in three adults receives the recommended amount of physical activity each week. Even a modest walking program can help increase your heart health, reduce stress and give you the extra energy to do the things you enjoy (see pages 217-220).

Safety

Do you wear a seat belt every time you drive or ride in a motor vehicle?

Yes _____ → Go to the next question.

No _____ → Buckle up!

Do you drink before you drive?

Yes _____ → Go to page 188.

No _____ → Go to the next question.

If you own firearms, do you lock them up and have trigger locks on them?

Yes _____ → Go to the next question.

No _____ → Keep firearms and ammunition under lock and key.

Have you done a home-safety survey in the past six months?

Yes _____ → Good for you! You'll reduce your risk of accidents and injuries.

No _____ → Use the home-safety checklist "Reduce your risk at home," page 231, to make your home safer.

Basic safety plan

1. Always wear your seat belt when traveling in a motor vehicle.
2. Do a home-safety review at least once a year.

Safety facts: If you're under age 35, the biggest threat to your life is a motor vehicle accident. About one-third of deaths from motor vehicle accidents in the U.S. are alcohol related.

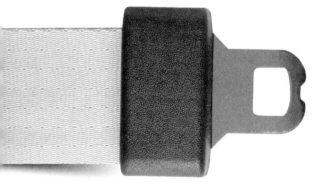
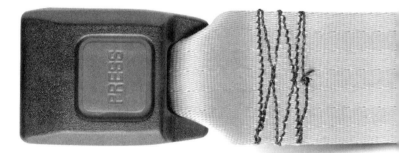

Emergencies and Urgent Care

Emergencies don't happen often, but when they do there's not much time to react. To be effective, you must know what to do when a person appears injured, seriously ill or in distress. Your skills may never be needed. However, you could someday save a life.

Take a certified first-aid training course to learn life-saving skills, such as CPR and the Heimlich maneuver, and how to recognize signs of a heart attack, shock and traumatic injury. Check with your local Red Cross, county emergency services, public safety office or the American Heart Association for information on first aid and related courses that are offered in your community.

- CPR
- Choking
- Heart attack
- Stroke
- Poisoning emergencies
- Severe bleeding
- Shock
- Allergic reactions
- Bites and stings
- Burns
- Cold-weather problems
- Cuts, scrapes and wounds
- Eye injuries
- Foodborne illness
- Heat-related problems
- Poisonous plants
- Tooth problems
- Trauma: Bones and muscles
- Trauma: Head injuries

CPR

Cardiopulmonary resuscitation (**CPR**) can save lives in many emergencies, including when someone's breathing or heartbeat has stopped, such as from a heart attack or near drowning. CPR can keep blood flowing to the brain and other vital organs until medical treatment can restore a normal heart rhythm.

Ideally, CPR involves chest compressions combined with mouth-to-mouth rescue breathing. But if you're untrained or unsure of your CPR skills, do hands-only CPR, unless the person in need is a child (see other exceptions on bottom of page 3).

Before you begin

Before starting CPR, assess the situation. Is the person conscious or unconscious?

- If the person is unconscious, tap or shake the shoulder and ask loudly, "Are you OK?" If there's no response, and another person is able to help you, one of you should call 911 or emergency medical help while the other begins CPR. If you're alone but have immediate access to a telephone, call the emergency number before starting CPR.
- If an automated external defibrillator (AED) is immediately available, bring it near the unconscious person. Voice prompts from the device will guide you step by step on its use. If advised to do so by the voice prompts, deliver one shock, and then begin CPR.
- If you're alone and the victim is an infant or a child age 1 to 8 years, perform two minutes of CPR before calling for help or getting the AED.

Think CAB

To remember the steps of CPR, think CAB — compressions, airway and breathing.

Compressions: Restore circulation

After you've delivered one shock from an AED or if an AED is unavailable, begin CPR by starting chest compressions:

1. Put the person on his or her back on a firm surface.
2. Kneel next to the person's neck and shoulders.
3. Place the heel of one hand over the center of the person's chest, between the nipples. Place your other hand on top of the first hand. Keep your elbows straight and position your shoulders directly above your hands.*
4. Use your upper body weight (not just your arms) as you push straight down on (compress) the chest 2 to 2.4 inches. Push hard at a rate of 100 to 120 compressions a minute.
5. If you haven't been trained in CPR, continue chest compressions until there are signs of movement or until emergency medical personnel take over. If you have been trained in CPR, continue below.

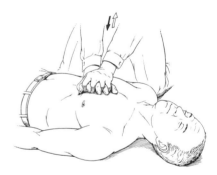

*Chest compression position on an adult (pictured). For a child age 1 to 8 years, use one or two hands (depending on the child's size) and breathe more gently. If you're alone, do two minutes of CPR before calling 911.

Airway: Clear the airway

1. Put your palm on the person's forehead and gently tilt the head back. Then with the other hand, gently lift the chin forward to open the airway.
2. Check for normal breathing, taking no more than five or 10 seconds. Look for chest motion, listen for normal breath sounds,

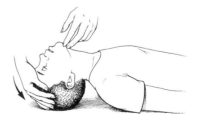

See back cover for online resource ⓘ

and feel for the person's breath on your cheek and ear. If the person isn't breathing normally and you are trained in CPR, begin mouth-to-mouth breathing. If you believe the person is unconscious from a heart attack and you haven't been trained in emergency procedures, skip mouth-to-mouth breathing and continue chest compressions.

Breathing: Breathe for the person

This can be mouth-to-mouth or mouth-to-nose if the mouth is seriously injured or can't be opened.

1. With the airway open (head tilted, chin lifted) pinch the nostrils shut and cover the person's mouth with yours, making a seal.
2. Prepare to give two breaths. Give the first breath, lasting one second. If the chest rises, give the second breath. If the chest doesn't rise, repeat the head-tilt, chin-lift maneuver, and then give the second breath. Thirty chest compressions followed by two rescue breaths is considered one cycle. Be careful not to provide too many breaths or to breathe with too much force.
3. Resume chest compressions at the same rate as before.
4. If the person has not begun moving after five cycles (about two minutes) and an automated external defibrillator (AED) becomes available, apply it now and follow the prompts. Administer one shock, and then resume CPR — starting with chest compressions — for two more minutes before administering a second shock. If an AED isn't available, go to step 5 below.
5. Continue CPR until there are signs of movement or until emergency medical responders can take over.

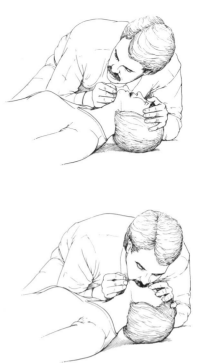

CPR for infants (under 12 months old)

Loudly call out the baby's name and gently tap a shoulder. Don't shake the child. If there's no response, have someone call for emergency help while you:

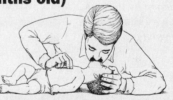

- Place the baby on his or her back on a firm, flat surface, such as a table or the floor.
- Imagine a horizontal line drawn between the baby's nipples. Place two fingers of one hand just below this line, in the center of the chest.
- Gently compress the chest about 1.5 inches. Count aloud as you push in fairly rapid rhythm (a rate of about 100 compressions a minute).
- After 30 compressions, gently tip the head back by lifting the chin with one hand and pushing down on the forehead with the other hand.
- In no more than 10 seconds, check for breathing: *Look* for chest motion, *listen* for breath sounds, and *feel* for breath on your cheek or ear.
- Cover the mouth and nose with your mouth.
- Prepare to give two gentle breaths. Use the strength of your cheeks to deliver puffs of air.

- After the first breath, watch to see if the chest rises. If it does, give a second breath. If it doesn't, repeat the head-tilt, chin-lift maneuver and give the second breath.
- If the baby's chest still doesn't rise, examine the mouth to make sure no foreign material is inside. If an object is seen, sweep it out with your finger. If the airway seems blocked perform first aid for a choking baby (see page 4).
- Give two rescue breaths after every 30 chest compressions given.
- Perform CPR for two minutes before making an emergency call for help.
- Continue CPR until you see signs of life or until emergency responders arrive.

Choking

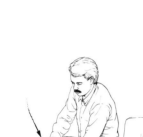

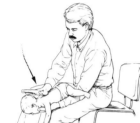

The universal sign for choking is hands clutched to the throat.

__Choking__ occurs when a foreign object becomes lodged in the throat or windpipe, blocking airflow. In adults, food often is the culprit. Young children may swallow small objects. Choking cuts off oxygen to the brain, so give first aid quickly.

The universal sign for choking is hands clutched to the throat. If the person doesn't give the signal, look for these indications:

- Inability to talk
- Difficulty breathing or noisy breathing
- Inability to cough forcefully
- Skin, lips and nails turning blue or dusky
- Loss of consciousness

Five-and-five approach

If choking occurs, the Red Cross recommends a "five-and-five" approach to first aid:
1. Give five back blows between the shoulder blades using the heel of your hand.
2. Deliver five abdominal thrusts (shown in the box below).
3. Alternate between five back blows and five abdominal thrusts until the blockage is dislodged.

If you're the only rescuer, do back blows and abdominal thrusts before calling 911 or emergency medical help. If another person is available, have that person call for help while you give first aid.

If the person becomes unconscious, perform CPR with chest compressions.

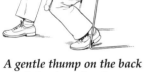

A gentle thump on the back can help clear the airway of a choking infant.

Children and infants

If the child is over 1 year, give abdominal thrusts only. If the infant is under 1 year, sit down and hold the infant facedown on your forearm, which should rest on your thigh. The infant's head should be slightly lower than the chest. Gently but firmly thump between the shoulder blades with the heel of your hand. If the object isn't released, hold the infant faceup on your forearm with the head lower than the trunk. Place two fingers at the center of the breastbone and give five quick chest compressions. Repeat the back thumps and chest compressions if breathing doesn't resume. Call for emergency help. If you open the airway but there's no breathing, begin CPR for infants (see page 3).

Abdominal thrusts (the Heimlich maneuver)

To perform abdominal thrusts, called the Heimlich maneuver:

__1. Stand behind the person.__ Wrap your arms around the waist. Tip the person forward slightly.

__2. Make a fist with one hand.__ Place it slightly above the person's navel.

__3. Grasp your fist with the other hand.__ Press hard into the abdomen with a quick, upward thrust, as if trying to lift the person up.

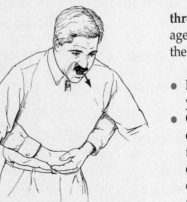

__4. Do five abdominal thrusts, if needed.__ If the blockage still isn't dislodged, repeat the five-and-five cycle above.

If you're alone and choking:
- __Place your fist__ slightly above your navel.
- __Grasp your fist with your other hand and shove your fist in and upward__ until the object dislodges. Or bend over a hard surface, such as a countertop or chair to produce this effect.

See back cover for online resource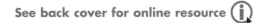

Heart attack

If you think you're having a **<u>heart attack</u>**, call 911 or emergency help immediately. Most people wait several hours after the start of symptoms before seeking treatment because they don't recognize symptoms or they deny them. Each year, more than a million Americans have a heart attack — and many die because of delayed treatment. In those who survive, most of the permanent damage to the heart happens in the first few hours.

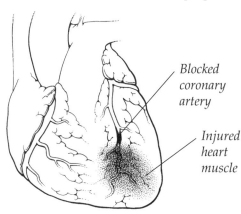

Blocked coronary artery

Injured heart muscle

A heart attack occurs when arteries become blocked. With each passing minute, more tissue is deprived of oxygen and deteriorates or dies.

Minutes matter

A heart attack occurs when a narrowed artery suddenly blocks the flow of blood and oxygen to the heart. This blockage is usually due to a buildup of fatty deposits called plaques. Without oxygen, cells are destroyed, causing pain or pressure. With each passing minute, more of the heart muscle is deprived of oxygen and deteriorates or dies.

Signs and symptoms vary

About half the people who have heart attacks have warning symptoms hours, days or weeks in advance. Signs and symptoms vary widely and may differ between men and women. Some people, especially those with diabetes, have "silent" heart attacks — mild symptoms or none at all. Not all the signs and symptoms below will occur, but the more symptoms you have, the more likely it's a heart attack.

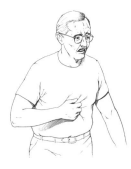

Signs and symptoms of a heart attack vary, but you may experience a squeezing sensation in your chest, with profuse sweating.

- **<u>Chest pain</u>**, pressure, tightness, squeezing or burning that lasts more than a few minutes (may come and go and be triggered by exertion and relieved by rest)
- Pain in one or both arms, neck or jaw, or between the shoulder blades (with or without chest pain)*
- Shortness of breath (with or without chest pain)*†
- Stomach pain or discomfort*
- Nausea or vomiting*
- Rapid, fluttering or pounding heartbeats
- Lightheadedness or dizziness
- Sweating
- Unusual fatigue for no apparent reason
- Anxiety or sense of doom

*These signs and symptoms are more common in women than in men. Most women have a type of chest discomfort with a heart attack, but it may not be the main symptom. †Shortness of breath without chest pain is a more common symptom of heart attack in people over age 65 and in people with diabetes.

Get help fast

Some heart attacks are sudden, but most start slowly, with mild pain or discomfort. Symptoms may come and go, over minutes or hours. But if you suspect you're having a heart attack, don't wait. Immediately call 911 or emergency medical help.

Paramedics can treat you on the way to the emergency department. If you can't access an emergency number, have someone drive you to the nearest hospital. Driving yourself can put others at risk.

What to do while waiting for help

If you're waiting for help:

- **Chew a regular-strength (325 milligrams, or mg) aspirin or four baby aspirin (81 mg each)** to help prevent blood clotting, if recommended by the emergency dispatcher. Chew aspirin even if you're on daily aspirin therapy. Chewing (versus swallowing) speeds absorption of the drug.
- **In addition to aspirin, if you have a prescription for nitroglycerin,** use as instructed by your doctor for emergencies. This medication can temporarily open blood vessels, improving blood flow to your heart.

If you're helping someone else while waiting for paramedics to arrive:

- **Have the person chew on aspirin** if recommended by the emergency dispatcher.
- **If the person becomes unconscious, begin CPR.** Even if you're not trained, you can do hands-only CPR (see pages 2-3). Most emergency dispatchers can instruct you in CPR until help arrives.

Medications

To prevent progressive damage, blood flow needs to be restored quickly. In addition to aspirin and nitroglycerin, medications given to treat a heart attack may include those below. Which medications you receive depend on your specific situation.

- **Thrombolytics.** Also called clot busters, these drugs help dissolve a blood clot that's blocking blood flow to your heart. The earlier you receive this drug, the greater the chance you'll survive and lessen the damage to your heart.
- **Platelet inhibitors.** Aspirin is a platelet inhibitor. This class of medications helps prevent new clots from forming. Medications such as clopidogrel (Plavix) and others are included in this category.
- **Other blood-thinning medications.** You'll likely be given other medications, such as heparin, to make your blood less "sticky" and less likely to form more dangerous clots. Heparin is given intravenously or by an injection under your skin.
- **Pain relievers.** If you're in a lot of pain, you may receive a pain reliever, such as morphine, to reduce your discomfort.
- **Cholesterol-lowering medications.** Examples include statins, niacin and other drugs to help lower your cholesterol.

Surgical and other procedures

In addition to medications, you may need one of these procedures:

- **Angioplasty and stenting.** Angioplasty, which is done as part of a cardiac catheterization (angiogram), uses balloons or devices called stents to unblock the artery. If angioplasty is delayed, benefits are reduced.
- **Coronary artery bypass surgery.** In rare cases, doctors may perform emergency bypass surgery at the time of a heart attack. Or they may suggest that you have this procedure after your heart has had time to recover from your heart attack.

Prevention

Adopting a healthy lifestyle is key to helping prevent a heart attack and lowering the risk of heart disease. You may also be advised to take a daily aspirin. You'll find both of these topics and more in the section on "Heart disease," pages 177-179.

Stroke

In the United States, **stroke** is the fifth-leading cause of death and a leading cause of adult disability.

A stroke is a "brain attack" — it occurs when the blood supply to a part of your brain is interrupted or severely reduced, depriving brain tissue of oxygen and nutrients. Almost 2 million brain cells die each minute during a typical stroke. So, as the American Heart Association emphasizes, "With a stroke, time lost is brain lost."

A stroke is a medical emergency, and prompt treatment is crucial. Early treatment can minimize damage to your brain and reduce your risk of complications.

Warning signs

To help yourself or someone else, the American Stroke Association, American Heart Association and others urge you to recognize stroke by thinking FAST.

- **Face.** Ask the person to smile. Does one side of the face droop?
- **Arms.** Ask the person to raise both arms. Does one arm drift downward? Or is the person unable to lift one arm?
- **Speech.** Ask the person to repeat a simple phrase. Is his or her speech slurred or strange?
- **Time.** If you observe any of these signs, call 911 or emergency medical help immediately.

Tell the 911 operator or emergency medical personnel that you think it's a stroke. If you're calling for another person, watch the person closely while waiting for an ambulance. Don't let the person eat or drink anything. If needed, take these actions:

- If the person stops breathing, begin CPR (see pages 2-3).
- If vomiting occurs, turn the person's head to the side. This can prevent choking.

Types of stroke

There are two main types of stroke:

- **Ischemic (is-KEE-mik).** Most strokes are ischemic strokes. They're caused by the buildup of fatty deposits called plaques. Growth of plaques can suddenly interrupt blood flow to the brain by blocking an artery. Or sometimes a clot breaks loose, blocking blood flow to the brain.
- **Hemorrhagic (hem-uh-RAJ-ik).** This type of stroke occurs when a blood vessel in your brain leaks or ruptures, causing bleeding in the brain. The most common cause of a hemorrhagic stroke is high blood pressure (hypertension), but it can also be caused by weak spots in your blood vessel walls (aneurysms) that develop with advancing age. Some aneurysms may form as a result of genetics. A less common cause of hemorrhage is the rupture of an arteriovenous malformation (AVM) — an abnormal tangle of thin-walled blood vessels, present at birth.

Although less common than ischemic strokes are, hemorrhagic strokes have a higher risk of death. Strokes in young adults are more likely to be hemorrhagic.

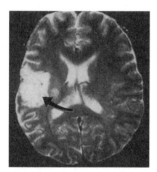

The arrow reveals an area of brain tissue damaged by a stroke, as shown on a magnetic resonance imaging (MRI) scan.

What's a TIA?

A transient ischemic attack (**TIA**), sometimes called a ministroke, is a temporary interruption of blood flow to part of your brain. TIA symptoms are similar to those of a stroke but resolve quickly, often within minutes. A TIA doesn't destroy brain cells or cause permanent disability, but each TIA increases your risk of stroke. If you think you've had a TIA, call your doctor. After a TIA, the risk of a stroke increases immediately and may be as high as 20 percent over the next three months. Depending on the cause, you may need medication to prevent blood clots or a procedure to remove fatty buildup in your arteries.

Stroke treatment

The success of treatment is often related to how soon medical care is given. Treatment depends on the type of stroke. After treatment, you may also be given preventive medications to reduce your risk of having another TIA or stroke.

- **Ischemic.** Therapy with clot busting drugs must start within three hours. You may be given aspirin in the emergency department, but don't take it before medical help arrives because aspirin can worsen a hemorrhagic stroke. Some people benefit from an injection of tissue plasminogen activator (TPA), but it does carry some risks. Your doctor may recommend clot removal surgery or other procedures to widen the inside of an artery leading to your brain.
- **Hemorrhagic.** Surgery may be used to treat a hemorrhagic stroke or prevent another one. The most common procedures — aneurysm clipping and arteriovenous malformation (AVM) removal — carry some risks. Your doctor may recommend one of these procedures if you're at high risk of spontaneous aneurysm or AVM rupture.

Can you prevent a stroke?

To help prevent a stroke or TIA, know your risk factors and take steps to adopt a healthy lifestyle:

- **Prevent or control high blood pressure.** High blood pressure significantly increases your risk of stroke. (See "High blood pressure," page 182.)
- **Don't smoke.** Smoking greatly increases your risk of stroke.
- **Lower your intake of cholesterol and fats.** Eating less cholesterol and fats, especially saturated and trans fats, may reduce the plaques in your arteries. If dietary changes aren't enough, your doctor may prescribe a cholesterol-lowering drug.
- **Maintain a healthy weight.** Being overweight contributes to other risk factors for stroke, such as high blood pressure, heart disease and diabetes.
- **Prevent or manage diabetes.** Having diabetes significantly increases your risk of stroke. (See "Diabetes," page 172.)
- **Get regular physical activity.** Physical activity and exercise lower your blood pressure and improve the overall health of your blood vessels and heart.
- **Drink alcohol in moderation, if at all.** Heavy alcohol consumption or binge drinking increases your risk of high blood pressure and stroke.

Risk factors beyond your control

While there are risk factors for stroke that you can't control, knowing that you're at higher than average risk can be beneficial. It highlights the importance of living a healthy lifestyle to reduce your risk.

- **Family history.** Your risk is greater if one of your parents, a brother or a sister has had a stroke or TIA. It's not clear whether the increased risk is inherited or due to family lifestyles.
- **Age.** Your risk of stroke increases as you age.

- **Sex.** More women than men die of stroke each year, in part because women are generally older than men when they have their strokes. But research continues about possible differences in medical care.
- **Race.** Black people have a higher incidence of stroke than white people do. The increase may be partly due to a higher incidence of high blood pressure and diabetes in that population.

Poisoning emergencies

Poisoning can be a serious medical emergency, and a person's condition can change quickly. Immediately call 911 or emergency medical help if you see the signs and symptoms listed below. Tell the 911 operator or emergency medical responders that you think the person has consumed poison.

Watch the person carefully while waiting for an ambulance. Don't let the person eat or drink anything. Take action if:

- **The person stops breathing.** Begin CPR (see pages 2-3).
- **Vomiting occurs.** Turn the person's head to the side to prevent choking.

If the person is going to the emergency department, take the container or any information about the poison with you and give it to the ambulance team.

If you suspect poisoning but the person isn't so ill that you need to call 911, call Poison Help in the U.S. at 800-222-1222. Call immediately, even if the person looks and feels fine. Many toxins have delayed life-threatening effects. Early treatment is critical. Don't give anything to the person unless the Poison Help representatitve advises you.

Signs and symptoms

- Unconsciousness
- Burns or redness around the mouth and lips, which can result from drinking certain poisons
- Breath that smells like chemicals, such as gasoline or paint thinner
- Burns, stains and odors on the person, on clothing, or on the furniture, floor, rugs or other objects in the surrounding area
- Empty medication bottles or scattered pills
- Vomiting, difficulty breathing, drowsiness, confusion
- Uncontrollably restless or agitated or having seizures

First aid	Below are first steps. Call Poison Help at 800-222-1222 for instructions. If you have the poison container, follow instructions on the label for accidental poisoning.

- **Swallowed poison.** Remove anything remaining in the person's mouth. Call Poison Help before giving fluids by mouth. For some poisons, fluids may make the situation worse. Don't administer ipecac syrup or do anything to induce vomiting. This can do more harm than good.
- **Poison in the eye.** Until help arrives, gently flush the eye for 20 minutes using slightly warm water in a shower. Or pour lukewarm water from a clean glass held about 3 inches above the eye. See "Chemical splash," page 24.
- **Poison on the skin.** Until help arrives, remove any contaminated clothing using gloves. Rinse the skin for 15 to 20 minutes by, for example, using a shower.
- **Inhaled poison.** Get the person to fresh air as soon as possible. Avoid breathing the fumes. Ventilate the area by opening windows or using fans.

Medications as poisons

Medications can be deadly. Overdoses of seemingly harmless medications such as aspirin and acetaminophen take many lives each year. Many prescription and over-the-counter drugs can be dangerous when taken in large doses.

Kids' care

Children under age 5 are often exposed to poisons because they're curious. If infants and toddlers live in or visit your home:

- Keep potential poisons in cabinets located up high, or with safety locks.
- Keep the Poison Help phone number handy: 800-222-1222.

Severe bleeding

To stop **severe bleeding**, follow these steps:

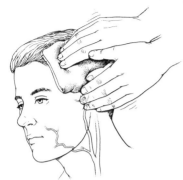

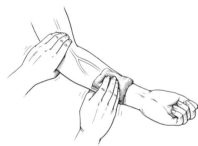

To stop bleeding, apply pressure directly to the wound using a clean cloth or a bandage.

If bleeding continues despite direct pressure to the wound, maintain pressure and also apply pressure to the nearest major artery above the level of the wound.

1. **Have the injured person lie down, and cover the person to prevent loss of body heat.** If possible, position the person's head slightly lower than the trunk or elevate the legs — this reduces the risk of fainting by increasing blood flow to the brain. If possible, raise the bleeding site.
2. **While wearing gloves, remove any obvious dirt or debris from the wound.** Don't remove any large or deeply embedded objects. Don't probe the wound or attempt to clean or rinse it out. Your main concern is to stop the bleeding.
3. **Apply pressure directly on the wound.** Use a sterile bandage or clean cloth and maintain pressure for at least 20 minutes without looking to see if the bleeding has stopped. Use your hands if nothing else is available. If possible, wear rubber or latex gloves or use a clean plastic bag for protection.
4. **Maintain pressure until the bleeding stops.** When it does, keep the bandage or cloth in place by taping, tying or wrapping. Bandages should be snug, but not loose or too tight. Don't apply a tourniquet except as a last resort.
5. **Don't remove the gauze or bandage.** If bleeding continues and seeps through the bandage or other material you're holding on the wound, add more absorbent layers on top of it.
6. **Squeeze a main artery if necessary.** If the bleeding still doesn't stop with direct pressure, apply pressure to the artery that delivers blood to the area of the wound. Pressure points of the arm are on the inside of the arm just above the elbow and just below the armpit. Pressure points of the leg are just behind the knee and in the groin. Squeeze the main artery in these areas against the bone. Keep your fingers flat. With the other hand, continue to put pressure on the wound itself.
7. **Immobilize the injured body part once the bleeding has been stopped.** Leave the bandages in place and call 911 or emergency medical help, or get the injured person to the emergency room.

Detecting internal bleeding

Internal bleeding (from a fall, for example) may not be immediately apparent. If you suspect internal bleeding, call 911 or emergency medical help immediately.

Signs and symptoms may include:
- Bleeding from any opening, such as ears, nose, mouth, rectum or vagina
- Vomiting or coughing up blood
- Bruising on the neck, chest, abdomen or side (between the ribs and hip)
- Wounds that have penetrated the skull, chest or abdomen

- Abdominal tenderness or severe pain, sometimes along with hardness or spasm of the abdominal muscles
- Limb deformity or exposed bone
- Shock, indicated by weakness, anxiety, thirst or skin that's cool to the touch, or other signs listed on the next page

While waiting for help, treat the person for shock (see page 11). Internal bleeding is extremely serious and can be life-threatening. Blood loss may be considerable, even without clear evidence of external bleeding.

Shock

<u>Shock</u> may result from trauma, heatstroke, allergic reaction, severe infection, poisoning or other causes. Various signs and symptoms may appear in a person who's in shock:

- **The skin is cool and clammy.** It may appear pale or gray.
- **The pulse may be weak and rapid.** Breathing may be slow and shallow, or rapid or deep breathing (hyperventilation) may occur. Blood pressure is low.
- **The eyes lack luster and seem to stare.** Sometimes the pupils are dilated.
- **The person may be conscious or unconscious.** If conscious, the person may feel faint or anxious and be very weak or confused. Shock sometimes causes a person to become irritable and restless, with slowed movement and responses.

If you suspect shock, even if the person seems normal after an injury:

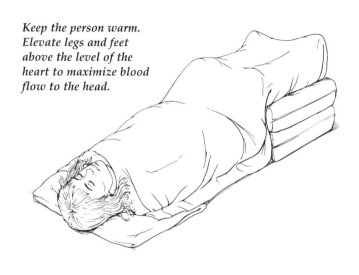

Keep the person warm. Elevate legs and feet above the level of the heart to maximize blood flow to the head.

1. **Call 911** or emergency medical help immediately.
2. **Have the person lie down** on his or her back with feet higher than the head. If raising the legs will cause pain or further injury, keep him or her flat. Keep the person still. Watch for signs of shock (above).
3. **Check for signs of circulation** (breathing, coughing or movement). If absent, begin CPR (see pages 2-3).
4. **Keep the person warm and comfortable.** Loosen belts and tight clothing. Cover the person with a blanket. Even if the person complains of thirst, give nothing by mouth.
5. **If the person vomits or bleeds from the mouth, turn the person on his or her side** to prevent choking.
6. **Seek or start treatment for injuries**, such as bleeding (see page 10) or broken bones.

Anaphylaxis can be life-threatening

The section on the next page focuses on allergic reactions. **Anaphylaxis** is a severe, life-threatening allergic reaction. It's infrequent, but each year hundreds of Americans die of allergic reactions.

Anaphylaxis can occur within seconds or minutes. Any allergen can cause the response, including insect venoms, pollens, latex, foods and drugs.

Signs and symptoms of anaphylaxis include:

- Constriction of airways with a swollen throat, which can cause wheezing and trouble breathing
- Shock associated with very low blood pressure
- Rapid pulse
- Skin reactions such as hives and intense itching, and flushed or pale skin
- Swelling of the lips and tongue
- Nausea, vomiting or diarrhea

If you see someone having an allergic reaction with signs of anaphylaxis:

- **Call 911** or emergency medical help immediately.
- **If the person isn't breathing or has no pulse, perform CPR** (see pages 2-3).
- **If the person is in shock,** follow steps 4 and 5 above.
- **If the person is carrying epinephrine (EpiPen, others)** — a medication to treat an allergic response — give it to the person right away. In the case of a severe reaction, a second dose may be recommended, if available.

Allergic reactions

An **allergy** is a reaction to a foreign substance (allergen) by the body's immune system. The reaction may take many forms, including rashes, nasal congestion, asthma and, rarely, a severe reaction (see box on anaphylaxis on page 11)) that can lead to shock and death. Common allergens include pollen (see "Respiratory allergies," page 158) and insect venom (see "Insect bites and stings," page 15). This section covers food and drug allergies.

■ Food allergies

Food allergies may be the most misunderstood of all allergies. About 1 in 3 Americans believes he or she is allergic to specific foods. However, 1 in 13 children has true food allergies. Most children eventually outgrow their food allergies.

The majority of food allergies are caused by certain proteins in cow's milk, eggs, peanuts, wheat, soy, fish, shellfish and tree nuts. But nearly all foods have the potential to cause an allergic reaction. Allergies to soy, eggs, wheat and milk occur mostly in children. Chocolate, long thought to cause allergies (particularly among children), is actually seldom a cause.

Signs and symptoms of food allergies include:
- Abdominal pain, diarrhea, nausea or vomiting
- Hives or swelling of the lips, eyes, face, tongue or throat (see page 123)
- Fainting
- Nasal congestion and asthma

Self-care

- Avoidance is the best way to prevent an allergic reaction.
- Read labels carefully and look for substances made from foods to which you're allergic. Example: Whey and casein are milk products used as additives.
- When choosing substitute foods, be careful to select foods that provide the necessary replacement nutrients.
- If you have a medical diagnosis of a food allergy, wear a medical alert bracelet or necklace, available in most drugstores. Ask your doctor about carrying emergency medications, such as self-injectable epinephrine (EpiPen), and know when and how to use it.
- Learn rescue techniques, and teach them to family members and friends.

Medical help

Food allergies can be diagnosed through a careful process that includes these steps:
1. History of your symptoms, including when they occur, which foods cause problems and the amount of food needed to trigger symptoms.
2. Food diary to track eating habits, symptoms and medication use.
3. Physical exam.
4. Skin prick tests using food extracts and a food-specific blood test that measures an antibody called immunoglobulin E (IgE). Neither test is 100 percent accurate. Both tests may be more helpful in determining foods to which you're not allergic.
5. Food challenge test, in which you're given suspected foods. The foods may be given in disguised form (blind challenge) or they may be given openly. These results are more conclusive than skin tests are, but food challenge tests take time and should not be used if you have a severe reaction to a particular food.

For mild reactions, your doctor may prescribe antihistamines or skin creams.

See back cover for online resource ⓘ

Caution	Severe reactions such as anaphylaxis (see page 11) and acute asthma can be life-threatening. Such reactions are rare. Most reactions are limited to rashes and hives. However, this doesn't mean they can be ignored, as later exposure to the foods may result in more symptoms.
Kids' care	Food allergies are more common in children than in adults. As the digestive system matures, it's less apt to allow absorption of foods that trigger allergies. Children typically outgrow allergies to milk, eggs, wheat and soy. Severe allergies and those due to peanuts, tree nuts, fish and shellfish are more likely to be lifelong.

■ Drug allergies

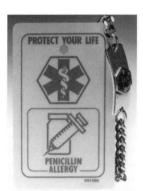

If you have a drug allergy, carry allergy identification at all times. Medical alert necklaces and bracelets are available at drugstores.

Many reactions thought to result from a **drug allergy** are actually side effects of a drug, such as an upset stomach or tiredness. Other effects, such as liver damage, are more severe. While rare, reactions such as rashes or difficulty breathing (anaphylaxis) may be an allergic response to the medication. Other reactions are poorly understood. Your doctor can determine the nature of the reactions and what to do about them.

Many people are allergic to penicillin drugs. While most reactions are minor skin rashes, they can lead to hives and immediate anaphylaxis.

Other drugs that are most likely to cause reactions include sulfas, aspirin, non-steroidal anti-inflammatory drugs (NSAIDs) such as ibuprofen and naproxen, and anticonvulsants. These are all common, effective, useful medications. Reactions occur in a minority of people. If you are taking one of the drugs and are not having problems, don't stop using it. In addition, contrast dyes used in some X-ray studies to help outline major organs may cause an allergic reaction.

Signs and symptoms of allergic reactions to drugs include:

- Rash, hives or generalized itching
- Wheezing and difficulty breathing
- Facial swelling
- Shock

Self-care	<ul><li>If you have a severe reaction, learn the names of related drugs and note what happened when you took the medication.</li><li>Report side effects or reactions to your doctor right away. Reactions can occur days after stopping use of a drug.</li><li>Ask your pharmacist or doctor to help determine if the symptoms that you developed after taking a drug are side effects or a true allergy.</li><li>Avoid drugs that have previously caused an allergic response.</li><li>Alert your health care providers of your sensitivity to a drug before treatment.</li><li>Wear a medical alert necklace or bracelet to indicate your allergy.</li></ul>
Medical help	See your doctor if you develop a rash, itching or hives or if you suspect other signs and symptoms you're having might be due to a drug you're taking. For life-threatening reactions, such as difficulty breathing, call 911 or emergency medical help. In some people, a penicillin allergy resolves over several years. Ask your doctor if you're a candidate for testing to find out if you still have an allergy. A penicillin allergy skin test may be an option.

Bites and stings

■ Animal bites

Household pets cause most **animal bites**. Cat bites or scratches cause a high risk of infection: Seek medical assessment. (See the rabies box below about wild animal bites.)

Self-care

- If the bite only breaks the skin, treat it as a minor wound. Wash the wound thoroughly with soap and water. Apply an antiseptic cream to prevent infection, and cover the wound with a clean bandage.
- If you haven't had a tetanus shot in the past five years, the bite breaks the skin, and your wound is deep or dirty, you may need a booster shot (see page 23).
- Report bites from aggressive or sick animals to local health authorities.
- Follow veterinary guidelines for vaccination of your pets.

Medical help

If the bite creates a deep puncture or the skin is badly torn and bleeding, apply pressure to stop the bleeding and see your doctor. If you haven't had a recent tetanus shot, seek medical care. Watch for signs and symptoms of infection. Swelling, redness around the wound or a red streak extending from the site, pus draining from the wound, or pain should be reported immediately to your doctor.

The risk of rabies

Bats, foxes, coyotes, raccoons, skunks and other wild animals may carry **rabies**. So can cats, dogs, ferrets and farm animals. Vaccinate your animals against rabies. If you wake up with a bat in your room, assume you've been exposed to saliva and that the bat has rabies.

Rabies is a deadly virus that affects your central nervous system. Transmitted to humans by saliva from the bite of an infected animal, the virus usually has an incubation period — the time from a bite until symptoms appear — of weeks to months. But in some cases it can range from days to years. If you think you've been exposed to rabies, thoroughly wash the wound with soap and water. Then immediately call your doctor or go to the emergency department. Once the earliest signs occur, death often follows without immediate medical care. Anyone exposed to rabies needs a series of shots.

After the incubation period, signs and symptoms may include fever, headache, insomnia, anxiety, hallucinations, agitation, foaming at the mouth, seizures or paralysis.

If you're bitten by a domestic dog, cat or ferret, the animal should be confined and observed for 10 days. Contact a veterinarian if the animal shows any sign of sickness. If a wild animal has bitten you, it should be euthanized and tested for rabies.

■ Human bites

There are two kinds of **human bites**. The first is what is usually thought of as a "true" bite — an injury that results from flesh being caught between the teeth. The second kind, called a "fight bite," occurs when a person is cut on the knuckles by an opponent's teeth. Treatment is the same in both cases. Human bites are dangerous because of the risk of infection. The human mouth is a breeding ground for bacteria.

Self-care

- Apply pressure to stop bleeding, wash the wound thoroughly with soap and water, and bandage the wound.
- Then visit an emergency room. You may need antibiotics to prevent infection or your tetanus shot updated (see page 23).

    See back cover for online resource (i)

■ Snakebites

Triangular head
Elliptical eyes
Nostrils
Pit
Fangs

Most snakes aren't venomous. However, because a few are (including rattlesnakes, coral snakes, water moccasins and copperheads), avoid picking up, handling or playing with any snake unless you're properly trained.

If you're bitten by a snake, it's important to determine whether the snake is venomous. Most venomous snakes have slit-like (elliptical) eyes. Their heads are triangular, with a depression (pit) midway between the eyes and nostrils.

Self-care

- If the snake isn't venomous, wash the bite thoroughly, cover it with an antiseptic cream and bandage it. In general, a **snakebite** is more scary than dangerous.
- Check on the date of your last tetanus shot (see page 23).

Medical help

If you suspect that the snake is venomous, seek emergency medical assistance immediately. Don't cut the wound or attempt to remove the venom. Don't use a tourniquet or apply ice. Immobilize the bitten arm or leg, elevate it if possible, and try to stay as calm as possible until medical help arrives.

■ Insect bites and stings

Usually **bites and stings** just cause an itching or stinging sensation and mild swelling that disappears within a day or so. However, about 1 person in 50 is allergic to the venom of bees, wasps, hornets, yellow jackets or fire ants.

Signs and symptoms of an allergic reaction usually appear within minutes after the sting or bite, but can take hours or even days. If you're mildly sensitive to the venom, hives, itchy eyes, pain and intense itching around the sting or bite are common. With a delayed reaction, fever, painful joints, hives and swollen glands may occur.

A severe allergic reaction (anaphylaxis) can be life-threatening. You may have severe hives and swelling of your eyes or lips or inside your throat. Throat swelling can cause breathing difficulty. Dizziness, mental confusion, abdominal cramping, rapid heartbeat, nausea, vomiting or fainting also may occur. See the box on anaphylaxis, page 11.

Mosquito bites may be merely annoying or potentially deadly if they carry serious viral diseases such as **West Nile virus**, **Zika virus** or **dengue fever**. Signs and symptoms may include severe headache, confusion, light sensitivity, widespread rash, bleeding or a high fever. Such symptoms require prompt medical attention.

To reduce your risk, avoid unnecessary outdoor activity when mosquitoes are most active, at dawn, dusk and early evening. Also, wear light-colored, long-sleeved shirts and long pants when outdoors. Use mosquito repellent that has been shown to be effective, such as one that contains DEET. Don't use DEET on the hands of young children or on infants under 2 months of age. Apply permethrin-containing mosquito repellent to your clothing, or buy clothing with permethrin in it.

For information on lice and scabies, see page 126.

Self-care

- Scrape or brush off the stinger with a straightedge. Don't pull out the stinger. This may release more venom. Wash the area with soap and water.
- Apply a cold pack or cloth filled with ice to reduce pain and swelling.
- Apply 0.5 or 1 percent hydrocortisone cream, calamine lotion or a baking soda paste to the bite or sting several times daily until your symptoms go away.
- Take an antihistamine (Benadryl, others) to reduce itching.

If you've experienced a severe reaction in the past, wear a medical alert bracelet or necklace, and always carry a self-injection allergy kit containing epinephrine.

Medical help

If your reaction to an insect bite is severe, call 911 or emergency medical help. The most severe allergic reactions to bee stings can be life-threatening. If you have any breathing problems, swelling of the lips, tongue or throat, faintness, confusion, rapid heartbeat, or hives after a sting, seek emergency care. Less severe allergic reactions include nausea, intestinal cramps, diarrhea or swelling larger than 2 inches wide at the site. See your doctor promptly if you have any of these symptoms.

Your doctor may prescribe shots that can help desensitize your body to insect venom, and an emergency kit containing antihistamine tablets and a syringe filled with epinephrine. Pressure injector units are available that deliver a pre-measured dose. Use medications within expiration dates. Regularly check the dates.

■ Spider bites

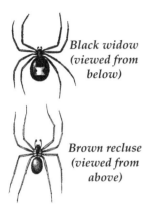

Black widow (viewed from below)

Brown recluse (viewed from above)

Only a few spiders are dangerous to humans. Two are the black widow spider (*Latrodectus mactans*), known for the red hourglass marking on its belly, and the brown recluse spider (*Loxosceles reclusa*), with its violin-shaped marking on its top.

These two spiders are more common in Southern states. Both prefer warm climates and dark, dry places where insects are plentiful. They often live in closets, woodpiles and outdoor toilets. Signs and symptoms of a black widow bite start with only slight swelling and faint red marks at the site, but within hours, they may include intense pain, stiffness, chills, fever, nausea and severe abdominal pain. A brown recluse bite starts with mild stinging, followed by local redness and intense pain within hours, and may include a mild fever, rash, nausea, fluid-filled blisters or listlessness.

If bitten by either of these spiders, seek emergency care immediately. In the meantime, wash the **spider bite** with soap and water. Apply a cloth dampened with cold water or filled with ice. If the bite is on a limb, slow the venom's spread by placing a snug (not tight) bandage over and above the bite and applying ice.

■ Tick bites

Some ticks carry infections, and their bites can transmit bacteria that cause illnesses such as **Lyme disease** (caused by the deer tick). Your risk of contracting one of these diseases depends on what part of the U.S. you live in, how much time you spend in wooded areas and how well you protect yourself.

Self-care

Actual size

Deer tick

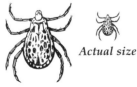

Actual size

Wood tick

- When walking in wooded or grassy areas, wear shoes, long pants tucked into socks and light-colored, long-sleeved shirts. Avoid low bushes and long grass.
- Tick-proof your yard by clearing brush and leaves. Keep woodpiles in sunny areas.
- Check yourself and your pets often for ticks after being in wooded or grassy areas. Shower immediately after leaving these areas because ticks often remain on your skin for many hours before biting.
- Insect repellents often repel ticks. Use products containing DEET or permethrin. Be sure to follow label precautions.
- If you find a tick, remove it promptly with tweezers by gently grasping it near its head or mouth. Don't crush the tick, but pull carefully and steadily.
- If possible, seal the tick in a jar. Your doctor may need to see it if you get a rash or get sick after a **tick bite**. If you discard the tick, burn or crush and flush it.
- Wash the area around the tick bite and your hands with soap and water.
- Call the doctor if you can't completely remove the tick or you don't feel well. Lyme disease can cause flu-like symptoms and a rash that looks like a target.

See back cover for online resource ⓘ

Burns

Burns can be caused by fire, the sun, chemicals, hot liquids or objects, steam, electricity, and other means. They can be minor medical problems or life-threatening emergencies.

Burn classifications

Distinguishing a minor burn from a more-serious burn involves determining the degree of damage to the tissues of the body. The following three categories and illustrations can help determine your response.

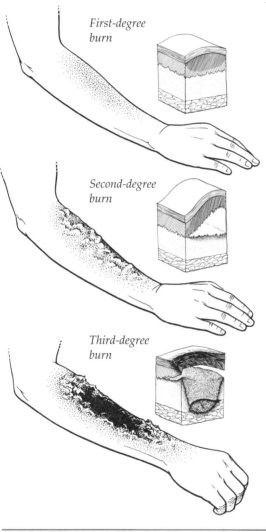

First-degree burn

Second-degree burn

Third-degree burn

First-degree

The least serious burns are those in which only the outer layer of skin (epidermis) is burned. The skin is usually reddened, and there may be swelling and pain, but the outer layer of skin hasn't been burned through. Unless such a burn involves substantial portions of the hands, feet, face, groin, buttocks or a major joint, it may be treated as a minor burn with the self-care remedies listed on page 18. Chemical burns may require additional follow-up. If the burn was caused by exposure to the sun, see "Sunburn," page 19.

Second-degree

When the first layer of skin has been burned through and the second layer of skin (dermis) also is burned, the injury is called a second-degree burn. Blisters develop, and the skin takes on an intensely reddened, splotchy appearance. Second-degree burns produce swelling and moderate to severe pain.

If a second-degree burn is limited to an area no larger than 3 inches wide, follow the home remedies listed on page 18. If the burned area of the skin is larger, or if the burn is on the hands, feet, face, groin, buttocks or over a major joint or encircles your limb, seek urgent care immediately.

Third-degree

The most serious burns involve all layers of the skin. Fat, nerves, muscles and even bones may be affected. Usually some areas are charred black or appear a dry white. There may be severe pain or, if nerve damage is substantial, no pain at all. It's important to take immediate action in all cases of third-degree burns.

Emergency treatment: All major burns

Seek emergency medical treatment immediately for major burns. Until an emergency unit arrives, follow these steps:
- **Don't remove burned clothing,** but do make sure that the person is no longer in contact with smoldering materials.
- **Make certain that the person burned is breathing.**
- **Cover the area of the burn** with a cool, moist sterile bandage or with a clean cloth.

Self-care: **Minor burns only**	For minor burns, including second-degree burns limited to an area no larger than 2 to 3 inches in diameter, take the following actions: • **Cool the burn.** Hold the burned area under cold running water until the pain subsides. If this step is impractical, immerse the burn in cold water or apply cold compresses. Cooling the burn reduces pain and swelling. • **Consider a lotion.** Once a burn is completely cooled, a lotion, such as one that contains aloe vera or a moisturizer prevents drying and increases your comfort. • **Bandage a burn.** Cover the burn with a sterile gauze bandage (not fluffy cotton). Wrap it loosely to avoid putting pressure on burned skin. Bandaging keeps air off the area, reduces pain and protects blistered skin. • **Take over-the-counter pain relievers** (see page 258). • **Watch for signs of infection.** Minor burns will usually heal in about one to two weeks without further treatment, but watch for indications of infection.
Caution	Don't use ice. Ice on a burn can cause frostbite and do more damage. Don't break blisters. Fluid-filled blisters protect against infection. If a blister breaks, clean the area daily by rinsing with water (mild soap is optional). Apply an antibiotic ointment. But if a rash appears, stop using the ointment.

■ Chemical burns

Self-care	• **Make sure the cause of the burn has been removed.** Flush the chemical off the skin surface with cool running water for at least 10 minutes. If the burning chemical is a powder-like substance such as lime, brush it off your skin before flushing. • **Treat the person for shock (see page 11).** Symptoms include fainting, pale complexion or breathing in a notably shallow fashion. • **Remove clothing or jewelry** that has been contaminated by the chemical. • **Wrap the burned area** with a dry, sterile dressing (if possible) or a clean cloth. • **If the person experiences increased burning after the initial flushing with water, flush the burn area with water again** for several more minutes. **Prevention** • When using chemicals, always wear protective eyewear and clothing. • Know about the chemicals you use. • At work, read appropriate Material Safety Data Sheets, or call Poison Help at 800-222-1222 to learn more about the substance.
Medical help	Minor **chemical burns** usually heal without further treatment. But seek emergency medical assistance if: • The chemical burned through the first layer of skin and the resulting second-degree burn covers an area more than 3 inches wide • The chemical burn occurred on the hands, feet, face, groin, buttocks, over a major joint or encircles your limb.
Caution	Common household cleaning products, particularly those that contain ammonia or bleach, and garden chemicals can cause serious harm to the eyes or skin. Read labels. They contain instructions for proper use and treatment recommendations.

Sunburn

Although the sun provides a welcome change from gray winter months, it can damage your skin and increase your risk of skin cancer. Symptoms of sunburn usually appear within a few hours after exposure, bringing pain, redness, swelling and occasional blistering. A sunburn can also cause a headache, fever and fatigue.

Self-care

- Take a cool bath or shower.
- Leave water blisters intact to speed healing and avoid infection. If they burst on their own, apply an antibacterial ointment on the open areas. If needed, cover with a nonstick sterile gauze bandage.
- Take an over-the-counter pain reliever, such as ibuprofen or aspirin (see page 258).
- Avoid products containing benzocaine (an anesthetic) because they can cause allergic reactions in many people.
- Drink plenty of fluids.

Prevention

- Try to avoid being outdoors from 10 a.m. to 4 p.m. when the sun's ultraviolet (UV) radiation is at its peak. Cover exposed areas, wear a broad-brimmed hat and use a sunscreen with a sun protection factor (SPF) of at least 30. Reapply after swimming and every two hours while out in the sun.
- Protect your eyes. Choose sunglasses that block 99 to 100 percent of UVA and UVB rays. Choose wraparound sunglasses or sunglasses that fit close to your face.

Medical help

If your sunburn begins to blister or you feel ill, see your doctor. Oral steroids such as prednisone are occasionally helpful.

Caution

A lifetime of overexposure to the sun's UV radiation can damage your skin and increase your risk of skin cancer. If you have severe sunburn or immediate complications (rash, itching or fever), contact your health care provider. Sunburn may also be accompanied by heat illness, such as heatstroke.

Electrical burns

Any electrical burn should be examined by a doctor. A burn may appear minor, but the damage can extend into deep tissues. A heart rhythm disturbance, cardiac arrest or other internal damage can occur if the amount of electrical current that passed through the body was large. Sometimes the jolt of electricity can cause a person to be thrown or to fall, causing fractures or other injuries. If the person who has been burned is in pain, is confused, or is experiencing changes in breathing, heartbeat or consciousness, call 911 or emergency medical help.

While waiting for medical help:

1. **Don't touch the person.** He or she may still be in contact with the electrical source. Touching the person may pass the current through you.
2. **Turn off the source of electricity, if possible.** If not, separate the person and the source using a *dry* nonconducting object made of wood, cardboard, plastic or fiberglass. Don't attempt a rescue if the voltage is over 600 volts, such as a downed power line. Stay at least 20 feet away.
3. **Check for signs of circulation (breathing, coughing or movement).** If absent, begin CPR immediately.

Cold-weather problems

Frostbite

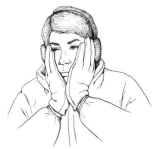

Cover your face if you feel the effects of frostbite.

Frostbite can affect any area of your body. Your hands, feet, nose and ears are most susceptible because they are delicate and often exposed.

In subfreezing temperatures, the tiny blood vessels in your skin tighten, reducing the flow of blood and oxygen to the tissues. Eventually, cells are destroyed.

The first sign of frostbite may be a slightly painful, tingling sensation. This often is followed by numbness. Your skin may be deathly pale and feel hard, cold and numb. Frostbite can damage deep layers of tissue. As deeper layers of tissue freeze, blisters often form. Blistering usually occurs over one to two days.

People with "hardening of the arteries" (atherosclerosis) or who are taking certain medications may be more susceptible to frostbite.

Self-care

- Carefully and gently rewarm frostbitten areas. Get out of the cold, if possible. If you're outside, place your hands directly on the skin of warmer areas of your body. Warm your hands by tucking them into your armpits. If your nose, ears or face is frostbitten, warm the area by covering it with your warm hands (but try to keep your hands protected).
- If possible, immerse your hands or feet in water that's warm — not hot — for 30 minutes.
- Don't use direct heat (such as heating pads).
- Don't rub the affected area. Never rub snow on frostbitten skin.
- Don't smoke cigarettes or drink alcohol. Nicotine causes blood vessels to tighten, impairing circulation. Alcohol impairs judgment, increasing re-exposure risk.
- If feet or hands are frostbitten, elevate them (to the level of your heart) after rewarming.
- Don't rewarm an affected area if there's a chance that it'll refreeze.

Follow-up

Frostbitten areas will turn red and throb, or burn with pain as they thaw. Even with mild frostbite, normal sensation may not return immediately. A nonprescription anti-inflammatory medication, such as ibuprofen, will help with pain and may lessen the damage. When frostbite is severe, the area will probably remain numb until it heals completely. Healing can take months, and the damage to your skin can permanently change your sense of touch. In severe cases, in which infection is present after the affected area has been rewarmed, antibiotics may be necessary. Bed rest and physical therapy may be appropriate. Don't smoke cigarettes during recovery. Once you've had frostbite — no matter how mild — you're more likely to have it again.

Emergency treatment

If numbness remains during rewarming, you develop blisters or the damage appears severe, seek medical care. A person with frostbite on the extremities may also have hypothermia (see page 21).

Kids' care

Watch for signs of chilling or cold injury — especially the face, hands and feet of infants and toddlers — while your child is outside. Watch for wet chin straps on caps or snowsuits because the skin under the strap can easily freeze. Teach your child to avoid touching cold metal with bare hands and licking cold metal objects.

See back cover for online resource

How to prevent cold-weather injuries

- **Stay dry.** Your body loses heat faster when your skin is dampened by rain, snow or perspiration.
- **Protect yourself from the wind.** Wind robs more heat from your body than does cold air alone. Exposed skin is particularly affected by wind.
- **Wear clothes that insulate, shield and breathe.** Dress in layers of light, loosefitting clothing to trap air for effective insulation. The outer layer should be windproof and water-repellent.
- **Cover your head, neck and face.** Wear two pairs of socks and boots that cover your ankles. Mittens protect hands better than gloves do.
- **Rewarm yourself.** If a part of your body becomes so cold that it starts to feel numb, rewarm it before continuing your activity.
- **Don't touch metal with bare skin.** Cold metal can absorb heat quickly.
- **Plan for trips and outdoor activities.** Carry an emergency kit.

■ Hypothermia

When your body is exposed for prolonged periods to cold temperatures or a cool, damp environment, its control mechanisms may fail to keep your body temperature normal. When more heat is lost than your body can generate, **hypothermia** can result. Wet or damp clothing can increase your chances of hypothermia.

Falling overboard from a boat into cold water is a common cause of hypothermia. An uncovered head or inadequate clothing in winter is another frequent cause.

The key symptom of hypothermia is a body temperature that drops to less than 95 F. Signs include shivering, slurred speech, an abnormally slow rate of breathing, skin that is cold and pale (although infants may have bright red skin), a loss of coordination, and feelings of tiredness, lethargy or apathy. The onset of symptoms is usually slow — there's likely to be a gradual loss of mental sharpness and physical ability. The person who has hypothermia, in fact, may be unaware that he or she is in a state requiring emergency medical treatment.

Older adults, the very young and very lean people are at particular risk. Other conditions that may predispose you to hypothermia are malnutrition, heart disease, an underactive thyroid, certain medications and excessive drinking of alcohol.

Emergency treatment

- After getting the person out of the cold, change the person into warm, dry clothing. If going indoors isn't possible, the person needs to be out of the wind, have his or her head covered, and be insulated from the cold ground.
- Seek emergency medical assistance. While waiting for help to arrive, monitor the person's breathing and pulse. If either has stopped or seems dangerously slow or shallow, start CPR immediately (see pages 2-3).
- In extreme cases, once the person has arrived at a medical center, blood rewarming, similar to the procedure in a heart bypass machine, is sometimes used to restore normal body temperature quickly.
- If emergency care isn't available, warm the person with a bath at 100 to 105 F, which is warm to the touch but not hot. Give warm, nutritional liquids.
- Companions may be able to share body heat.

Caution

Don't give the person alcohol. Give warm nonalcoholic, caffeine-free drinks, unless he or she is vomiting.

Cuts, scrapes and wounds

Everyday cuts, scrapes and wounds often don't require a trip to the emergency room. Yet proper care is essential to avoid infection or other complications.

◼ Simple wounds

The following guidelines can help you in caring for simple wounds.

Self-care

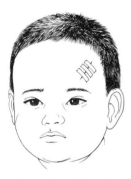

A few strips of surgical tape (Steri-Strips) may be used to close a minor cut. But if the mouth of the wound is not easily closed, seek a doctor's care. Proper closure will help minimize scarring.

- **Stop the bleeding.** Minor <u>cuts and scrapes</u> usually stop bleeding on their own. If not, apply gentle pressure with a clean cloth or bandage.
- **Keep the wound clean.** Rinse with clear water. Clean the area around the wound with soap and a washcloth. Keep soap out of the wound, as it can cause irritation. If dirt or debris remains in the wound after washing, use tweezers cleaned with alcohol to remove the particles. If debris still remains embedded in the wound, don't attempt to remove the particles by yourself — contact your health care provider. Thorough wound cleaning reduces the risk of infection and tetanus. There's no need to use hydrogen peroxide, iodine or an iodine-containing cleanser, which can be irritating to tissue already injured.
- **Consider the source.** Puncture wounds or other deep cuts, animal bites or particularly dirty wounds put you at higher risk of infections, including tetanus. If the wound is serious, you may require antibiotics or an additional tetanus booster (see page 23).
- **Prevent infection.** After you clean the wound, if desired, apply a thin layer of an antibiotic cream or ointment (such as Neosporin or Polysporin) to help keep the surface moist. The products don't make the wound heal faster, but they can discourage infection and allow your body's healing factors to close the wound more efficiently. However, certain ingredients in some ointments can cause a mild rash in some people. If a rash appears, stop using the ointment.
- **Cover the wound.** Exposure to air will speed healing, but bandages can help keep the wound clean, keep harmful bacteria out and protect the wound from additional irritation. Blisters that are draining are vulnerable and should be covered until a scab forms.
- **Change the dressing to help prevent infection.** Do this at least once a day or whenever it becomes wet or dirty. If you're allergic to the adhesive in tapes, switch to sterile gauze and paper tape or pressure netting to hold the dressing in place. These supplies generally are available at pharmacies.

Medical help

If bleeding persists — if the blood spurts or continues to flow after several minutes of direct pressure — emergency care is necessary.

Are stitches needed? A deep (all the way through the skin), gaping or jagged-edged wound with exposed fat or muscle will require stitches to hold it together for proper healing. Strips of surgical tape may be used to close a minor cut, but if the torn skin isn't easily closed, seek medical care. Proper closure will help minimize scarring (see page 23), speed healing and reduce the risk of infection.

See back cover for online resource ⓘ

Caution Watch for signs of infection. Every day that a wound remains open, the risk of infection increases. See your health care provider if your wound isn't healing steadily or if you notice any redness, drainage, warmth or swelling.

A shot in the arm: Tetanus vaccine

A cut, laceration, puncture, bite or other wound, even if minor, can lead to a **tetanus** infection. Tetanus is a serious bacterial disease caused by a toxin that leads to stiffness of your jaw muscles and other muscles, sometimes called lockjaw. Tetanus can cause severe muscle spasms, make breathing difficult and, ultimately, threaten your life.

Spores of tetanus bacteria, *Clostridium tetani*, usually are found in the soil, but can occur virtually anywhere. If deposited in a wound, bacteria can produce a toxin that interferes with the nerves controlling your muscles.

Immunization is vital *before* an injury (see page 227). The tetanus vaccine usually is given to children as a diphtheria, tetanus and acellular pertussis (DTaP) shot. Adults generally need a tetanus-diphtheria (Td) booster every 10 years. If the wound is serious, your doctor may recommend an additional booster even if your last one was within 10 years, as well as an injection of anti-tetanus antibody. A booster is given if you have a deep or dirty wound and your most recent booster was more than five years ago. Boosters should be given within two days of the injury.

■ Puncture wounds

A **puncture wound** doesn't usually result in excessive bleeding. Often, in fact, little blood flows, and the wound seems to close almost instantly. This doesn't mean that treatment is unnecessary. Puncture wounds may require medical attention.

A puncture wound — such as from stepping on a nail, glass, tack or wood splinter — may be dangerous because of the risk of infection. The object that caused the wound may carry spores of tetanus or other bacteria, especially if the object has been exposed to dirt. For a simple wound, follow the self-care steps and advice on seeking medical help on page 22. A deep puncture wound may need to be cleaned by a doctor.

What about scarring?

No matter how you treat cuts, all deep wounds that penetrate deeper than the first layer of skin form a scar when healed. Even superficial wounds can change skin tone or form a scar if infection or re-injury occurs.

When a healing wound is exposed to sunlight, it can darken permanently. This darkening can be prevented by covering the area with clothing or a sunblock (SPF over 30) whenever you're outside during the first six months after the wound occurred.

A scar usually thickens about two months into the healing process. Within six months to a year, the scar tissue thins out.

Scar tissue that continues to enlarge and thicken is called a keloid. Surgical incisions, vaccinations,

burns or even a scratch can cause keloids. The tendency to develop keloids is often inherited, and the darker the skin, the greater the likelihood for keloids. Keloids are most common on the shoulders or chest.

Keloids are harmless. But if they itch or look unattractive, doctors can sometimes remove small keloids by freezing them with liquid nitrogen, then injecting them with cortisone. Or they may use topical medicines, surgery or other types of scar revision. Sometimes keloids stop growing, but they rarely disappear by themselves.

Ask a dermatologist or plastic surgeon to evaluate your scar and advise treatment if it looks bad to you. Keloids can recur after treatment.

Eye injuries

Consider some common objects in your home — paper clips, pencils, tools and toys. Used without care, they pose a threat to your windows on the world — your eyes.

Eye injuries are common, and some are serious. Fortunately, you can prevent most injuries by taking simple steps. (See pages 76-81 for common eye problems.)

■ Corneal abrasion (scratch)

The most common types of eye injury involve the cornea — the clear, protective tissue over the front of the eye that covers the iris and pupil. The cornea can be scratched or cut by contact with dust, dirt, sand, wood shavings, metal particles or even an edge of a piece of paper. Usually the scratch is superficial, and this is called a **corneal abrasion**. Some corneal abrasions become infected and result in a corneal ulcer, which is a serious problem.

Everyday activities can lead to corneal abrasions. Examples are playing sports, doing home repairs or being scratched by children who accidentally brush your cornea with a fingernail.

Because the cornea is extremely sensitive, abrasions can be painful. A scratched cornea might make you feel like you have sand in your eye. Excessive eye watering, blurred vision, light sensitivity, pain or redness in or around the eye may indicate a corneal abrasion.

Self-care

In case of injury, seek prompt medical attention. In addition:
- Don't rub your eye. This action can worsen a corneal abrasion.
- If you have a corneal abrasion and there is no foreign body in your eye, do *not* rinse with water. If you do have a foreign body in your eye, see page 25.
- Do not apply patches or ice packs to the eye.

■ Chemical splash

Other common injuries to the cornea include "splash accidents" — contact with chemicals ranging from antifreeze to household cleaners.

Self-care

If a chemical splashes into your eye:
- Flush your eye immediately: Run lukewarm water over your eye or splash your eye with clean water. Any source of clean drinking water will do if you have a **chemical splash**. Continue to flush your eye for 20 minutes, particularly if your eye is exposed to household cleaners that have ammonia. Many work sites have eye-rinse stations for this purpose.
- After flushing your eye thoroughly, close your eyelid and cover it with a loose, moist dressing. If the chemical is hazardous, or you have pain or vision changes (or other symptoms), seek emergency medical care. If you're not sure whether a substance is harmful to the eye, call Poison Help at 800-222-1222.

Caution
- Don't rub your eye.
- Don't apply patches or ice packs to your eye.

See back cover for online resource (i)

■ Foreign object in the eye

If you or someone else has a **foreign object in the eye**, below are guidelines for action.

Self-care

To remove a small foreign object from your eye, flush the eye with a small amount of clean water using a small cup.

Clearing your own eye
- If it's a minor issue, such as small particles of dust, blinking several times may remove the particles. If this doesn't work:
- Try to flush the object out of your eye with clean, lukewarm water or saline solution. Use an eyecup or small clean glass. Position the glass with its rim resting on the bone at the base of your eye socket and pour the fluid in, keeping the eye open.

Clearing someone else's eye
- Wash your hands. Seat the person in a well-lighted area.
- Examine the eye to find the object. Gently pull the lower lid down and ask the person to look up. Then hold the upper lid while the person looks down.
- If the object is floating in the tear film or on the surface of the eye, try flushing it out. If you're able to remove the object, flush the eye with a saline solution or clean, lukewarm water.
- If the object is large and makes closing the eye difficult, cover it with a paper cup taped to the face and forehead. *Seek emergency medical care immediately.*

Caution
- Don't rub the eye, and don't apply patches or ice packs to the eye.
- Don't try to remove an object that's embedded in the eyeball.
- Don't try to remove a large object that makes closing the eye difficult.

Emergency care

Seek emergency medical help when:
- You can't remove the object
- The object is embedded in the eyeball
- The person with the object in the eye is experiencing abnormal vision
- Pain, redness or vision problems persist

Common sense can save your sight

- **Wear goggles** while working with industrial chemicals, power tools and even hand tools. Some of the most serious eye injuries occur while people are using hammers. Also wear a safety helmet when appropriate.
- **Wear safety glasses** for sports such as racquetball, basketball, squash and tennis. Also wear appropriate headgear, such as a batter's helmet for baseball and a face mask for hockey.
- **Carefully follow the instructions for using detergents, ammonia and cleaning fluids.** When using fluids in spray containers, always point the nozzles away from your eyes. Store household chemicals safely and out of children's reach.

- **Supervise children at play.** Remove any toys that could lead to an eye injury. Examples are BB guns, plastic swords and spring-loaded toys that shoot darts. Don't allow children to have fireworks.
- **Don't lean over a car battery** when attaching jumper cables.
- **Pick up rocks and sticks** before mowing your lawn. While mowing, watch for trees with low-hanging branches.
- **Carefully follow instructions** for removing and applying contact lenses. Also, investigate any pain or eye reddening that occurs while you're wearing contact lenses.

Foodborne illness

Foodborne illness, also called food poisoning, is a growing problem in the United States. And our global food supply contributes to widespread outbreaks.

Foods naturally contain small amounts of bacteria. But when food is improperly grown, poorly handled, improperly cooked or inadequately stored, bacteria can multiply in great enough numbers to cause illness. Parasites, viruses and chemicals also can contaminate food, but foodborne illness from these sources is less common.

If you eat contaminated food, whether you become ill depends on the organism, the amount of exposure, your age and your health. The immune systems of older adults may not respond as quickly and effectively to infectious organisms as they used to. Young children are at increased risk of illness because their immune systems haven't developed fully. If you're pregnant or you've had an organ transplant, you may be at higher risk. Conditions such as diabetes, AIDS and cancer treatment also reduce immune response, making you more susceptible to foodborne illness.

Signs and symptoms may start within hours after consuming contaminated food or water, or they may begin days later. Signs or symptoms may include nausea, vomiting, diarrhea, abdominal pain, stomach cramps, fatigue or fever.

Self-care	• If you have nausea and vomiting, see "Self-care," page 66. For diarrhea, see "Self-care," page 59. If you have both, use the self-care tips for vomiting first. • Don't use anti-diarrheal medications unless recommended by your doctor. These drugs may slow elimination of the bacteria and toxins from your system. • Mild to moderate illness often resolves on its own in one or two days.
Medical help	If symptoms last more than 48 hours, or are severe, or you belong to one of the high-risk groups noted above, seek prompt medical attention to avoid dehydration.
Caution	Botulism is a potentially fatal food poisoning. It results from eating foods containing a toxin formed by certain spores in food. Botulinum toxin is most often found in home-canned foods, especially green beans and tomatoes. Symptoms usually begin 12 to 36 hours after eating the contaminated food. Symptoms include a headache, blurred or double vision, muscle weakness, and, eventually, paralysis. Some people report nausea, vomiting, constipation, urinary retention and reduced salivation. These symptoms require immediate medical attention.

Handling food safely

- **Plan ahead.** Thaw meats and other frozen foods in the refrigerator, not on the countertop.
- **When shopping,** don't buy food in cans or jars with dented or bulging lids.
- **When preparing food,** wash your hands with soap and water. Rinse produce thoroughly or peel off the skin or outer leaves. Wash knives and cutting surfaces frequently, especially after handling raw meat and before preparing other foods. Launder kitchen linens frequently.

- **When cooking,** use a meat thermometer. Cook red meat to an internal temperature of 160 F, poultry to 165 F. Cook fish until it flakes easily with a fork. Cook eggs until the yolks are firm.
- **When storing food,** check expiration dates. Refrigerate perishables within two hours of purchase. Use or freeze fresh poultry, fish and ground meat within one to two days and red meats within three to five days. Refrigerate or freeze leftovers within two hours of serving.

See back cover for online resource (i)

Troublesome bacteria and how you can stop them

Keep hot food hot. Keep cold food cold. Keep everything — especially your hands — clean. Use soap when washing. If you follow these basic rules, you'll be less likely to become ill from the troublesome bacteria listed here.

Bacteria	How spread	Symptoms	To prevent
Campylobacter jejuni	Contaminates meat and poultry during processing if feces contacts meat surfaces. Other sources: unpasteurized milk, untreated water.	Severe diarrhea (sometimes bloody), abdominal cramps, chills, headache. Onset: 2 to 5 days. Lasts 2 to 10 days.	Cook meat and poultry thoroughly. Wash knives and cutting surfaces after contact with raw meat. Don't drink unpasteurized milk or untreated water.
Clostridium perfringens	Meats, stews, gravies. Commonly spread when serving dishes don't keep food hot enough or food is chilled too slowly.	Watery diarrhea, nausea, abdominal cramps. Fever is rare. Onset: up to 16 hours. Lasts 1 to 2 days.	Keep foods hot. Hold cooked meats above 140 F. Reheat to at least 165 F. Chill foods quickly. Store in small containers.
Escherichia coli O157:H7	Contaminates beef during slaughter. Spread mainly by undercooked ground beef. Other sources: unpasteurized milk and unpasteurized apple cider, water or crops that are contaminated.	Watery diarrhea may turn bloody within 24 hours. Severe abdominal cramps, nausea, occasional vomiting. Usually no fever. Onset: 1 to 8 days. Lasts 5 to 10 days.	Cook beef to internal temperature of 160 F. Don't drink unpasteurized milk or unpasteurized apple cider. Wash hands after bathroom use.
Noroviruses (Norwalk-like viruses)	Consuming contaminated food or liquids; touching contaminated surfaces or objects.	Nausea, vomiting, diarrhea, stomach cramps, low-grade fever, chills. Onset: 12 to 48 hours. Lasts 12 to 60 hours.	Wash hands after bathroom use. Wash fruits and vegetables. Disinfect surfaces.
Salmonella	Raw or contaminated meat, poultry, milk, egg yolks. Survives inadequate cooking. Spread by knives, cutting surfaces or an infected person with poor hygiene.	Severe diarrhea, watery stools, nausea, vomiting, temperature 101 F or higher. Onset: 1 to 3 days. Lasts 4 to 7 days.	Cook meat and poultry thoroughly. Don't drink unpasteurized milk. Don't eat raw or undercooked eggs. Keep cutting surfaces clean. Wash hands after bathroom use.
Staphylococcus aureus	Spread by hand contact, coughing and sneezing. Grows on meats and prepared salads, cream sauces, cream-filled pastries.	Explosive, watery diarrhea, nausea, vomiting, abdominal cramps, lightheadedness. Onset: 1 to 6 hours. Lasts 1 to 2 days.	Don't leave high-risk foods at room temperature for more than 2 hours. Wash hands and utensils before preparing food.
Vibrio vulnificus	Raw oysters and raw or undercooked mussels, clams, whole scallops.	Chills, fever, open wound. Onset: 1 to 7 days. Can be fatal if immunity is low.	Don't eat raw oysters. Make sure all shellfish is thoroughly cooked.
Listeria monocytogenes	Hot dogs, luncheon meats, unpasteurized milk and cheeses, unwashed raw vegetables.	Abdominal cramps, nausea, diarrhea, vomiting, fever. Onset: 9 to 48 hours, or after weeks if invasive disease.	Heat meats thoroughly. Avoid unpasteurized milk and milk products. Wash raw vegetables.

Heat-related problems

Under normal conditions, your body's natural control mechanisms — skin and perspiration — adjust to the heat. These systems may fail if you're exposed to high temperatures for prolonged periods.

Working out in hot or humid conditions can overstress your body's temperature-regulation system, causing an excessive increase in body temperature. Heat-related problems may include heat cramps, dehydration, heat exhaustion and heatstroke.

Heat cramps

Heat cramps are painful muscle spasms. They usually occur after vigorous activity in a hot environment. They develop when sweating depletes your body of salt (sodium) and water. The muscles of the arms, legs and abdomen are most often affected.

Heat exhaustion

Signs and symptoms of heat exhaustion include cool, clammy and pale skin, heat cramps, a weak pulse, nausea, chills and dizziness, weakness, or disorientation. You may have a headache and be short of breath.

Heatstroke

Heatstroke can be life-threatening. Your skin becomes hot, flushed and dry. You stop perspiring and have a fever. Your body temperature can quickly reach dangerous levels of 104 F or higher. You may feel confused and may even faint. Other signs include a rapid heartbeat, rapid and shallow breathing, confusion, and increased or reduced blood pressure.

Young children, older adults and people who are obese are particularly at risk of heatstroke. Other risk factors include dehydration, alcohol use, heart disease, certain medications and vigorous exercise. People born with an impaired ability to sweat also are at higher risk.

Self-care

To avoid heat-related conditions:
- Avoid going outside during the hottest part of the day, noon to 4 p.m.
- Drink plenty of fluids, especially water and sports drinks. Avoid alcohol and caffeine.
- Wear light-colored, lightweight loosefitting clothing made of breathable fabric.
- Reserve vigorous exercise or activities for early morning or evening. If possible, exercise in the shade.
- Allow yourself time to adjust to higher temperatures.
- Talk to your doctor if you take medications. Certain medications, such as diuretics and antihistamines, may make you more susceptible to heat-related illness.
- Avoid hot and heavy meals.

Medical help

If you suspect a heat-related illness, get out of the heat, drink fluids, elevate your feet above your head, and either wet and fan your skin or immerse yourself in cool water. If you suspect heatstroke, call 9ll or emergency medical help immediately.

See back cover for online resource

Poisonous plants

Poison ivy

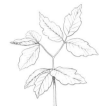
Poison oak

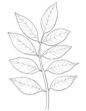
Poison sumac

When it comes to poison oak and ivy, it's wise to heed these words of advice: "Leaves of three, let them be." With their leaves usually grouped three to a stem, poison ivy and poison oak are two of the most common causes of an allergic skin reaction called *contact dermatitis*.

Contact with poison ivy and poison oak usually causes red, swollen skin, blisters and severe itching. This reaction typically develops within two days after exposure, but it may start within a few hours or it may take several days. The rash is usually gone in a couple of weeks but may last longer in people who are more sensitive to poison ivy. It may leave scars.

The rash is caused by exposure to resin, a colorless, oily substance in these plants. Resin transfers easily from clothing or from pet hair to your skin. The rash may be in a line or patchy, due to the way the plant sweeps across your skin. Don't burn poisonous plants because the resin in the smoke can irritate or injure your eyes or nasal passages.

It may take only a tiny amount of resin to cause a reaction. Sensitivity to poison ivy varies. The rash doesn't spread as a result of washing or scratching open the blisters. The resin isn't in blister fluid. However, it can be spread by accidentally rubbing the resin on other areas of the skin before all the resin is washed off.

These plants also can cause a reaction: sumac, heliotrope (found in the deserts of the Southwest), ragweed, daisies, chrysanthemums, sagebrush, wormwood, celery, oranges, limes and potatoes. Wild parsnip causes a burn-like reaction.

Self-care

- Washing the harmful resin off the skin with soap as soon as possible after exposure may avert a skin reaction. Be sure to wash under your fingernails.
- Don't try to remove the resin by taking a bath. That can spread the resin to other areas of your body. Shower with a mild soap and water for at least 15 minutes.
- Try not to scratch. Take cool showers. Over-the-counter products (OTC), such as calamine lotion and hydrocortisone cream, can ease itching, as can an OTC antihistamine, such as diphenhydramine (Benadryl, others). Or try tub soaks with baking soda ($1/2$ to 1 cup) or colloidal oatmeal (such as Aveeno).
- Cover open blisters with sterile gauze to prevent infection.
- Avoid exposure to the sun after encountering wild parsnip. Treat the rash as you would a sunburn (see page 19.)
- Wash any clothing or jewelry that may have been in contact with the plant. Also wash footwear and shoelaces. Bathe pets that may have plant oils on their fur.

Prevention

- Learn to recognize poisonous plants and wear protective clothing when appropriate to avoid exposure. Poison ivy leaves are oval or spoon-shaped. Poison oak leaves resemble oak leaves. The colors of the leaves of these plants change from green in the summer to orange and red in the fall.
- If there's a risk of exposure, consider applying an over-the counter skin cream containing bentoquatam as a barrier. (If your child is under 6 years old, check with the doctor first.)

Medical help

If you have a severe reaction, or your eyes, face or genital area is involved, contact your doctor, who may prescribe cortisone or an oral antihistamine. If you have an infected open cut, you may need an antibiotic. To reduce scarring, see page 23.

Tooth problems

▮ Toothache

Dental cavities can lead to toothaches.

<u>Tooth decay</u> (cavities) is the primary cause of <u>toothaches</u>. Tooth decay mainly is caused by bacteria and carbohydrates. Bacteria are present in a thin, almost invisible film on your teeth called plaque.

Decay can occur faster in people with dry mouth, people who drink a lot of soft drinks or sports drinks, people who suck on hard candies or cough drops, those who eat a lot of high-sugar foods, and those who abuse methamphetamine.

Decay-producing acid — which forms soon after you eat — forms in plaque and attacks the tooth's outer surface. The erosion caused by the plaque leads to the formation of tiny openings (cavities) in the tooth surface. The first sign of decay may be a sensation of pain when you eat something sweet, very cold or very hot.

Self-care

Until you're able to get to the dentist, try these self-care tips:
- Take an over-the-counter (OTC) pain reliever.
- Sparingly apply an OTC gel containing benzocaine directly to the irritated tooth and gum to relieve pain.
- Prevention is the best way to avoid tooth decay and cavities by regular brushing and flossing. Most bottled water doesn't contain fluoride — ask your dentist (and your child's dentist) how much fluoride is needed and how to get it.

Caution

Facial or jaw swelling, pain when you bite, a foul-tasting discharge, gum redness, or a fever indicate infection. See your dentist as soon as possible. If you have a fever with the pain, seek emergency care.

▮ Tooth loss

Whenever a tooth is accidentally knocked out, appropriate care is required immediately. Today, permanent teeth that are knocked out sometimes can be reimplanted if you act quickly. A broken tooth, however, cannot be reimplanted.

Emergency treatment

If a permanent tooth is knocked out, save the tooth (see tips below) and contact your dentist immediately. If it's after office hours, call your dentist's emergency number. If he or she is unavailable, go to the nearest emergency room. Successful reimplantation depends on several factors: prompt insertion (within 30 minutes if possible) and proper storage and transportation of the tooth. Keeping it moist is essential.

Self-care

To preserve the tooth and treat yourself until you get to the dentist:
- Handle the tooth by the top (crown) only.
- Do not rub it or scrape it to remove dirt — rinse in cold water.
- Rinse your mouth with water, and apply pressure to stop bleeding.
- Place the tooth in milk, a saltwater solution ($1/4$ teaspoon salt to 1 quart water) or tucked inside the cheek. If these options aren't possible, place the tooth in water or a clean moist cloth.

With contact sports, you can often prevent <u>tooth loss</u> by wearing a mouth guard, fitted by your dentist. Seeing your dentist regularly is also important.

Trauma: Bones and muscles

Trauma is any injury resulting from external force or violence. A broken bone, a severe blow to the head and a knocked-out tooth are all considered trauma.

Fractures, severe sprains, dislocations and other serious bone and joint injuries are trauma emergencies and usually require medical care.

■ Dislocations

A **dislocation** is an injury in which the end of a bone in a joint are forced from its normal position. In most cases, a blow, fall or other trauma causes the dislocation.

Indications of a dislocation include:

- An injured joint that's visibly out of position, misshapen and difficult to move
- Swelling and intense pain at a joint

The dislocation should be treated as quickly as possible, but don't try to return the joint to its proper place. Splint the affected joint in the position it's in. Treat it as you would a fracture. Seek immediate medical attention. Placing a covered ice pack on the injured joint will help reduce swelling by controlling internal bleeding and buildup of fluids. (For information on a dislocated elbow in a child, see page 93.)

■ Fractures

A **fracture** is a broken bone. It requires immediate medical attention. If you suspect a fracture, protect the affected area from further damage. Don't try to realign the broken bone. Instead, immobilize the injured bone — including the joint above and below the injury — with a firm pillow or other firm item. If you've been trained in how to splint and professional help isn't readily available, apply a splint to the area.

If bleeding occurs with the broken bone, apply pressure to stop the bleeding. If possible, elevate the site of bleeding to lessen the blood flow. Maintain pressure for at least 15 minutes. If bleeding continues, reapply pressure until it stops.

If the person appears faint, pale or is breathing in a notably shallow and rapid fashion, treat for shock: Lay the person down, elevate the legs and cover him or her with a blanket to keep warm. Lay the person on the uninjured side if vomiting occurs.

To make a splint, use rigid material such as wood, plastic or metal. The splint should be longer than the bone it's splinting and extend above and below the injury. Pad the splint wherever possible.

Signs and symptoms

Signs and symptoms of a fracture may include:

- Swelling or bruising over a bone.
- Deformity of the affected limb.
- Localized pain that is intensified when the affected area is moved or pressure is put on it.
- Loss of function in the area of the injury.
- A broken bone that has poked through soft tissues and is sticking out of the skin. This open fracture could get infected, so cover it with sterile gauze before applying the splint.

For more information on fractures, see page 89.

 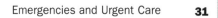

■ Sprains

A sprain occurs when a violent twist or stretch causes a joint to move outside its normal range. **Sprains** are the result of overstretched ligaments. Tearing of the ligaments may occur. The usual indications of a sprain are the following:

- Pain and tenderness in the affected area
- Rapid swelling and possible discoloration of the skin
- Impaired joint function

Most minor sprains can be treated at home. However, if a popping sound and immediate difficulty in using the joint accompany the injury, seek emergency medical care. For more information on sprains, see page 88.

Trauma: Head injuries

Some head injuries require hospitalization. However, most head injuries are minor. Simple cuts and bruises can often be treated with basic first-aid techniques.

In all cases of worrisome **head injury**, don't move the neck because it may be injured. Wait for trained emergency personnel who can move the person safely. Move the person only if he or she is in grave danger, keeping the head and neck stable with your hands. Serious head injuries requiring emergency care are described below.

Concussion. When the head sustains a hard blow as the result of being struck or from a fall, a **concussion** may result. The impact creates a sudden movement of the brain within the skull. Some concussions cause you to lose consciousness, but most do not. People with concussions are often described as dazed or confused. Loss of memory, repetitive speech, a headache, dizziness and vomiting also may occur.

Blood clot on the brain. This occurs when a blood vessel ruptures between the skull and the brain. Blood then leaks between the brain and skull and forms a blood clot (hematoma), which presses on the brain tissue. Symptoms occur from a few hours to several weeks to months after a blow to the head. There may be no open wound, bruise or other outward sign. Signs and symptoms include a headache, nausea, vomiting, alteration of consciousness and pupils of unequal size. There may be progressive lethargy, unconsciousness and death if the condition isn't treated.

Skull fracture. This type of injury isn't always apparent. Look for:

- Bruising or discoloring behind the ear or around the eyes
- Blood or clear, watery fluids leaking from the ears or nose
- Pupils of unequal size
- Deformity of the skull, including swelling or depressions

Emergency treatment

Call 911 or your local emergency number if any of these occur:

- Severe head or facial bleeding
- Change in level of consciousness, even if only briefly
- Irregular or labored breathing or stopping of breathing
- Confusion, loss of balance, weakness in an arm or leg, or slurred speech
- Vomiting more than once

Caution

Until emergency help arrives, do *not* move the person. Keep the person lying down. Watch for normal breathing and alertness. If there is no pulse and no breathing, begin CPR (see pages 2-3). Stop any bleeding by using firm pressure.

General Symptoms

- **Dizziness and fainting**
- **Fatigue**
- **Fever**
- **Pain**
- **Sleep disorders**
- **Sweating and body odor**
- **Unexpected weight changes**

Dizziness, fainting, fatigue, fever, pain, difficulty sleeping, sweating and unexpected weight changes: In medicine, these conditions are called general symptoms because they tend to affect your entire body rather than a particular body part or system. In this section, the common causes for each of these general symptoms are explained, along with self-care tips and advice on when to seek medical care.

Dizziness and fainting

Dizziness has many causes. Fortunately, most dizziness is mild, brief and harmless. It can be caused by many things, including medications, infections and stress. The word *dizziness* actually describes various sensations.

Vertigo and imbalance

Vertigo is the sensation that you or your surroundings are rotating. You may feel that the room is spinning, or you may sense the rotation within your own head or body. Vertigo usually is associated with problems in your inner ear. The inner ear has an ultrasensitive device for sensing movement. Viral illness, trauma or other disturbance can result in the device sending a false message to your brain.

Imbalance is the sensation that you must touch or hold on to something to maintain your balance. Severe imbalance may make it difficult to stand without falling.

Lightheadedness and fainting

Lightheadedness includes feelings of being woozy, floating or near fainting. Fainting is a sudden, brief loss of consciousness. It occurs when your brain doesn't receive enough blood and the oxygen it carries. Once you're lying flat, blood flows to your brain and you regain consciousness within about a minute. Fainting may be caused by medical disorders, including heart disease, severe coughing spells and circulatory problems. In other cases, fainting may be related to:

- Medications for high blood pressure and erratic heartbeats
- Excessive sweating, vomiting or diarrhea resulting in fluid loss and dehydration
- Extreme fatigue
- Upsetting news or an unexpected or unusual stress such as the sight of blood

A rapid drop in blood pressure, called **orthostatic hypotension** (or postural hypotension), occurs when you get up quickly from a sitting or reclining position. Everyone experiences this reaction to a mild degree. You feel lightheaded or slightly faint, and it usually passes within seconds. The reaction may also occur after a hot bath or in people taking blood pressure medication. When it leads to fainting or blackouts, it's more serious.

Self-care

If you feel faint or dizzy, lie down or sit down. If you lie down, elevate your legs slightly to return blood to your heart. If you can't lie down, then sit down, lean forward and put your head between your knees.

Prevention

- Stand and change positions slowly — particularly when turning from side to side or when changing from lying down to standing. Before standing up in the morning, sit on the edge of the bed for a minute or two.
- Pace yourself. Take breaks when you are active in heat and humidity. Dress appropriate to the conditions to avoid overheating.
- Drink enough fluids to avoid dehydration. Aim to drink at least 48 to 64 ounces a day, unless your doctor tells you to limit fluids.
- Avoid caffeine, smoking, alcohol and illegal drugs.
- Don't drive a car or operate dangerous equipment if you feel dizzy.
- Check your medications. You may need to ask your doctor about adjustments.

See back cover for online resource (i)

Medical help

Mild symptoms that persist for weeks or months may be due to nervous system diseases. Sudden nausea, vomiting, dizziness or vertigo, and double vision are symptoms that require emergency attention, and may be due to bleeding in the brain.

Because problems of dizziness and balance can have many different causes, a diagnosis usually requires a complete medical history and several tests. Treatments for sudden onset of vertigo may include medication and avoiding positions or movements that cause dizziness. Your doctor may also suggest an inner ear positioning treatment (vestibular rehabilitation).

Seek emergency medical care if:

- There was any loss of consciousness
- Fainting or dizziness is accompanied by symptoms such as pain in the chest or head, trouble with breathing, numbness or continuing weakness or paralysis, irregular heartbeat, new confusion, decreased responsiveness, memory loss, seizure, trouble talking, problems with vision or coordination, blood in stools (sometimes indicated by black tarry stools) or other signs of blood loss, or nausea or vomiting

Until medical help arrives, if the person is lying down, position him or her on the back. If you believe the person is about to vomit, roll him or her onto the side. Raise the legs above the level of the head. If a person faints and remains seated, quickly lay him or her flat. Loosen tight clothing. Listen for breathing sounds. If they're absent, the problem is more serious than fainting, and CPR must be started. (See "CPR," page 2.)

If it's not an emergency, contact your health care provider if:

- The condition is severe, prolonged (more than a few days or a week) or recurrent
- You're taking medication for high blood pressure

How your body maintains balance

Maintaining balance requires a complex networking of several different parts of your body. To maintain balance, your brain must coordinate a constant flow of information from your eyes, nerves, muscles and tendons, and inner ear. All of these parts of the body work together to help keep you upright and provide you with a sense of stability when you're moving.

Many problems with dizziness are caused by problems within your inner ear. However, problems in any part of the system that controls your balance can cause dizziness and imbalance.

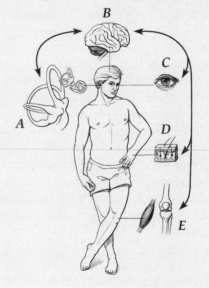

A. *The inner ear contains your primary balance structure.*

B. *The brain relays and interprets information to and from your body.*

C. *The eyes record your body's position and surroundings.*

D. *When you touch things, sensors in your skin give you information about your environment.*

E. *Muscles and joints report bodily movement to your brain.*

Fatigue

Almost everyone experiences **fatigue** at some time. After putting in a long weekend of yard chores or a hectic day with the children or at the office, it's natural to feel tired. This kind of physical and emotional fatigue is normal, and you can usually restore your energy with rest or exercise.

If you feel tired all the time, or if the exhaustion is overwhelming, you may begin to worry that your condition is more serious than just fatigue. When fatigue isn't accompanied by other symptoms, a specific cause often can't be determined. A common cause of chronic fatigue is lack of regular exercise (deconditioning). This problem can be remedied easily by gradually increasing your activity and beginning an exercise program.

Fatigue can be the result of physical or emotional problems. Physical fatigue is usually more pronounced later in the day, and it often resolves with a good night's sleep. Emotional fatigue often peaks first thing in the morning and gets better as the day progresses.

Common causes

Common causes of physical fatigue include:
- Poor eating habits
- Lack of sleep
- Being out of shape
- Warm working or living quarters
- Carbon monoxide poisoning
- Over-the-counter medications, including pain relievers, cough and cold medicines, antihistamines and allergy remedies, sleeping pills, and motion sickness pills
- Prescription drugs such as tranquilizers, muscle relaxants, sedatives, birth control pills and blood pressure medications
- Dehydration

Fatigue can also be an early symptom of these conditions:
- A low red blood cell count (anemia)
- Low thyroid activity (hypothyroidism)
- Various acute or chronic infections
- Heart disease
- Sleep disorder
- Electrolyte imbalance (when the levels of salts in your blood, such as sodium, potassium and other minerals, are too high or too low)
- Cancer
- Diabetes
- Alcoholism
- Rheumatoid arthritis

Many of these illnesses are accompanied by other signs and symptoms such as muscle aches, pain, nausea, weight loss, cold sensitivity and shortness of breath.

Common causes of emotional fatigue include:
- Overextending yourself, especially if you can't say no
- Boredom or lack of stimulation from family, friends or co-workers
- A major crisis (losing a spouse or a job), a move or a family difficulty
- Depression
- Loneliness
- Unresolved past emotional issues
- Repressing anger instead of expressing it

See back cover for online resource ⓘ

Self-care

Before you talk to a health care provider, consider the possibility that your fatigue may go away if you try some of these lifestyle changes:

- Get an adequate night's sleep — seven to eight hours of uninterrupted sleep. (See "Self-care," page 44.)
- Follow a sleep schedule. Go to bed and wake up at the same time each day.
- Give yourself a break. Ask others to pitch in.
- Organize your daily schedule and prioritize activities.
- Identify your stressors and try to reduce your stress level. (See "Keeping stress under control," page 221, and "Stress relievers," page 243.)
- Get more physical activity and exercise, starting gradually. If you're over age 40, consult your doctor before beginning a vigorous exercise program. (See "Physical activity and fitness," page 215.)
- Increase your exposure to fresh air at home and at work.
- Eat a balanced diet with plenty of fruits, vegetables and whole grains. Steer clear of high-fat foods. Eat a healthy breakfast. Don't skip meals.
- Create a plan to lose weight if you're overweight. But avoid very low calorie diets that don't provide enough nutrients and increase fatigue.
- Drink plenty of water. If your urine is clear or pale yellow, you're probably getting enough. If it's dark yellow, you probably need to drink more water.
- Review your medications (over-the-counter and prescription) to determine if fatigue is a side effect.
- Quit smoking.
- Reduce or eliminate use of alcohol, caffeine or other substances known to affect sleep or cause fatigue.

Medical help

If fatigue persists even when you rest enough and it lasts for two weeks or longer, you may have a problem that requires medical care. See your health care provider.

Kids' care

Sleep requirements vary by age. Consult a health care provider if fatigue interferes with the usual activities that your child likes to do.

What is chronic fatigue syndrome?

Chronic fatigue syndrome, also known as systemic exertion intolerance disease, is a poorly understood condition that can completely drain your energy and may last for years. People who were previously healthy and full of energy may experience intense fatigue, pain in joints and muscles, painful lymph glands, and headaches.

Experts haven't determined the causes of chronic fatigue syndrome, although there are likely many. Theories include infections, hormonal imbalances, and psychological, immunological or neurological abnormalities.

Treatment for chronic fatigue syndrome is aimed at relieving your symptoms. Anti-inflammatory pain relievers, such as ibuprofen (Advil, Motrin IB, others), often are prescribed, but they rarely help. Low doses of certain antidepressants may help relieve pain and depression often present with a chronic illness, as well as promote better sleep.

Because people with chronic fatigue syndrome may become out of shape, which perpetuates the fatigue, physical activity or physical therapy are crucial. These can help prevent or decrease muscle weakness caused by prolonged inactivity. In addition, you may benefit from cognitive behavioral therapy to help you deal with the illness and the limitations it creates.

Fever

Even when you're well, your temperature varies, and that variation is normal. The average healthy temperature is 98.6 F (37 C). But your normal temperature may differ by a degree or more — in the morning it's generally lower, and in the afternoon it's somewhat higher. Normal temperature also varies monthly by menstrual cycle.

Temperatures up to 100.4 F (38 C) typically are normal in healthy people. Check family members' temperatures when they're healthy. Discover their normal range. A temperature of 100.4 F (38 C) or higher is a **fever**.

What is the cause?

A fever itself isn't an illness, but it is often a sign of one. A fever tells you that something is happening inside your body.

Most likely, your body is fighting an infection caused by either bacteria or a virus. The fever may even be helpful in fighting the infection. Rarely, it's a sign of a reaction to a medicine, a malignancy or an inflammatory condition. Sometimes you don't know why you have a fever. But don't automatically try to lower your temperature. Decreasing it may mask symptoms and delay identifying the cause.

If you think the cause is something other than a viral illness, consult your health care provider. Common causes of a fever include the following:

- An infection, such as a kidney infection (frequent or painful urination), strep throat or tonsillitis (often with a sore throat), sinus infection (pain above or beneath the eyes), bronchitis or pneumonia (a cough and chest congestion), and dental abscess (tender area in the mouth)
- Infectious mononucleosis, accompanied by fatigue
- An illness you picked up in a foreign country
- Heat exhaustion or severe sunburn

Caution

Don't give aspirin to anyone under 18 years old, unless specifically recommended by the child's doctor. Rarely, aspirin causes a serious or even fatal disease called Reye's syndrome if given to children during a viral infection.

Self-care

You can try a number of things to make yourself or your child more comfortable during a fever (also see "Kids' care" on the next page):

- **Drink plenty of fluids.** A fever can cause fluid loss and dehydration. Drink water, juices or rehydration drinks such as Gatorade or Pedialyte (for infants).
- **Rest.** It's necessary for recovery, and activity can raise your body temperature.
- **Take acetaminophen or ibuprofen.** Use according to the label instructions or as recommended by your doctor. Don't use acetaminophen (Tylenol, others) and ibuprofen (Advil, Motrin IB, others) at the same time or alternate doses unless instructed to do so by your doctor. Avoid taking too much. High doses or long-term use may cause liver or kidney damage, and acute overdoses can be fatal. If you're not able to get your child's fever down, don't give more medication: Call your doctor instead. For temperatures below 102 F (38.9 C), don't use fever-lowering drugs unless advised by your doctor. Sometimes a low-grade fever helps the body eliminate a virus, such as a cold.
- **Soak in lukewarm water.** Especially for high temperatures, a lukewarm five- to 10-minute soak or giving your child a sponge bath can be cooling. Do not use alcohol. If the bath causes shivering, stop the bath and dry your child. Shivering raises the body's internal temperature — shaking muscles generate heat.

    See back cover for online resource

Medical help

Call your doctor in any of the following situations, especially if you have a productive cough, pain in the side, red skin, painful urination or diarrhea:

- Temperature of more than 104 F (40 C)
- Temperature of more than 102 F (38.9 C) for 48 hours or more
- Fever for over three days or one that returns after it was gone for 24 hours

A fever is only one sign of an illness. In particular, older adults or anyone with lowered immunity may run a fever when ill. Tell the doctor what contagious diseases people around you have had, including flu, colds, measles and mumps.

Call 911 (or a local emergency number) immediately if any of these also occur:

- Severe headache or unusual eye sensitivity to bright light
- Severe swelling of the throat, difficulty breathing or difficulty swallowing
- Significant stiff neck and pain when the head is bent forward
- Persistent vomiting or severe diarrhea
- Mental confusion or extreme listlessness or irritability

Kids' care

Call 911 or your local emergency number if your baby has a fever along with a bulging soft spot on the head. Call your health care provider immediately if your baby is 3 months or younger with a rectal temperature of 100.4 F (38 C) or higher.

Children under 6 may have a rapid rise or fall in temperature along with a seizure (febrile seizure). Typically the seizure lasts less than five minutes with no lasting effects. If a seizure happens, lay your child on his or her side where falling can't occur. Don't put anything in the mouth or try to stop the seizure. Promptly seek medical care. Call 911 if it's the first febrile seizure or it lasts over five minutes.

Sometimes a low-grade fever accompanies teething or a recent immunization. A fever with ear pulling may occasionally indicate a middle ear infection. Ask your doctor for advice and whether medication is needed.

Have your child drink water, juice or suck on frozen fruit pops. For children under age 1, use a rehydration drink such as Pedialyte. Pedialyte ice pops also are available. (Also see "Self-care," page 38, for more on children.)

Taking temperatures

Don't use mercury thermometers — recycle them to prevent accidental exposure to this toxin. There are several types of electronic digital thermometers for use with children. Options include:

Rectal thermometer. Provides the best reading for infants and for children up to 4 years old.

- Clean end of thermometer with rubbing alcohol or soap and water. Place a small amount of lubricant, such as petroleum jelly, on the end.
- Lay the child on his or her stomach.
- Turn on the thermometer and carefully insert the end one-half to 1 inch into the anal opening.
- Hold the thermometer and child still for about one minute, until you hear the beep.
- Remove the thermometer and check the reading.

Oral thermometer. Generally an effective method for children age 4 and older.

- Clean end of thermometer with rubbing alcohol or soap and water.
- Turn the switch on and place the sensor under the tongue toward the back of the mouth.
- Hold the thermometer in place about one minute, until you hear the beep.
- Remove the thermometer and check the reading.

Ear thermometer. Tympanic thermometers, which measure temperature inside the ear, are an option for children 3 months to 4 years.

- Gently place the end of the thermometer in the ear canal — make sure the placement is correct.
- Press start button. Reading appears in seconds.

Temporal artery (forehead) thermometer. By sweeping it across the forehead, this thermometer uses an infrared scanner to measure temperature. It's appropriate for children 3 months and up.

Pain

Physical pain is a part of life. Maybe you've slammed your finger in a door, burned your hand touching the hot handle of a pan on the stove or twisted your ankle while playing your favorite sport. The result is a sensation of pain. Pain can be acute or chronic.

Acute pain is temporary pain. It may be mild and last just a moment, such as from a sting. Or it can be severe and last for weeks or months, depending on the severity of the injury and how long it takes to heal — such as from a burn, pulled muscle or broken bone.

Chronic pain is persistent pain that lasts long after the normal healing process, or when there doesn't seem to be any past injury or bodily damage causing ongoing pain. Generally, chronic pain is considered to be pain that lasts more than three to six months. Many older adults have trouble sleeping due to chronic pain.

Chronic pain can be overwhelming. But you can learn ways to manage your pain so that your life can be more fulfilling and enjoyable, and you can still carry out your daily activities. Your attitude about pain, along with medications and therapies, can help you to manage it. An important part of managing your pain is understanding it.

Why doesn't the pain stop?

When your body is injured or infected, special nerve endings in your skin, joints, muscles or internal organs send messages to your brain telling it that there has been damage or an unpleasant stimulus to your body. Specialized nerve fibers instantly tell your brain where the pain is, how badly it hurts and the nature of the pain, such as burning, aching or stinging. Your brain then "reads" these pain signals and sends back a message to stop you from doing whatever is causing the pain. If you're touching something hot, for example, your brain will send a message to your muscles to contract so that you will pull back your hand.

Your brain also sends a message to your nerve cells to stop sending pain signals once the cause of the pain goes away (for example, when your injury starts to heal). But sometimes this mechanism fails, like a gate that's blocked open. For some reason, your nervous system continues to fire pain signals to your brain for months or even years after the injury, resulting in chronic pain.

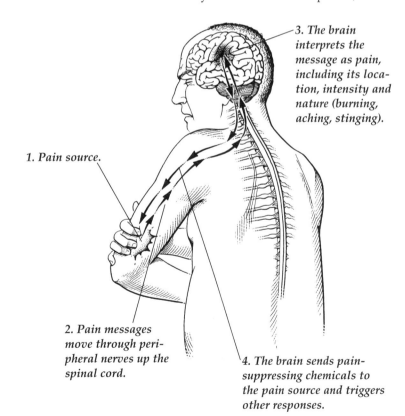

1. Pain source.

2. Pain messages move through peripheral nerves up the spinal cord.

3. The brain interprets the message as pain, including its location, intensity and nature (burning, aching, stinging).

4. The brain sends pain-suppressing chemicals to the pain source and triggers other responses.

The role of emotions and behavior in pain

Pain isn't only a physical experience but also an emotional one. People may perceive pain differently and react in different ways.

When you experience pain for a long time, you may find yourself overwhelmed by intense, often negative, emotions, including panic, fear, grief, anxiety and anger. Chronic pain can cause frustration and irritability, and can lead to feelings of depression and loss of hope. Like the pain that causes them, these emotions can linger and transform you into a different person.

Changes in your behavior, expressed through words and actions, can affect your sense of self-worth and your relationships. These changes can also affect your body, sapping your energy and intensifying your pain.

Finding positive ways to cope with your pain can have both physical and emotional benefits.

■ Common forms of chronic pain

General Symptoms

Chronic pain can become debilitating, but there are many ways to effectively manage pain. The key to pain control is a careful review of causes and a coordinated approach to management. Early and effective treatment of acute pain, such as after an operation or after a bout of shingles, often can prevent chronic pain. If you already have chronic pain, various treatments exist. Some common forms of chronic pain are listed below.

Back pain. Low **back pain** is the most common cause of job-related disability in the United States and a leading contributor to missed work. Lingering back pain may be related to a variety of causes, including muscle strain and spasm, poor body mechanics, physical deconditioning, spinal changes, such as a herniated disk, and degenerative diseases, such as osteoarthritis. (See "Back and neck," page 50.)

Headache. The most common type of head pain is the so-called **tension-type headache.** However, doctors aren't certain it's caused by actual muscle tension. The start or worsening of tension headaches isn't always related to stressful events. The throbbing pain of a **migraine** may be related to changes in blood vessels located in your head. Genetics, medication, alcohol, certain foods, exertion, and anxiety or depression may provoke a migraine. (See "Headache," page 82.)

Arthritis. Arthritis is the general name for inflammation of one or more joints. **Osteoarthritis** usually affects cartilage in joints of the knees, hands, hips and spine. **Rheumatoid arthritis** involves inflammation of tissue around and in the joints. It typically affects the hands and feet. (See "Arthritis," page 161.)

Fibromyalgia. Fibromyalgia syndrome is a collection of symptoms that includes widespread pain and tenderness. It differs from arthritis in that the pain is in muscles and tissues near the joints instead of in the joints themselves. Symptoms may flare and then subside, but they usually don't disappear completely. (See "Fibromyalgia," page 91.)

Neuropathy. Neuropathic pain is caused by damage to your peripheral nerves — those nerves that extend from your spinal cord into your arms and hands and your legs and feet. **Peripheral neuropathy** may occur after an injury or as a result of a long-term disease, such as diabetes. It can be one of the most difficult types of pain to treat.

Irritable bowel syndrome. This is a complex disorder of the lower intestinal tract that causes pain, bloating, and recurrent bouts of diarrhea or constipation. (See "Irritable bowel syndrome," page 65.)

Stimulating your natural painkillers

Studies show that aerobic exercise can stimulate the release of endorphins, your body's own natural painkillers. Endorphins are morphine-like pain relievers that send "stop pain" messages to your nerve cells. Duration of exercise seems to be more important than intensity. Doing low-intensity aerobic exercises for 30 to 45 minutes at a time five or six days a week may produce an effect. Be sure to build up slowly. Even three or four days of exercise a week may have some effect.

If you want to start an exercise program that's more vigorous than walking, have a medical evaluation if:
- You're older than age 40
- You've been sedentary
- You have risk factors for coronary artery disease
- You have chronic health problems

Self-care

After serious diseases have been excluded or treated, the following options may help you better manage chronic pain:

- **Stay physically active.** Focus on the things you can do. Try new hobbies and leisure activities. Exercise daily. An activity that initially causes some pain doesn't necessarily cause further damage or worsen chronic pain. If you have arthritis, exercise can improve the range of motion in your joints. Exercises for your back and abdominal muscles may help relieve or even prevent back pain. Begin slowly. Work up to 20 to 30 minutes three or four times a week.
- **Stay connected with others.** People with a solid support system — who have family and friends who care about them — generally cope better than others who have chronic pain. Stay connected with family and friends. For example, attend family gatherings, stay involved with children's or grandchildren's activities, and attend social events with friends. Get involved in your community, church or other volunteer activities.
- **Focus on wellness.** Maintain a healthy weight, get enough sleep (and sleep on a regular schedule), and eat healthy foods. The best way to increase nutrients in your diet and limit fat and calories is to eat more plant-based foods: vegetables, fruits and whole grains.
- **Learn how to stress less and relax more.** When you're in pain, you're less able to handle the stress of everyday living. Stress may also cause you to do things that intensify your pain, such as tense your muscles. In short, pain causes stress, and stress intensifies pain. But stress is your response to an event, not the event itself. Take steps to better manage your stress and learn relaxation skills, such as relaxed-breathing exercises, progressive muscle relaxation and visual imagery. Even a good massage can promote muscle relaxation and general comfort. (See "Keeping stress under control," page 221.)

Medical help

If your pain changes in character — for example, it escalates from mild to severe — or if you develop new symptoms — such as tingling or numbness — it might be a good idea to see your doctor to have your condition re-evaluated.

Using pain-relieving medications safely

Some over-the-counter medications can be effective for reducing chronic pain. Medications such as aspirin, ibuprofen and acetaminophen help control pain in various ways by interfering with the manner in which pain messages are developed, transmitted or interpreted.

For safe use of pain medications:

- Read the label and follow all instructions, cautions and warnings. Never use more than the maximum recommended dose.
- Unless a doctor recommends it, adults should not use pain medication for more than 10 days in a row. The limit for children and teenagers is five days.
- Don't take aspirin, ibuprofen or naproxen during the last three months of pregnancy unless your doctor recommends it. Aspirin can cause bleeding in both the mother and the child. Children shouldn't take aspirin unless directed to do so by a doctor.
- If you're allergic to aspirin, check with your doctor or pharmacist about which pain relievers you can use safely. (For more on pain medications, see pages 257-258.)

■ Treatment for chronic pain

Advances in medicine have created a wide range of options for helping you manage chronic pain:

Surgery. In some situations, surgery may help relieve or reduce the pain. Many times, though, surgery isn't an option.

Interventional approaches. For some forms of chronic pain, a doctor may attempt to control the pain with X-ray-guided injections of medication at or near the site of the pain, but typically other forms of treatment are tried first. Other interventional approaches include implanting small devices in your body, such as a nerve stimulator or medication pump, to help control pain.

Medication. Many types of drugs are used to help control chronic pain, based on the severity of the pain and the disease or disorder causing it.

Physical therapy. Physical therapy programs focus on reducing pain through a regular exercise program that includes flexibility, aerobic and strengthening exercises. Physical therapy is primarily based on proper body mechanics — using your muscles and joints correctly to limit pain.

Cognitive and behavioral therapies. These approaches focus on understanding the behaviors, actions, feelings and relationship problems that often accompany chronic pain, and developing positive ways to deal with them.

Integrative therapies. These include a variety of practices such as yoga, massage, meditation and acupuncture.

Rehabilitation. Rehabilitation therapy may involve a specific program to regain motor function or assistance in learning new skills.

Interdisciplinary pain treatment programs. Sometimes referred to as multidisciplinary pain rehabilitation programs, these programs incorporate a variety of nonsurgical treatments — including many of those listed above — delivered in a coordinated manner in an outpatient setting to help find the source of pain, manage pain and improve functioning.

FOR MORE INFORMATION
- American Chronic Pain Association, 800-533-3231, *https://theacpa.org*
- American Pain Society, 847-375-4715, *http://americanpainsociety.org/*

Sleep disorders

▊ Insomnia

The most common of 70 or more sleep disorders is **insomnia**. Insomnia includes difficulty going to sleep, staying asleep or going back to sleep when you awaken early. It may be temporary or chronic. Insomnia may be either a symptom of another disorder or, in some cases, a separate disease. Common causes include the following:

- Stress related to work, school, health or family concerns
- Behavioral insomnia, which may occur when you worry excessively about not being able to sleep well and try too hard to fall asleep
- Depression and anxiety
- Use of stimulants (caffeine or nicotine), herbal supplements and certain over-the-counter and prescription medications
- Alcohol
- Change in environment or work schedule
- Long-term use of sleep medications
- Chronic medical problems, including fibromyalgia or complex diseases of the nerves and muscles

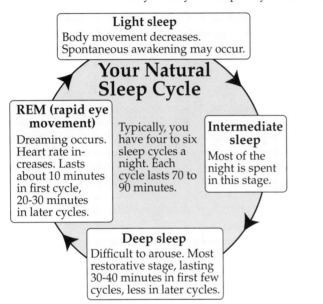

Light sleep
Body movement decreases. Spontaneous awakening may occur.

Your Natural Sleep Cycle

REM (rapid eye movement)
Dreaming occurs. Heart rate increases. Lasts about 10 minutes in first cycle, 20-30 minutes in later cycles.

Typically, you have four to six sleep cycles a night. Each cycle lasts 70 to 90 minutes.

Intermediate sleep
Most of the night is spent in this stage.

Deep sleep
Difficult to arouse. Most restorative stage, lasting 30-40 minutes in first few cycles, less in later cycles.

Self-care

- Establish and follow a ritual and sleep schedule for going to bed.
- Avoid strenuous exercise right before bedtime.
- Avoid taking work materials to bed or using the internet or your cellphone right before bedtime.
- Take a warm bath one to two hours before bedtime.
- Avoid or limit caffeine, alcohol and nicotine. Caffeine after lunchtime and using nicotine can keep you from falling asleep at night. Alcohol, while it may initially make you feel sleepy, can cause unrestful sleep and frequent awakenings.
- Avoid large meals and beverages before bedtime. Eating too much late in the evening can interfere with sleep. Drink fewer fluids before bedtime to avoid the need to urinate in the middle of the night.
- Keep your sleeping environment dark, quiet and comfortably cool. If necessary, use eye covers and earplugs. Some people feel that subtle background noises, such as from a fan, help them sleep.
- Try relaxation techniques (see page 223).
- Avoid medications with caffeine or other stimulants, such as pseudoephedrine. Check labels and ask your doctor if your medications may interfere with sleep.
- If you still can't sleep after 30 minutes, get up. Stay up until you feel tired, and then return to bed. But, as a result, do not shift your rising time.
- Keep a sleep diary. If, after a week or two, you still can't sleep, see your doctor.
- If pain limits your ability to sleep, ask your doctor for advice.

See back cover for online resource ⓘ

Kids' care

Bed-wetting (enuresis) can wake children up at night. Before age 7, the nighttime bladder control simply may not be established yet. If bed-wetting continues, treat the issue with patience and understanding. Ask your child's doctor for advice.

Nightmares may be a response to stress or trauma that occurs during waking hours. Calmly reassure your child after an incident.

Night terrors are relatively rare, and they tend to run in families. Sleepers may awaken screaming, with no recollection of a dream. Emotional tension increases night terrors. They're usually not a cause for concern, but ask the doctor about it.

Sleepwalking tends to run in families and involves walking around while asleep. If it involves dangerous activities, prevent your child from wandering to unsafe areas, such as by locking outside doors. Ask the doctor for advice.

Should you nap, or not?

Don't nap if sleeping at night is a problem. Otherwise, if a nap refreshes you:

- **Keep it short.** Limit your nap to 20 or 30 minutes. Longer naps are more likely to interfere with your nighttime sleep.

- **Just rest if you can't nap.** Lie down for a short time and focus your mind on something else.
- **Don't rely on naps to keep you going.** It's important to get enough sleep at night to avoid building a sleep deficit.

■ Other sleep disorders

If your breathing repeatedly stops and starts during sleep, you may have **sleep apnea**. If you snore loudly or have severe daytime drowsiness, see your doctor. You may not realize that you have sleep apnea. This is a serious medical condition that increases the risk of high blood pressure, heart problems and strokes. When the muscles that support the soft tissues in your throat relax, your airway is narrowed or closed, causing obstructive sleep apnea. Losing weight, sleeping on your stomach or side, and avoiding alcohol before bedtime may help. Your doctor may advise wearing a mask over your nose that delivers pressurized air while you sleep to keep the airway open.

Grinding or clenching your teeth during sleep (bruxism) may be associated with stress. Your dentist can check whether your bite needs adjustment and provide you with a plastic dental guard to prevent further damage. Attempt to deal with the source of your tension. Learn relaxation skills (see page 223).

Excessive sleepiness may be controlled by getting plenty of sleep at night, taking a daytime nap and following a regular sleep schedule. Eat light or vegetarian meals and consider using caffeinated drinks (such as coffee or tea) early in the day. But ongoing daytime sleepiness may indicate a sleep disorder such as sleep apnea. Ask your doctor for advice.

Restless legs syndrome (RLS) is the irresistible urge to move your legs and can occur shortly after you go to bed or throughout the night, interfering with your ability to sleep. Get up and walk around. Try muscle relaxation techniques and a warm bath before bedtime. See a doctor if you have severe symptoms. Also ask about getting your iron levels checked, as iron deficiency can cause or worsen RLS.

FOR MORE INFORMATION

- National Sleep Foundation, *https://sleepfoundation.org*
- Restless Legs Syndrome Foundation, 512-366-9109, *https://www.rls.org*

General Symptoms

Sweating and body odor

Sweating is the body's normal response to the buildup of body heat. Sweating varies widely from person to person. Many women perspire more heavily during menopause. Drinking hot beverages, or those containing alcohol or caffeine, can cause temporary increases in sweating.

For most of us, sweating is only a minor nuisance. But for some people, sweaty armpits, feet and hands are a major dilemma. Sweat is basically odorless, but it may take on an unpleasant or offensive odor when bacteria multiply and break down the body's secretions into odor-causing byproducts. Sweating and odor may be influenced by mood, activity, hormones and some foods, such as caffeine.

A "cold sweat" is usually the body's response to a serious illness, anxiety or severe pain. A cold sweat should receive immediate medical attention if there are signs of lightheadedness or chest and stomach pains.

Self-care

- **Wear clothing made of natural materials,** especially cotton, next to the skin.
- **Bathe daily.** Antibacterial soaps may help, but they can be irritating.
- **Try over-the-counter products,** such as antiperspirant sprays and lotions, that contain aluminum chlorohydrate or buffered aluminum sulfate.
- **For sweaty feet,** choose shoes made of natural materials that breathe, such as leather. Wear the right socks. Cotton and wool socks can help keep your feet dry because they absorb moisture. Change your socks or hosiery once or twice a day, drying your feet thoroughly each time. Dry your feet thoroughly after a bath. Microorganisms thrive in the damp spaces between your toes. Use over-the-counter foot powders to help absorb sweat. Air out your feet. Go without shoes when it's sensible. But when you can't, slip out of them from time to time. Women should try pantyhose with cotton soles.
- **For sweaty armpits,** use antiperspirants. If irritation remains a problem, a 0.5 percent hydrocortisone cream (available without a prescription) can help, but ask your doctor how long you can use this.
- **Apply antiperspirants nightly** at bedtime to sweaty palms or soles of feet. Try perfume-free antiperspirants.
- **Try iontophoresis (i-on-toe-fuh-REE-sis).** This procedure, in which a low current of electricity is delivered to the affected body part with a battery-powered device, may help. But it may be no more effective than a topical antiperspirant.
- **Eliminate caffeine and other stimulants** from your diet, as well as foods with strong odors, such as garlic and onions.

Medical help

Your doctor may recommend a prescription antiperspirant. Repeated injections of botulinum toxin may decrease sweat gland activity. In rare cases, surgical removal of sweat glands may help if excessive sweating occurs just in your armpits. In severe cases, endoscopic thoracic sympathectomy may be considered — a procedure done by neurosurgeons that cuts nerves (which stimulate excess sweat) near the spine.

Consult your doctor if there's an increase in sweating or nighttime sweating without an obvious cause. Infections, thyroid gland dysfunction and certain forms of cancer may produce unusual sweating patterns.

Excessive sweating associated with shortness of breath requires immediate action. This could be a sign of a heart attack.

Occasionally, a change in odor signals a disease. A fruity smell may be a sign of diabetes, or an ammonia-like smell could be a sign of liver disease.

Unexpected weight changes

In most cases, the reasons for change in weight are obvious. Changes in diet or activity are the usual explanations. Physical illness also can affect your weight. An unexpected weight change of 5 to 10 percent of your body weight in six months or less is significant. If you lose or gain weight and can't point to a reason, or if you are losing or gaining weight very rapidly, talk to your health care provider.

■ Weight gain

Weight gain is common in adulthood. The increase in weight is usually a gradual creep — a few pounds a year. Careful diet and regular exercise can stop this trend.

If you've experienced a rapid gain, consider these possible causes:

1. **Diet changes.** Increased intake of alcohol or soda; a new favorite high-fat food such as ice cream, sweet rolls or fried foods; increased snacking; or a switch to fast foods or prepared foods.
2. **Decrease in activity.** An injury restricting movement, a switch from an active to a sedentary job, or a change in a routine such as using stairs or walking to work.
3. **New medication.** Some antidepressants and some hormones, including estrogen, progesterone and cortisone, as well as other medications.
4. **Changes in mood.** Excessive anxiety, stress or depression, which can affect activity and food intake. (See "Depression," page 200.)
5. **Fluid retention.** Medical conditions such as heart or kidney failure or thyroid conditions that cause fluid buildup. (Have you noticed puffiness of the tissues — tight rings or shoes, progressive swelling of the ankles as the day progresses, unusual shortness of breath, or new, frequent trips to the bathroom at night?)

Self-care

If item 1 or 2 above applies to you, change your diet and increase activity. (See "Weight," page 206, "Healthy eating," page 210, and "Physical activity," page 215.) If the changes don't work in four to six weeks, or if you're taking a new medication, have mood changes or fluid retention (items 3, 4 or 5 above), see your doctor.

■ Unexplained weight loss

<u>Unexplained weight loss</u> of 10 percent or more of your body weight over six months or less may be a cause for concern. Consider the following possibilities:

1. **A change in diet,** such as skipping meals, eating on the run, a significant reduction in fat intake, a change in meal preparation methods, a change in routines around mealtime or eating alone, can cause weight loss.
2. **A change in activity,** such as a job change, a new exercise program, a busy or hectic schedule, or a seasonal variation, can cause weight loss.
3. **A decrease in appetite,** perhaps due to stress, anxiety or an underlying medical condition, can cause weight loss.
4. **A new medication,** including some antidepressants or stimulants — prescription or over-the-counter (caffeine, herbs) — can cause weight loss.
5. **Mood changes,** such as depression, can cause weight loss.
6. **Other conditions,** including dental problems; uncontrolled diabetes with thirst or

increased urination; an overactive thyroid gland (hyperthyroidism); digestive disorders, such as malabsorption or an ulcer with abdominal pain; inflammatory bowel diseases, such as Crohn's or colitis, causing diarrhea and bloody stools; cancer; and infections, such as human immunodeficiency virus (HIV), AIDS or tuberculosis.

Self-care

If item 1 or 2 (bottom of page 47) applies, but not the other items, change your diet. Eat three balanced meals a day. For snacks, or when you can't eat a good meal, try a nutritional supplement drink (ask your doctor or dietitian for suggestions). Powders that you mix with milk are simple, fairly balanced and less expensive than ready-to-drink supplements. If you haven't reversed the weight-loss trend in two weeks, or you have a new medication or mood changes, see your doctor right away.

Kids' care

Weight loss or failure to grow in children may be caused by a digestive problem that prevents important nutrients from being digested or absorbed. Loss of these nutrients can lead to stunted growth and other problems. Your child also may have another underlying medical condition or an eating disorder. If your child has unexplained weight loss, consult your child's health care provider.

Eating disorders: Anorexia, bulimia and binge eating

<u>Anorexia nervosa</u> is an eating disorder that leads to severe weight loss as a result of restricted food intake or of binging and purging (self-induced vomiting or laxative abuse). A person with **bulimia nervosa** is often at normal weight but uses binge eating and purging to control weight. In a **binge-eating disorder** the person frequently consumes unusually large amounts of food.

Eating disorders are most common in teen girls and young women, but they can occur in males and older adults.

Anorexia

Signs and symptoms:
- Extreme weight loss and thin appearance
- Unrealistic fear of becoming fat
- Excessive dieting, exercise or both
- Refusal to eat and denial of hunger
- Absence of menstrual periods
- Hair that thins, breaks or falls out
- Preoccupation with food and calories
- Binge eating and purging through vomiting or misuse of laxatives, diuretics or enemas

The cause of anorexia is unclear, but biological and psychological factors may be involved. Left untreated, anorexia can lead to death. Treatment involves psychotherapy, diet counseling and family counseling in most cases. Hospitalization may be needed in severe cases. Recurrence is typical over the years, so ongoing or periodic therapy may help.

Bulimia

Signs and symptoms:
- Recurrent episodes of binge eating
- Self-induced vomiting or laxative abuse
- Weight usually within fairly normal range
- Fear of becoming fat

Bulimia involves eating large amounts of food and then purging by vomiting or abusing laxatives. It's also a form of semistarvation. Purging depletes water and potassium from the body and can lead to death. People with bulimia often become depressed because they judge themselves harshly. Treatment usually includes behavior modification, psychotherapy and, in some cases, antidepressant medication. Hospitalization may be needed in severe cases.

Binge-eating disorder

Signs and symptoms:
- Eating large amounts of food rapidly, even when you're full, and frequently eating alone
- Feeling that your eating is out of control
- Hoarding food and hiding empty containers
- Frequent dieting without weight loss

Treatment usually includes psychotherapy, whether in individual or group sessions, to teach you how to exchange unhealthy habits for healthy ones. If depression is a factor, antidepressants may be recommended.

See back cover for online resource ⓘ

Common Problems

- Back and neck
- Digestive system
- Ears and hearing
- Eyes and vision
- Headache
- Limbs, muscles, bones and joints
- Lungs, chest and breathing
- Nose and sinuses
- Skin, hair and nails
- Throat and mouth
- Men's health
- Women's health

Most pains and illnesses aren't serious. Often, simple remedies in combination with time can help resolve the problem and save you a trip to the doctor. Of course, if the problem persists or if simple remedies don't help, you need to seek medical care.

This section is mainly organized by body system. Each section includes several illnesses or symptoms with self-care advice and suggestions on when to see your doctor. Children's health ("Kids' care") also is included where appropriate throughout the section.

Back and neck

Almost everyone has a back problem at some time. Back pain sends many people to health care providers each year. Fortunately, you can do things to prevent back problems. And you can do them most effectively if you know a little bit about your back.

Your back supports your body. It holds and protects your spinal cord and nerves that send signals back and forth from your brain to the rest of your body. And it serves as a place of attachment for muscles and ligaments of the back.

Anatomy

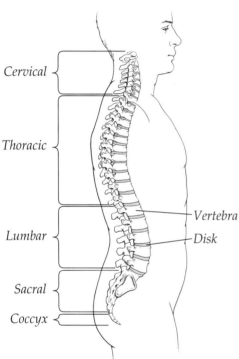

Cervical

Thoracic

Lumbar

Sacral

Coccyx

Vertebra

Disk

Your spine, sometimes called your backbone, isn't one bone, but many. If you look at a healthy spine from the side, it curves inward at the neck and lower back and outward at the upper back and pelvis.

Vertebrae. The backbone (vertebral column) is composed of bones called vertebrae, which are held together by tough, fibrous bands called ligaments. The adult vertebral column consists of seven neck (cervical) vertebrae, 12 middle back (thoracic) vertebrae and five lower back (lumbar) vertebrae. The lumbar vertebrae are the largest because they bear most of the body weight. The sacrum, made from five vertebrae that are fused together, is below the lumbar vertebrae. The last three vertebrae, also fused together, form the tailbone (coccyx).

Spinal cord. The spinal cord, part of the central nervous system, extends from the base of the skull to the lower back through the bony spinal canal. Two nerves (spinal nerves) are sent out at each vertebral level. In the upper lumbar part of the back where the spinal cord ends, a group of nerves (cauda equina) continue down the spinal canal. The spinal nerves exit from openings (foramina) on each side of the vertebrae, one leading to the right side of the body and the other to the left. In all, there are 31 pairs of these spinal nerves in the back and neck.

Disks. Between the vertebrae, and close to the point of exit of each pair of spinal nerves, are intervertebral disks. These disks prevent the hard and bony vertebrae from hitting one another when you walk, run or jump. They also allow the spine to move in all directions — twisting, bending and extending. A disk is made up of a ring of tough, fibrous tissue that has a jellylike substance in the center.

Muscles. Muscles are like elastic bands up and down your back that support your spine. They contract or relax to help you stand, twist, bend or stretch. Tendons connect muscles to bones. The muscles of your abdomen and trunk support, protect and move your spine.

Pain issues

With age your spine may become stiff, disks become worn, and the spaces between vertebrae may narrow. These changes are part of the aging process, but they're not necessarily painful. As the cartilage that cushions joints wears out, bones can rub together, and you may experience the pain of arthritis. Often, though, it's hard to pinpoint the cause of back pain because of the back's complexity.

Common back and neck problems

Your lower back, a pivot point for turning at your waist, is vulnerable to muscle strains.

Your lower back carries most of your weight. Among people age 40 and older, it's the site of most **back pain**. However, strains and sprains can injure any part of your neck or back.

Causes of back and neck pain include:

- Improper lifting (see "Lifting properly," page 54)
- A sudden, strenuous physical effort; an accident, sports injury or fall
- Lack of muscle tone
- Excess weight, especially around your middle
- Your sleeping position, especially if you sleep on your stomach
- Sitting in one position for a long time; poor sitting and standing postures
- A pillow that forces your neck into an awkward angle
- Holding the telephone with your shoulder
- Carrying a heavy briefcase, purse or shoulder bag or backpack
- Sitting with a thick wallet in your back pocket
- Holding a forward-bending position for a long time
- Daily stress and tension
- Relaxation of muscles and ligaments during pregnancy

'No pain, no gain' — Not true!

You may feel sore immediately after you've injured a muscle, or it may take several hours. An injured muscle may uncontrollably tighten or "knot up" (a muscle spasm). Your body is telling you to slow down and prevent further injury. A severe muscle spasm may last 48 to 72 hours, followed by days or weeks of less severe pain. Strenuous use of an injured muscle during the next three to six weeks may bring back the pain. However, most back pain is gone within a few weeks.

As you age, muscle tone and strength tends to decrease, and your back is more prone to aches or injury. Maintaining your flexibility and strength and keeping your abdominal muscles strong are your best bets to avoid back problems. Spending 10 to 15 minutes a day doing gentle stretching and strengthening exercises can help.

Self-care

Healing will occur most quickly if you can continue your usual activities in a gentle manner while avoiding what may have caused the pain in the first place. Avoid long periods of bed rest, which can worsen your pain and make you weaker.

With proper care of a strain or sprain, you should notice improvement within the first two weeks. Most forms of acute back pain improve in four to six weeks. Sprained ligaments or severe muscle strains may take up to 12 weeks to heal. Once you have back pain, you're more prone to experience repeated painful episodes.

Follow these home care steps:

- Use cold packs initially to relieve pain. Wrap an ice pack or a bag of frozen vegetables in a piece of cloth. Hold it on the sore area for 15 minutes four times a day. To avoid frostbite, never place ice directly on your skin.
- You may be most comfortable lying with your back on the floor, hips and knees bent, and legs elevated. Get plenty of rest, but avoid prolonged bed rest — more than a day or two may slow recovery. Moderate movement keeps your muscles strong and flexible. Avoid the activity that caused the sprain or strain. Avoid heavy lifting, pushing or pulling, repetitive bending, and twisting.

Self-care

- After 48 hours, you may use heat to relax sore or knotted muscles. Use a warm bath, warm packs, a heating pad or a heat lamp. Be careful not to burn your skin with extreme heat. But if you find that cold provides more relief than heat does, you can continue using cold, or try a combination of the two methods.
- Gradually begin gentle stretching exercises. Avoid jerking, bouncing, or any movements that increase pain or require straining.
- Use over-the-counter pain medications (see page 258).
- Massage may be helpful, especially for muscle spasms, but avoid placing any pressure directly on your spine.
- If you must stand or sit much of the day, consider using a support brace or corset. Worn properly, they may relieve your pain and provide warmth, comfort and support. However, relying on this type of support for a long time prevents you from using, stretching and exercising your muscles and can unintentionally lead to muscle weakness.

Medical help

Although uncommon, back or neck pain can result from serious problems such as cancer, infection, inflammatory arthritis and other diseases. Pain that worsens or remains constant for a month or more should be investigated by a doctor.

Seek medical care immediately if your pain:

- Is severe, progressive or prolonged (lasting more than one month).
- Results from an injury. Don't try to move someone who has severe neck pain or can't move his or her arms or legs after an accident. Moving the person can cause further injury.
- Produces weakness, pain or numbness in one or both legs or arms.
- Is new and is accompanied by an unexplained fever or weight loss.
- Is constant and worse at night.
- Is accompanied by poorly controlled blood pressure, an abdominal aortic aneurysm, cancer, or a sudden loss of bowel or bladder control.

The nerves to most of your body travel through your back. Sometimes, back or neck pain may be caused by a problem somewhere else in your body. Your health care provider may do testing to determine the cause of your pain.

Kids' care

Low back pain is unusual in children before their teen years. Common causes for back pain are sports injuries, falls or heavy backpacks. Be sure that your children's athletic programs:

- Use the proper protective equipment
- Have competent coaches
- Use sufficient warm-up and conditioning activities

If your injured child hasn't been unconscious, can move freely, and has no numbness or weakness, use the self-care tips listed on page 51 and above. Be careful to avoid excessive heat or cold. Check proper children's doses for over-the-counter medicines. Don't give children aspirin.

If the pain is unrelated to an injury or other known cause, your health care provider may want to check for an infection (especially if your child has a fever) or for factors in your child's development that may cause the pain.

Warning signs of serious back problems in children include constant pain that lasts for several weeks or occurs at night; pain that interferes with school, play or sports; and pain that occurs with stiffness and fever.

Other back and neck problems

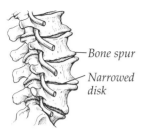

Osteoarthritis

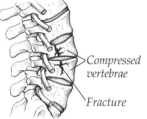

Osteoporosis

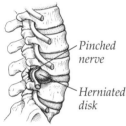

Herniated disk

Back and neck problems often don't result from a single incident. They may be the product of a lifetime of stress and strain on your back and neck. If you have chronic back pain, your health care provider may look for the following conditions.

Osteoarthritis, the most common form of arthritis, typically occurs in older adults. Aging causes the protective tissue that covers the surface of vertebral joints to deteriorate. Disks between vertebrae become worn, and the spaces between the bones narrow. Bony outgrowths called spurs can develop, which may or may not cause pain. Gradually, your spine can stiffen and lose flexibility.

Osteoporosis is the weakening of your bone structure as calcium in your bones decreases. Weakened vertebrae become compressed and fracture easily. Medication may slow or halt this process. People over 50, especially women, are at greatest risk.

A **bulging disk** is one in which the tough outer layers of the disk simply bulge into the spinal canal. Bulging disks are common, often painless, and usually considered part of the normal aging process. A **herniated disk** (also called a ruptured or slipped disk) is one in which the disk has cracked and some of the soft inner part has leaked out. It can cause pain when it puts pressure on nearby nerves, such as the sciatic nerve (sciatica), which extends down the back of the leg. Symptoms may resolve over days or weeks. Sometimes, the condition becomes chronic and may lead to weakness or numbness in the legs. Similar problems may occur in the neck, causing pain, weakness, numbness and tingling in the arms or legs or both.

Surgery

Surgery is usually reserved for times when a nerve is pinched and threatens to cause permanent weakness or is affecting bowel or bladder control. Back pain without nerve injury isn't usually treated with surgery. Arm or leg weakness or pain that persists for more than six weeks despite other treatment may be relieved with surgery.

Preventing back injuries in the workplace

You can avoid many back problems by following these guidelines:
- Change positions often.
- Avoid high heels. If you stand for long periods, rest one foot on a small box or stool from time to time.
- Use adjustable equipment. Find comfortable (rather than extreme) positions.
- Don't bend continuously over your work. Hold reading materials at eye level.
- Avoid excessive repetition. Take frequent, short breaks to stretch or relax — even 30 seconds every 10 to 15 minutes helps.
- Avoid unnecessary bending, twisting and reaching.
- Stand up to answer your phone. If you're on the phone a lot, get a headset.
- Adjust your chair so that your feet are flat on the floor. Change leg positions often.
- Use a chair that supports your lower back's curve or place a rolled towel or pillow behind your lower back. The seat of your chair shouldn't press on the back of your knees.
- Lift objects properly (see page 54) and carry them close to your body.
- Keep fit. Poor physical fitness, excess weight and smoking increase your risk of back injury and decrease your body's ability to heal itself.

Preventing common backaches and neck pains

Regular exercise is your most powerful weapon against back and neck problems. Proper exercise can help you:
- Maintain or increase flexibility of muscles, tendons and ligaments
- Strengthen the muscles that support your back
- Increase muscle strength in your arms, legs and lower body to reduce the risk of falls and other injuries and allow optimal posture for lifting and carrying
- Improve your posture and increase bone density
- Shed excess pounds that stress your back

If you are older than age 40 or have an illness or injury, check with your health care provider before you begin an exercise program. If you're out of condition, start slowly. Exercises that are good for your back include:
- Abdominal and leg-strengthening exercises.
- Nonjarring exercise on a stationary bike, treadmill or cross-country skiing machine. Bicycling is good, but be sure your bike seat and handlebars are properly adjusted to keep you in a comfortable position.

Even after episodes of low back or neck pain, proper exercise can significantly reduce your risk of pain flare-ups. If you have back problems or are out of shape, avoid activities that involve quick stops and starts and a lot of twisting. High-impact activities on hard surfaces — such as jogging, tennis, racquetball and basketball — may cause wear and tear to your back. Try to avoid falling and avoid contact sports.

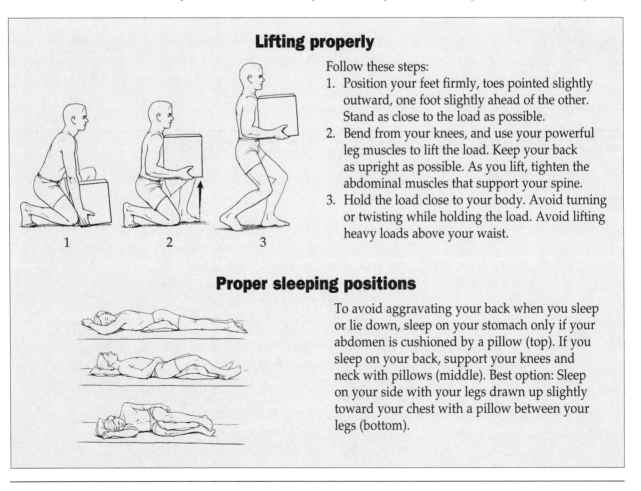

Lifting properly

Follow these steps:
1. Position your feet firmly, toes pointed slightly outward, one foot slightly ahead of the other. Stand as close to the load as possible.
2. Bend from your knees, and use your powerful leg muscles to lift the load. Keep your back as upright as possible. As you lift, tighten the abdominal muscles that support your spine.
3. Hold the load close to your body. Avoid turning or twisting while holding the load. Avoid lifting heavy loads above your waist.

Proper sleeping positions

To avoid aggravating your back when you sleep or lie down, sleep on your stomach only if your abdomen is cushioned by a pillow (top). If you sleep on your back, support your knees and neck with pillows (middle). Best option: Sleep on your side with your legs drawn up slightly toward your chest with a pillow between your legs (bottom).

Your daily back routine

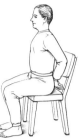

These exercises stretch and strengthen your back and supporting muscles. Exercising should be comfortable and not cause pain. Try to work at least 15 minutes of back exercise into your daily routine. Do each exercise three or four times, then increase your goal over time. (If you've hurt your back before or you have health problems such as osteoporosis, talk to your doctor before doing these exercises.)

Shoulder blade squeeze. Sit upright in a chair. Keep your chin tucked in and shoulders down. Pull your shoulder blades together and straighten (but don't arch) your upper back. Hold a few seconds. Return to starting position. Repeat several times.

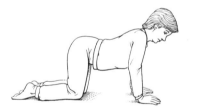

Knee-to-chest stretch. Lie on your back on the floor or other firm surface with your knees bent and feet flat. Pull your left knee toward your chest with both hands. Hold for 15 to 30 seconds. Return to starting position. Repeat with opposite leg. Repeat with each leg three or four times.

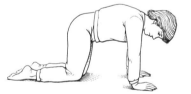

Half situp. Lie on your back on the floor or other firm surface with your knees bent and feet flat. With your arms outstretched, reach toward your knees with your hands until your shoulder blades no longer touch the ground. Don't grasp your knees. Hold for a few seconds and slowly return to the starting position. Repeat several times.

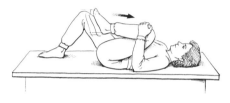

Cat stretch. Step 1. Get down on your hands and knees. Slowly let your back and abdomen sag toward the floor.

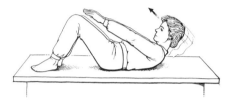

Cat stretch. Step 2. Slowly arch your back away from the floor. Repeat steps 1 and 2 several times.

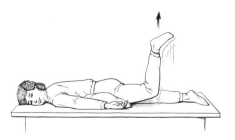

Leg lifts. Step 1. Lie facedown on a firm surface with a large pillow under your hips and lower abdomen. Keeping your knee bent, raise your leg slightly off the surface and hold about five seconds. Repeat several times with each leg.

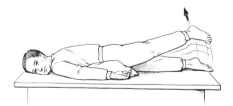

Leg lifts. Step 2. With your leg straight, raise one leg slightly off the surface and hold for about five seconds. Repeat several times with each leg.

Common Problems

Common Problems **55**

Digestive system

Your digestive tract is an extremely complex system. Problems can occur anywhere along this tract, upsetting its delicate balance. Because of the complexity of this system, don't attempt to diagnose new problems, such as unexplained pain or bleeding, on your own.

Digestion begins when you chew your food. The food is broken into smaller pieces by your teeth and, at the same time, is mixed with saliva secreted by your salivary glands. Your saliva contains an enzyme that begins to change starches (carbohydrates) into sugars.

Food is propelled down your esophagus to the stomach and then on through the intestines by muscular contractions. This process, called digestion, is aided by digestive juices (acid, bile and enzymes) from the stomach, gallbladder and pancreas. They break down food and allow the nutrients to be absorbed. Undigested food and bacteria are eliminated as feces from the rectum.

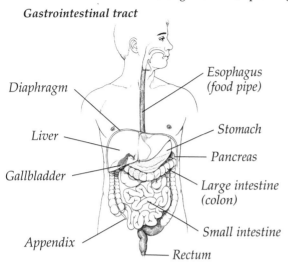

Gastrointestinal tract

Diaphragm

Liver

Gallbladder

Appendix

Esophagus (food pipe)

Stomach

Pancreas

Large intestine (colon)

Small intestine

Rectum

■ Abdominal pain and discomfort

Pain in your abdomen can feel widespread or in a specific area and range from mild to severe. It can be constant or come and go. In some cases, pain may be related to overeating. In others, it can be an early warning sign of a more serious disorder that may require medical treatment.

Fortunately, many forms of discomfort respond well to a combination of self-care and supervised medical treatment. See the following pages if your pain accompanies any of these conditions: constipation, page 58; diarrhea, page 59; excessive gas, page 60; gastritis, page 61; or hemorrhoids, page 62.

Caution

Although most abdominal pains aren't serious, seek medical attention if you experience any of the following: intense pain lasting longer than a minute or pain that seems to be worsening, or pain accompanied by shortness of breath, dizziness, chest pain, a temperature of 101 F or more, or bloody diarrhea.

What is appendicitis?

Your appendix is a worm-shaped structure that projects out from the large intestine. This tiny structure can become inflamed, swollen and filled with pus. This condition is called appendicitis.

Appendicitis typically causes acute pain that starts around your navel and settles in the lower right side of your abdomen. These symptoms generally progress over 12 to 24 hours. You may also experience a loss of appetite, nausea, vomiting, and the urge to have a bowel movement or pass gas.

Although appendicitis can affect people of all ages, it usually occurs between the ages of 10 and 30.

An infected appendix may burst and cause a serious infection. Seek immediate medical attention if you suspect you have appendicitis.

■ Colic

Generations of families have dealt with **colic**. This frustrating and largely unexplainable condition affects babies who otherwise seem healthy. Colic usually peaks at six weeks of age and disappears in the baby's third to fifth month.

Colic is a difficult experience for everyone. One doctor describes colic as "when the baby's crying — and so is the parent."

Although the term *colic* is used widely for any fussy baby, true colic is determined by the following:

- **Predictable crying episodes.** A colicky baby cries about the same time each day, usually in the evening. Colic episodes may last minutes or two or more hours.
- **Activity.** Many colicky babies pull their legs to their chests or thrash around during crying episodes as if they are in pain.
- **Intense or inconsolable crying.** Colicky babies cry more than usual and are extremely difficult — if not impossible — to comfort.

Doctors call colic a "diagnosis of exclusion," which means other possible problems are ruled out before determining the baby has colic. The parent of a colicky infant, therefore, can be assured that the crying is probably not a sign of a serious medical problem.

Studies of colic have focused on several possible causes: allergies, an immature digestive system, gas, hormones, mother's anxieties and handling. Still, it's unclear why some babies have colic and others don't.

Self-care

If your health care provider determines that your baby has colic, these measures may help you and your child find some relief:

- Lay your baby tummy-down on your lap or arms and sway your baby gently and slowly. This may help him or her pass stool or gas.
- Rock, cuddle or walk your baby. Avoid fast, jiggling movements.
- Play a steady, uninterrupted "white noise" near your baby. Motors with soft noise, such as that in a clothes dryer, may work.
- Put your baby in an infant swing.
- Give your baby a warm bath or lay him or her tummy-down on a warm water bottle.
- Try singing or humming while walking with or rocking the baby. A soothing song can have a quieting effect on both parent and baby.
- Offer a pacifier. Even if you're breast-feeding, it's OK to try a pacifier.
- Experiment with food. Dietary changes can sometimes be helpful, but it's best to work with your doctor.
- Take your baby for a car ride.
- Leave your baby with someone else for 10 minutes and walk alone.

Medical help

At this time, there are no medications to relieve colic safely and effectively. In general, consult with your health care provider before giving your baby any medication.

If you're worried that your baby is sick or if you or others caring for the baby are becoming frustrated or angry because of the crying, call your doctor or bring the baby to the doctor's office or emergency department.

Common Problems

Constipation

People who experience **constipation** have infrequent bowel movements (generally, fewer than three stools a week), pass hard stools or strain during bowel movements. The normal frequency for bowel movements varies widely — from three a day to three a week. You also may have a bloated sensation and occasional crampy discomfort. This common problem is often improperly treated.

Constipation is a symptom, not a disease. It's the perception of difficult passage of stool. Contributing factors to constipation include not drinking enough fluids, a diet low in fiber, irregular bowel habits, older age, lack of activity, pregnancy and illness. Various medications also can cause constipation.

Although constipation may be extremely bothersome, the condition itself usually is not serious. If it persists, however, constipation can lead to complications such as hemorrhoids and cracks or tears in the anus (fissures).

Self-care

To lessen your chances of constipation:
- Eat on a regular schedule (including breakfast), and eat plenty of high-fiber foods, including fresh fruits, vegetables, and whole-grain cereals and breads
- Drink plenty of water or other liquids daily
- Increase your physical activity
- Don't ignore the urge to have a bowel movement
- Don't rely on certain laxatives (see below)

Medical help

Contact your doctor if your constipation is severe or it lasts longer than three weeks. In rare cases, constipation may signal more-serious medical conditions such as cancer and hormonal disturbances.

Kids' care

Constipation isn't usually a problem among infants, especially if they're breast-feeding. A healthy breast-fed infant may have as few as one bowel movement a week.

Young children sometimes experience constipation because they neglect to take time to use the bathroom. Toddlers also may become constipated during toilet training because of a fear or unwillingness to use the toilet. Stress or anxiety sometimes plays a role in a change in bowel habits. However, as few as one bowel movement a week may be normal for your child.

If constipation is a problem, have your child drink plenty of fluids to soften stools. Warm baths also may help relax your child and encourage bowel movements. Avoid use of laxatives in children unless advised by your health care provider.

Overuse of certain laxatives can be harmful

Excessive use of certain laxatives can be harmful and make your constipation worse. Stimulant laxatives (such as Ex-lax and Senokot) are the harshest and not for long-term use. Overuse can:
- Cause your body to flush out vitamins and other nutrients before they're absorbed and disrupt the normal balance of salts and nutrients.
- Interfere with other medications you're taking.
- Cause lazy bowel syndrome, a condition in which your bowels don't function properly

because they rely on the laxative to stimulate elimination. So when you stop using these laxatives, your constipation may worsen.

The effectiveness of each laxative type varies from person to person. In general, bulk-forming laxatives, also called fiber supplements (such as Citrucel and Metamucil), are the gentlest on your body and safe to use long term.

See back cover for online resource ⓘ

■ Diarrhea

Symptoms of **diarrhea** include loose, watery stools, often with abdominal cramps. You also may notice abdominal pain and other flu-like signs and symptoms, such as low-grade fever, achy or cramping muscles, and headache.

Diarrhea may be acute or chronic. Acute diarrhea is something that nearly everyone experiences at some time, and it usually clears up within days. The most common cause of acute diarrhea is a viral infection of the digestive tract. Bacteria and parasites also can cause diarrhea, sometimes with bloody stools and high fever. Infection-induced diarrhea can be extremely contagious. Nausea and vomiting may precede it. Diarrhea also can be a side effect of many medications, particularly antibiotics.

Chronic diarrhea generally lasts longer than four weeks and may signal a serious underlying medical problem such as chronic infection, inflammatory bowel disease, irritable bowel syndrome (IBS), microscopic colitis or certain kinds of cancer.

Diarrhea also can be a sign of lactose intolerance or from the use of products made with artificial sweeteners, such as sorbitol and mannitol. In these cases, the diarrhea usually improves with a change in diet.

Self-care

Although uncomfortable, diarrhea caused by infections typically clears on its own without antibiotics. Over-the-counter medications such as Imodium A-D, Pepto-Bismol and Kaopectate may slow diarrhea, but they won't speed recovery. To prevent dehydration and reduce symptoms while you recover:
- Drink plenty of clear liquids, including water, clear sodas (caffeine-free), broths and weak tea.
- Add semisolid and low-fiber foods gradually as your bowel movements return to normal. Try soda crackers, toast, eggs, rice or chicken.
- Avoid dairy products, fatty foods or highly seasoned foods for a few days.
- Avoid caffeine, alcohol and nicotine.

Medical help

Contact your health care provider if diarrhea persists beyond a week or if you become dehydrated (excessive thirst, dry mouth, little or no urination, severe weakness, dizziness, or lightheadedness) or you see blood in your stool or the toilet bowl. Also seek medical attention if you have severe abdominal or rectal pain, a temperature of more than 101 F, or signs of dehydration despite drinking fluids.

Your doctor may prescribe antibiotics to shorten the duration of diarrhea caused by some bacteria and parasites. However, not all diarrhea caused by bacteria requires treatment with antibiotics, and antibiotics don't help viral diarrhea, which is the most common kind of infectious diarrhea.

Kids' care

Diarrhea is common in infants and can cause dehydration. Contact your health care provider if diarrhea persists for more than 12 hours and if your baby:
- Hasn't had a wet diaper in eight hours
- Has a temperature of more than 102 F
- Has bloody stools
- Has a dry mouth or cries without tears
- Is unusually sleepy or drowsy or unresponsive

■ Excessive gas and gas pains

Belching
Belching (burping) is your body's way of getting rid of excess air from your stomach. You may swallow too much air if you eat or drink too fast, talk while you eat, drink carbonated beverages, or drink through a straw. Some people swallow air as a nervous habit. Indigestion and heartburn may be relieved by belching (see page 64).

Passing gas (flatulence)
Most intestinal gas (flatus) is produced in the colon. Gas buildup in the colon is typically caused by the fermentation of food, such as plant fiber. Gas can also form when your digestive system doesn't completely break down certain food components, such as gluten or sugar. Other examples of sources include changes in intestinal bacteria, medications and swallowed air.

Bloating and gas pains
When gas isn't expelled by belching or flatulence, it can build up in the stomach and intestines and lead to **bloating**. Bloating often occurs with abdominal pain, either mild and dull or sharp and intense. Passing gas may relieve the pain. Bloating is also related to conditions such as irritable bowel syndrome or lactose intolerance.

Any of the sources of intestinal gas (above) can lead to **gas pains**. Gas pains can also result from stress and anxiety and from diarrhea.

Self-care

To reduce belching, try these tips:
- Eat and drink slowly and avoid gulping. Limit drinking through a straw.
- Cut down on carbonated drinks and beer.
- Avoid chewing gum or sucking on hard candy.
- Don't smoke cigarettes, pipes or cigars.
- Manage stress, which may aggravate the nervous habit of swallowing air.
- Check dentures. A poor fit may cause swallowing of excess air when eating.
- Avoid lying down immediately after you eat and treat heartburn.

To reduce flatulence, try these tips:
- Avoid foods that affect you the most. Common offenders include beans, peas, lentils, cabbage, onions, broccoli, cauliflower, bananas, raisins, prunes, whole-wheat bread, bran cereals or muffins, and carbonated drinks.
- Temporarily cut back on high-fiber foods. Add them back gradually over weeks.
- Try adding Beano to high-fiber foods to reduce the amount of gas they make.
- Try low-lactose or lactose-free dairy products, if dairy products are a problem.
- Eat fewer fatty foods, which slow digestion.
- Eat slowly and get moving, such as taking a short walk after you eat.
- Try an over-the-counter remedy. Products such as Lactaid or Dairy Ease can help digest lactose. Products with simethicone can break up the bubbles in gas.

To reduce bloating, try these tips:
- Eat fewer fatty foods, which delay stomach emptying.
- Eat fewer gas-producing foods, such as baked beans, broccoli, Brussels sprouts, cabbage, cauliflower, carbonated drinks, apples, chewing gum and hard candy.

See back cover for online resource ⓘ

Gallstones

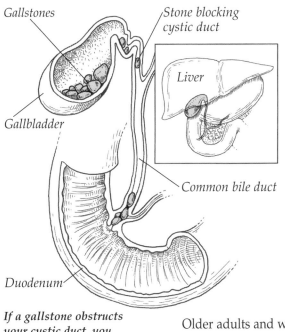

Gallstones

Stone blocking cystic duct

Liver

Gallbladder

Common bile duct

Duodenum

If a gallstone obstructs your cystic duct, you may experience a gallbladder attack.

Many Americans have **gallstones**, but gallstones may not cause symptoms. Stones that block the ducts that connect your gallbladder with your liver and small intestine can be painful and potentially dangerous.

Your gallbladder stores bile, a digestive fluid produced in the liver. Normally, the bile passes through ducts from the gallbladder into the small intestine and helps digest fats. A healthy gallbladder has balanced amounts of bile acids and cholesterol. When the concentration of cholesterol becomes too high, gallstones may form.

Gallstones can cause intense and sudden pain that may last for hours. The pain usually begins shortly after eating, in your right upper abdomen. It may shift to your back or right shoulder blade. You may also have a fever and nausea. After your pain subsides, you may notice a mild aching sensation or soreness in your right upper abdomen. If a gallstone blocks your bile duct, your skin and the whites of your eyes may turn yellow (jaundice). You may also develop a fever or pass pale, clay-colored stools.

Older adults and women tend to be at higher risk, especially women who are pregnant or taking estrogen or birth control pills. Your risk also may be higher if:

- You are overweight or have recently lost weight
- You have a family history of gallstones or a disorder of the small intestine

Self-care	Avoid rich, fatty foods and eat smaller meals to reduce episodes of gallbladder pain.
Medical help	Contact your health care provider if you have recurrent or intense pain. Seek prompt medical attention if you develop yellowing skin or a fever during an attack.

Gastritis

Gastritis is an inflammation of your stomach lining. Upper abdominal discomfort, nausea and vomiting are common symptoms. Gastritis may cause bleeding that appears in vomit or turns your stools black. Most often, gastritis is mild and poses no danger. Gastritis may occur when acid damages your stomach lining. Excessive smoking, alcohol and medications such as aspirin can cause gastritis. Some infections, such as *Helicobacter pylori* (*H. pylori*) infection, also can cause gastritis. In some cases, gastritis can lead to ulcers and an increased risk of stomach cancer.

Self-care	<ul><li>Avoid smoking, alcohol, and foods and drinks that irritate your stomach.</li><li>Try taking over-the-counter antacids or medicines such as Pepcid, Prilosec and Zantac. **Caution:** Excessive use of antacids containing magnesium can cause diarrhea. Calcium- or aluminum-based antacids can lead to constipation.</li><li>Use pain relievers that contain acetaminophen (see page 258). Avoid aspirin, ibuprofen, ketoprofen and naproxen sodium. They can cause or worsen gastritis.</li></ul>
Medical help	If your discomfort lasts longer than one week, contact your health care provider.

■ Hemorrhoids and rectal bleeding

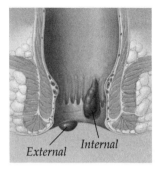

External   *Internal*

Internal hemorrhoids are usually painless, but they can bleed. External hemorrhoids may cause discomfort, pain or itching.

By age 50, about half of all people have experienced symptoms of **hemorrhoids** to some extent. Itching, burning and pain around the anus may signal their presence. You may also notice small amounts of bright red blood on your toilet tissue or in the toilet bowl.

Hemorrhoids occur when veins in your rectum become enlarged. They usually form over time as you strain to pass hard stools or sit for prolonged periods on the toilet. Hemorrhoids may be internal, developing above or inside the anal canal, or external, protruding outside the anal opening. Lifting heavy objects, obesity, pregnancy, childbirth, stress and diarrhea also can increase the pressure on these veins and lead to hemorrhoids. This condition seems to run in families.

In addition to hemorrhoids, bleeding from the rectum can occur for other reasons, some of which can be serious. Passing hard, dry stools may scrape the anal lining. An infection of the lining of the rectum or tiny cracks or tears in the lining of your anus called anal fissures also can cause rectal bleeding. With these types of problems, you may notice small drops of bright red blood on your stool, on your toilet tissue or in the toilet bowl.

Black, tarry stools, maroon stools or bright red blood in your stools can signal more-extensive bleeding elsewhere in your digestive tract. Small sacs that protrude from your large intestines (diverticula), ulcers, small growths (polyps) and cancer can all cause bleeding. Sharp pain with bleeding can be caused by a fissure or tear in the anal tissue.

Self-care

Although uncomfortable, hemorrhoids are not a serious medical condition. Most hemorrhoids respond well to the following self-care measures:

- Drink plenty of water each day and eat high-fiber foods such as wheat-bran cereal, whole-wheat bread, fresh fruit and vegetables.
- Bathe or shower daily to cleanse the skin around your anus gently with warm water. Soap isn't necessary and may aggravate the problem.
- Avoid sitting for prolonged periods. If sitting for work is necessary, take short walks or breaks to decrease the pressure.
- Try not to strain during bowel movements or sit on the toilet too long — limit your time there to five to 10 minutes, if possible.
- Take warm baths or sitz baths to relieve irritation. Use hypoallergenic wipes or moistened toilet paper to wipe. Avoid excessive wiping. Blot dry.
- Apply ice packs.
- For flares of pain or irritation, apply over-the-counter creams, ointments or pads containing witch hazel or a topical numbing agent. Keep in mind that these products help relieve only mild itching and irritation.
- Try fiber supplements (Citrucel, Metamucil, others) to keep stools soft and regular.

Medical help

Hemorrhoids become most painful when a clot forms in the enlarged vein. If your hemorrhoids are extremely painful, your health care provider may prescribe a cream or suppository containing hydrocortisone to reduce inflammation. Some troublesome internal hemorrhoids may require surgery or other procedures to shrink or eliminate them.

Diagnosing the cause of rectal bleeding can be difficult. See your health care provider for evaluation. Seek immediate emergency care if you notice large amounts of rectal bleeding, lightheadedness, weakness or rapid heart rate (more than 100 beats a minute).

See back cover for online resource ⓘ

■ Hernias

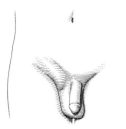

An inguinal hernia can cause a bulge at the junction of your thigh and groin. Bulges can be round or oval.

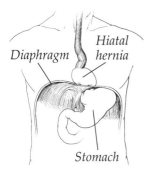

In a hiatal hernia, a portion of the stomach protrudes through the diaphragm into the chest cavity.

A hernia occurs when one body part protrudes through a gap into another body area. Some hernias cause no pain or noticeable signs.

Types of hernias

<u>Inguinal hernia</u> is the medical name for a hernia in the groin area. This type of hernia — which is more frequent in men than in women — accounts for about 75 percent of all hernias. An inguinal hernia occurs along the inguinal canal, an opening in the abdominal muscles. In men, the canal is the spermatic cord's passageway between the abdominal cavity and the scrotum. In women, it's the passageway for a ligament that helps hold the uterus in place. With an inguinal hernia, you may be able to see and feel the bulge created by the protruding tissue or intestine. It's often located at the junction of your thigh and groin. Sometimes in men the protruding intestine enters the scrotum. This can be painful and cause the scrotum to swell. The first sign of an inguinal hernia may be a bulge or lump in your groin. You may notice discomfort while bending over, coughing or lifting, and a heavy or dragging sensation.

A strangulated hernia occurs when the tissue bulging through the abdominal wall becomes pinched and the blood supply is cut off. The affected tissue dies and then swells, causing extreme pain and a potentially life-threatening situation. Seek immediate medical attention if you think you have a strangulated hernia.

A <u>hiatal hernia</u> occurs at the spot called the hiatus, which is an opening in your diaphragm through which your food pipe (esophagus) passes into your stomach. If this opening is too large, your stomach may protrude (herniate) through it into your chest cavity, creating a hiatal hernia. Hiatal hernias are common, occurring most often in people older than 50. Most small hiatal hernias cause no problems. If you have a large hernia that causes stomach acids to back up into your esophagus, you may experience heartburn, belching, chest pain and nausea. Symptoms may worsen when you lean forward, strain, lift heavy objects or lie down. Obesity aggravates these symptoms.

Self-care

For an inguinal hernia
You can't prevent or cure a hernia through self-care. Once you've had the lump evaluated and know it's a hernia, if your hernia doesn't cause you discomfort, you don't need to take any special precautions. Don't rely on a corset or truss for support — it won't protect against complications or correct the problem.

For a hiatal hernia
- Lose weight if you're overweight.
- Follow self-care precautions for heartburn on page 64.

Medical help

If your hernia is painful or bothersome, contact your doctor to discuss whether medications or other treatment or surgery may be necessary.

Caution

If you can't reduce the hernia by lying down and pushing on the lump, the blood supply to this segment of bowel may be cut off. Signs and symptoms of this complication include nausea, vomiting and severe pain. Left untreated, intestinal blockage or, in rare cases, a life-threatening infection may result. If you have any of these signs or symptoms, contact your doctor.

Common Problems

■ Indigestion and heartburn

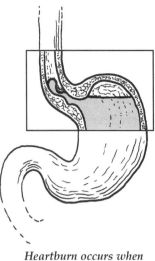

Heartburn occurs when stomach contents back up into your esophagus, causing irritation.

Indigestion, also called an upset stomach or dyspepsia, is a general term that describes discomfort in your upper abdomen that may occur after eating. Indigestion isn't a disease. It's a collection of symptoms, such as nausea and a bloated or full feeling that belching may relieve. The cause of indigestion is sometimes difficult to pinpoint. In some people, eating certain foods or drinking alcohol may trigger it.

A common form of indigestion is the burning sensation called **heartburn**. As many as 10 percent of adults have heartburn at least once a week. Often due to gastro-esophageal reflux disease (GERD), heartburn occurs when stomach contents back up into your food pipe (esophagus). A sour taste and the sensation of food coming back into your mouth may accompany the burning sensation behind your breastbone.

Why do these contents back up? Normally, esophageal muscles contract in sequence, sending food through the esophagus to the stomach. If the muscle is weak, stomach contents can wash back up (reflux), irritating the esophagus.

Various factors can cause reflux. A hiatal hernia increases your chances of experiencing reflux. Being overweight puts too much pressure on your abdomen. Some medications, foods and beverages can relax the esophageal sphincter muscle or irritate the esophagus. Overeating or lying down after a meal also can lead to reflux.

Self-care

Changing what and how you eat is the first step to prevent heartburn.
- Slim down if you're overweight. Losing 5 to 10 percent of your body weight can reduce symptoms (and lower your risk of heart and blood vessel disease).
- Eat small, frequent meals.
- Avoid foods and drinks that relax the esophageal sphincter or irritate the esophagus (such as fatty foods, alcohol, caffeinated or carbonated beverages, decaffeinated coffee, peppermint, spearmint, garlic, onion, cinnamon, chocolate, citrus fruits and juices, and tomato products).
- Stop eating two to three hours before you lie down or go to bed.
- Elevate the head of your bed.
- Quit smoking; eliminate nicotine use.
- Don't wear tight clothing and tight belts.
- Avoid excessive stooping or bending or heavy exertion for an hour after eating.
- Over-the-counter antacids can relieve mild heartburn by neutralizing stomach acids temporarily. However, prolonged or excessive use of antacids containing magnesium can cause diarrhea. Calcium- or aluminum-based products can lead to constipation.

Medications such as Pepcid, Prilosec and Zantac may relieve or prevent heartburn symptoms by reducing the production of stomach acid. These medications are available in over-the-counter and prescription strengths. Follow medication instructions about eating and drinking to maximize their effectiveness.

Medical help

Most problems with indigestion and heartburn are occasional and mild. But if you have severe or daily discomfort, don't ignore your symptoms. Left untreated, chronic heartburn can cause scarring in the lower esophagus. This can make swallowing difficult. In rare cases, severe heartburn can lead to a condition called Barrett's esophagus, which may increase your risk of cancer.

Heartburn and indigestion symptoms may indicate a more serious underlying disease. Contact your health care provider if your symptoms are persistent or severe, or if you have difficulty swallowing.

See back cover for online resource ⓘ

Irritable bowel syndrome

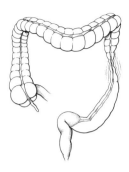

A spasm in the bowel wall may cause abdominal pain and other unpleasant symptoms commonly associated with IBS.

Irritable bowel syndrome (IBS), sometimes known as spastic bowel or spastic colon, is a common medical problem that's not completely understood. IBS is stressful, painful, disruptive and at times embarrassing. But it does not indicate cancer, and it's not life-threatening.

You're more likely to have IBS if you are young, are female (about twice as many women as men have the condition) and have a family history of IBS. Researchers are studying whether family history relates to a genetic inheritance, to a shared environment or to a combination of both.

It's not known what causes IBS, but the condition affects muscle contractions in the intestines and colon. If you have IBS, the contractions can feel stronger, last longer and are often relieved — at least temporarily — by passing stool. Triggers for IBS can range from gas or pressure on your intestines to certain foods, medications or emotions.

Signs and symptoms of IBS vary widely and can resemble those of many other diseases. Abdominal pain or discomfort, diarrhea or constipation, bloating, abdominal gas, and mucus in the stool are all signs and symptoms of IBS. You may experience only mild signs and symptoms, but for some, these problems are disabling. IBS tends to be a chronic condition, with periods of more-severe symptoms alternating with periods of low-level symptoms or no symptoms.

Self-care

You may be able to improve your symptoms by managing your diet, lifestyle and stress:

- Avoid or eat smaller portions of foods that consistently aggravate your symptoms. Common culprits include alcohol, chocolate, caffeinated beverages, carbonated drinks, and sugary drinks and sweeteners. High-fructose foods or sweeteners such as sorbitol or mannitol can aggravate symptoms.
- Eat high-fiber foods, such as fresh fruits, vegetables and whole-grain foods. Add fiber gradually to minimize problems with gas and bloating.
- Drink plenty of fluids — at least eight to 10 glasses a day.
- Try using fiber supplements, such as Citrucel or Metamucil, to help relieve your constipation and diarrhea.
- Reduce your stress through regular exercise, sports or hobbies that help you relax.
- Try over-the-counter medications such as Imodium A-D or Kaopectate to help relieve diarrhea.

Medical help

If self-care doesn't help, your doctor may recommend prescription medications designed to relieve muscle spasms, abdominal pain and other symptoms. If depression or anxiety plays a role in your symptoms, treating this problem may be helpful.

Because the symptoms of IBS may mimic those of more-serious medical problems such as cancer, gallbladder disease and ulcers, contact your doctor for evaluation if self-care measures don't help within a couple of weeks. Some red flags that might require additional testing include new onset after age 50, weight loss, rectal bleeding, fever, nausea or recurrent vomiting, abdominal pain (especially if it's not completely relieved by a bowel movement), or persistent diarrhea.

Common Problems

Nausea and vomiting

Nausea and vomiting are common and uncomfortable signs and symptoms of a wide variety of disorders, many of which aren't serious.

Feeling queasy and throwing up can signal a viral infection called **gastroenteritis**. Diarrhea, abdominal cramps, bloating and fever also may accompany this condition. Other causes include food poisoning, pregnancy, some medications and gastritis (see page 61). Nausea and vomiting also occur in **gastroparesis**, a condition in which your stomach doesn't empty properly.

Self-care

If gastroenteritis is the culprit, nausea and vomiting may last from a few hours to two or three days. Diarrhea and mild abdominal cramping also are common. To keep yourself comfortable and prevent dehydration while you recover, try the following:

- Stop eating and drinking for a few hours until your stomach has settled.
- Try ice chips or small sips of weak tea, clear soda (such as 7Up or Sprite) and broths, or noncaffeinated clear sports drinks to prevent dehydration. Consume 2 to 4 quarts (eight to 16 glasses) of liquid for no longer than 24 hours, taking frequent, small sips.
- Add semisolid and low-fiber foods gradually and stop eating if the vomiting returns. Try soda crackers, gelatin, toast, eggs, rice or chicken.
- Avoid dairy products, caffeine, alcohol, nicotine, or fatty or highly seasoned foods for a few days.

Medical help

Vomiting can lead to complications such as dehydration (if vomiting is persistent), food in the windpipe (aspiration) or, in rare instances, a torn blood vessel in the food pipe that causes bleeding. Infants, older adults and people with suppressed immune systems are particularly vulnerable to complications. Contact your health care provider if you're unable to drink anything for 24 hours, if vomiting persists beyond two or three days, if you become dehydrated, or if you vomit blood. Warning signs of dehydration include excessive thirst, dry mouth, little or no urination, severe weakness, dizziness, or lightheadedness. Vomiting also can be a warning of more-serious underlying problems such as gallbladder disease, ulcers or bowel obstruction.

Kids' care

Most babies spit up at least occasionally. But vomiting is more forceful and disturbing to your baby and can lead to dehydration and weight loss if it's persistent.

To prevent dehydration, let the baby's stomach rest for 30 to 60 minutes and then offer small amounts of liquid. If you're breast-feeding, let your baby nurse smaller amounts more frequently. Offer bottle-fed babies a small amount of formula or an oral electrolyte solution such as Pedialyte or Enfamil Enfalyte.

If the vomiting doesn't recur, continue to offer small sips of liquid or the breast every 15 to 30 minutes. Contact your health care provider if vomiting persists for more than 12 hours or if your child:

- Hasn't had a wet diaper in eight hours
- Has diarrhea or bloody stools
- Has a dry mouth or cries without tears
- Is unusually sleepy or drowsy or unresponsive

A few newborn babies have a disorder called **pyloric stenosis**, which can cause repeated, forceful and persistent vomiting. This condition usually appears after the third week of life and requires surgical correction.

See back cover for online resource

Peptic ulcers

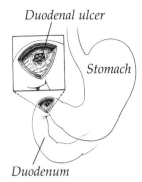

Duodenal ulcer

Stomach

Duodenum

The most common form of peptic ulcer occurs in the duodenum and is called a duodenal ulcer.

Peptic ulcers are sores in the inner lining of your stomach (gastric ulcer) or the uppermost section of your small intestine called the duodenum (duodenal ulcer).

Most peptic ulcers are caused by a bacterium called *Helicobacter pylori (H. pylori). H. pylori* infection is one of the risk factors for stomach cancer. Stomach ulcers can also be caused by excessive use of aspirin or aspirin-like medications. Contrary to popular belief, there's no evidence that stress causes ulcers, but it may aggravate symptoms.

Ulcers can cause considerable distress. Symptoms may include a burning feeling beneath your breastbone in your upper abdomen, gnawing hunger pangs, or pain and nausea. At times, ulcers can also cause belching or bloating. These symptoms typically occur when your stomach is empty. Although eating may relieve the symptoms, they often resume one to two hours later. In severe cases, ulcers may bleed and cause you to vomit blood or pass black, tarry stools. In rare cases, an ulcer may perforate the wall of your stomach or duodenum, causing severe abdominal pain.

Self-care

Dietary, lifestyle and medication choices may help prevent or control ulcers.
- If you're using pain relievers, use acetaminophen (Tylenol, others). Aspirin, ibuprofen, ketoprofen and naproxen sodium can cause ulcers.
- Avoid alcohol and caffeinated foods, beverages and medications.
- Stop smoking.
- Eat small meals and avoid letting your stomach remain empty for long periods.
- Avoid spicy or fatty foods if they seem to make your symptoms worse.
- Take nonprescription antacids to neutralize stomach acids or medications such as Pepcid, Prilosec OTC or Zantac to stop the production of stomach acid.

Medical help

Some ulcers disappear with self-care or with over-the-counter medication. If your symptoms don't improve after a week or if you have troublesome, recurrent ulcers, see your doctor. You may have diagnostic tests, such as a stool antigen test, an X-ray or an endoscopy — a procedure used to visually examine your upper digestive system with a tiny camera on the end of a long flexible tube.

Bleeding ulcers can cause serious blood loss. Seek help immediately if you vomit blood, pass black, tarry stools or have severe pain.

Treatment for peptic ulcers

Because many ulcers stem from *H. pylori* bacteria, the treatment approach is to kill the bacteria and reduce the level of acid in your digestive system to relieve pain and encourage healing.

This typically involves taking three drugs: two antibiotics to kill the bacteria and a proton pump inhibitor, such as Prilosec, Prevacid, Aciphex, Nexium or Protonix, to reduce stomach acid. The antibiotics are usually taken for two weeks. Other medications prescribed with the antibiotics generally are taken for a longer period.

FOR MORE INFORMATION
- National Institute of Diabetes and Digestive and Kidney Diseases Health Information Center, 800-860-8747, *www.niddk.nih.gov/health-information/digestive-diseases*

See back cover for online resource (i)

Ears and hearing

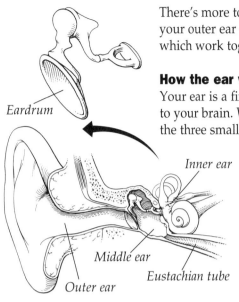

Eardrum

Inner ear

Middle ear

Eustachian tube

Outer ear

There's more to the ear than meets the eye. The part of your ear that's visible — your outer ear — is connected inside your head to your middle ear and inner ear, which work together to allow you to hear and help you maintain balance.

How the ear works

Your ear is a finely tuned organ that's specially designed to send sound impulses to your brain. When sound waves travel through the ear canal, your eardrum and the three small bones to which it's attached vibrate. This vibration moves through the middle ear to your inner ear, triggering nerve impulses to your brain, where you perceive them as sound.

Air reaches your middle ear through the eustachian tube. The middle ear must maintain the same pressure as the air outside your ear to allow your eardrum and ear bones to vibrate freely and conduct sound waves. If the middle ear has fluid in it, the eardrum and the bones can't move well. This is why an ear infection can cause temporary hearing problems.

Some common causes of ear pain and ear problems are described in this section.

■ Airplane ear

The medical name for **airplane ear** is ear barotrauma or barotitis media. It means an injury caused by changes in pressure. It can occur if you fly or scuba dive, especially if you have a stuffy nose, nasal allergy, cold or throat infection. You may have pain in one ear, a slight hearing loss or a stuffy feeling in your ears. It's caused by your eardrum bulging outward or retracting inward as a result of a change in air pressure. Having a severe cold or ear infection may be a reason to change or delay a flight.

Self-care

- Try taking a decongestant an hour before takeoff and an hour before landing. This may prevent blockage of your eustachian tube. However, if you have heart disease, a heart rhythm disorder or high blood pressure, or if you've experienced possible medication interactions, avoid taking an oral decongestant.
- During flight, suck candy or chew gum to encourage swallowing, which helps open your eustachian tube.
- If your ears plug as the plane descends, inhale and then gently exhale while holding your nostrils closed and keeping your mouth closed. If you can swallow at the same time, it's more helpful.
- Consider using earplugs designed specifically to help prevent or reduce ear pain and discomfort during airplane travel.

Medical help

If your symptoms don't disappear within a few hours, see your doctor.

Kids' care

For babies and young children, make sure they are drinking fluids (swallowing) during ascent and descent. Give the child a bottle or pacifier to encourage swallowing. Decongestants should not be used in infants or young children.

See back cover for online resource ⓘ

Foreign objects in the ear

Objects stuck in your ear can cause pain and hearing loss. Usually you know if something is stuck in your ear, but small children may not be aware of it.

Self-care

If an object becomes lodged in the ear, follow these steps:
- Don't attempt to remove the foreign object by probing with a cotton swab, matchstick or any other tool. To do so is to risk pushing the object farther into the ear and damaging the fragile structures of the middle ear.
- If the object is clearly visible, is pliable and can be grasped easily with tweezers, gently remove it.
- Try using the pull of gravity: Tilt the head to the affected side. Don't strike the person's head, but shake it gently in the direction of the ground to try to dislodge the object.
- If the foreign object is an insect, tilt the person's head so that the ear with the offending insect is upward. Try to float the insect out by pouring mineral oil, olive oil or baby oil into the ear. The oil should be warm but not hot. As you pour the oil, you can ease the entry of the oil by straightening the ear canal. Pull the earlobe gently backward and upward. The insect should suffocate and may float out in the oil bath.
- Don't use oil to remove any object other than an insect. Don't use this method if there's any suspicion of a perforation in the eardrum (pain, bleeding or discharge from the ear).

Medical help

If these methods fail or the person continues to experience pain in the ear, reduced hearing or a sensation of something lodged in the ear, seek medical assistance.

Ruptured eardrum

Eardrum

Rupture

An eardrum may rupture (tear) after an infection or from trauma. Signs and symptoms of a **ruptured eardrum** are earache, partial hearing loss, and slight bleeding or discharge from your ear. With an infection, the pain often resolves once the eardrum ruptures, releasing infected fluid or pus. Usually, the rupture heals by itself without complications and with little or no permanent hearing loss. Large ruptures may cause recurring infections. If you suspect that you have ruptured an eardrum, see your doctor as soon as possible. Meanwhile, try the self-care tips below.

Self-care

- Relieve pain with aspirin or another pain medication that is safe for you.
- Place a warm (not hot) heating pad over your ear.
- Don't flush your ear.

Medical help

Your doctor may prescribe an antibiotic to make sure that no infection develops in your middle ear. Sometimes a paper patch is placed over your eardrum to seal the opening while it heals. Your eardrum will often heal within three months. If it hasn't healed in that time, you may require a minor surgical procedure to repair the tear.

■ Ear infections

For many parents of young children, coping with ear infections is almost as routine as changing wet diapers. It's estimated that 5 out of 6 children will have at least one **middle ear infection** (otitis media) by age 3. Many have multiple episodes. Ear infections are one of the most common illnesses in babies and young children.

Millions of children see a health care provider for middle ear infections each year, and millions of children receive antibiotic prescriptions — many of which aren't really needed. Most ear infections don't lead to permanent hearing loss. Some infections that aren't treated, however, can spread to other parts of the ear, including the inner ear. Untreated infections of the middle ear can damage the eardrum, ear bones and inner ear structure, causing permanent hearing loss.

An ear infection often begins with a respiratory infection such as a cold. Colds cause swelling and inflammation in the sinuses and eustachian tubes. Children's eustachian tubes are shorter and narrower than are adults'. This makes it more likely that inflammation will block the tube completely, trapping fluid in the middle ear. This trapped fluid causes an earache and creates an ideal environment for bacteria to grow. The result is a middle ear infection.

Fluid (shown in blue) is trapped in the middle ear.

Self-care	• Consider an over-the-counter pain reliever such as ibuprofen (Advil, Motrin, others) or acetaminophen (Tylenol, others). If your child is younger than age 2, consult your health care provider. • Place a warm (not hot) moist cloth or heating pad (on lowest setting) over the ear.
Medical help	Contact your child's doctor if pain lasts more than a day or so or it's associated with fever. In many cases, children's ear infections resolve on their own, without using antibiotics. But antibiotics may be used if your child is under 2 years old, has recurrent middle ear infections or has a high-risk medical condition. Keep immunizations up to date: Some may help reduce the risk of middle ear infections.

The pros and cons of ear tubes

Children's chronic ear fluid is sometimes treated by surgically inserting a small plastic tube through the eardrum in order to remove chronic fluid and mucus from the middle ear. Surgery is not common for adults.

Pros of the procedure
• Hearing should improve immediately.
• Ear tubes allow ventilation of the middle ear, which reduces the risk of permanent changes in the lining of the middle ear that can occur with a lengthy infection.

Cons of the procedure
• It requires brief general anesthesia.
• Your child should avoid getting water in the ear while the tube is in place — often for 6 months or longer.
• In rare cases, severe scarring or a permanent hole in the eardrum may result.

See back cover for online resource (i)

Common questions about ear infections in kids

What are the risk factors for infections?

Although all children are susceptible to ear infections, those at higher risk are children who:

- Are male
- Have siblings with a history of recurrent ear infection
- Have their first ear infection before they're 4 months old
- Are in group child care
- Are exposed to tobacco smoke
- Are of American Indian, Alaskan or Inuit descent
- Have frequent upper respiratory tract infections
- Have medical conditions that predispose them to middle ear infections
- Were bottle-fed instead of breast-fed

What are the symptoms?

In addition to an earache or a feeling of pressure and blockage in the ear, some children may experience temporary hearing loss. Be aware of other signs and symptoms of an ear infection, such as irritability, a sudden loss of appetite, the development of a fever a few days after onset of a cold, nausea, vomiting or a preference for sleeping in an upright position. Your child may also have discharge in the ear or may tug at the ear.

Does your child need an antibiotic?

Because most ear infections clear on their own, your health care provider may first recommend a wait-and-see approach, especially if your child has few symptoms. In other cases, your doctor may opt to prescribe an antibiotic to treat the infection. Within two to three days of beginning the medication, symptoms usually improve.

Be sure to follow instructions carefully for giving the antibiotic. Continue to give the medication to your child for the entire recommended time. If you stop giving your child the antibiotic when symptoms improve, you may allow stronger remaining bacteria to multiply and cause another infection. Surviving bacteria may carry genes that make them drug resistant.

If symptoms don't go away or if your child is younger than 15 months, schedule a follow-up visit as recommended by your health care provider. If your child is older and symptoms have resolved, a recheck may not be necessary, especially if infections haven't been recurrent.

What can you do?

Although an ear infection isn't an emergency, the first 24 hours are often when your child's pain and irritability are the worst. Follow the self-care tips on page 70. To make your child more comfortable, don't underestimate the benefits of extra cuddling.

What about recurrent infections?

Time and the use of antibiotics usually resolve ear infections. But sometimes ear infections can become a chronic problem. If so, ask your health care provider about the possibility of ear tubes. Persistent fluid buildup may cause temporary or even permanent hearing loss. This can lead to delayed speech development.

Can you prevent infections?

Preventing ear infections is difficult, but consider these approaches to help reduce your child's risk:

- Breast-feed rather than bottle-feed your baby for as long as possible.
- When bottle-feeding, hold your baby in an upright position.
- Avoid exposing your child to tobacco smoke.
- Keep your child's immunizations up to date. Certain vaccines, such as the pneumococcal vaccine, can reduce the risk of middle ear infections.

Do children outgrow ear infections?

As your child matures, the eustachian tubes become wider and more angled, making it easier for secretions and fluid to drain out of the ear. Although ear infections still may occur, they probably won't develop as often as during the first few years of life.

What are medical researchers working on to help treat ear infections?

Research on many different types and doses of antibiotic therapy and other medications continues. Refining immunizations (developing new and better ones) will likely be the best route to reducing frequency of ear infections.

■ Ringing in your ear

A ringing or buzzing in your ear when no other sounds are present can have many causes, including earwax, a foreign object, infection or exposure to loud noise. It may also be caused by high doses of aspirin or large amounts of caffeine. This condition, called **tinnitus**, uncommonly is a symptom of more-serious ear disorders, particularly if it's accompanied by other symptoms such as hearing loss or dizziness.

Self-care

- If aspirin was recommended to you in high doses, ask your doctor about alternatives. If you're taking aspirin on your own, try lower doses or another over-the-counter pain medication.
- Avoid nicotine, caffeine and alcohol, which may aggravate the condition.
- Try to determine a cause, such as exposure to loud noise, and avoid or block it if possible.
- Wear earplugs or some other form of hearing protection if you have excess noise exposure, such as when you're working with yard equipment (leaf blowers or lawn mowers).
- Cover up the ringing sound with another, more acceptable sound, such as music. Try listening to a radio as you fall asleep).
- Give a masker a try. A masker is a device that fits in your ear and produces low-level noise, such as white noise or nature sounds.

Medical help

If tinnitus worsens, persists, or is accompanied by hearing loss or dizziness, consider evaluation by your health care provider. He or she may choose to pursue further evaluation. Although most causes of tinnitus are benign, it can be a difficult and frustrating condition to treat.

■ Swimmer's ear

This is an infection of your outer ear canal. In addition to pain or itching, you may see a clear drainage or yellow-green pus and experience temporary hearing loss. **Swimmer's ear** is the result of having persistent moisture in the ear or, sometimes, from swimming in polluted water. Other similar inflammations or infections may occur from scraping your ear canal when you clean your ear or from hair sprays or hair dyes. Some people are prone to bacterial or fungal infections.

Self-care

If the aching is mild and there's no drainage from the ear, do the following:
- Place a warm (not hot) heating pad over your ear.
- Take ibuprofen (Advil, Motrin IB, others) or another pain medication.
- To prevent swimmer's ear, try to keep ear canals dry, avoid substances that might irritate your ear and don't clean inside the ear canal unless you're instructed to do so by your health care provider.

Medical help

Seek medical care if you have severe pain or swelling of the ear, a fever, drainage from the ear, or an underlying disease such as diabetes. Your doctor may clean your ear canal with a suction device or a cotton-tipped probe. Your doctor may also prescribe eardrops or medications to control infection and reduce pain. Keep your ear dry while it's healing.

See back cover for online resource

■ Wax blockage

Earwax (cerumen) is a helpful and natural part of your body's defenses. It protects your ear canal by trapping dirt and slowing the growth of bacteria. At times, you may produce too much earwax, blocking your ear canal, which gives you hearing loss or a feeling of fullness in the affected ear or causes ear noise (tinnitus). **Earwax blockage** occurs when earwax accumulates in your ear and becomes too hard to wash away naturally. Earwax blockage can also cause gradual hearing loss as the wax accumulates.

Self-care

If you're having signs and symptoms of earwax blockage, talk to your doctor for advice on self-care. If your eardrum doesn't contain a tube or have a hole (perforation) in it, these self-care measures may help you remove excess earwax that's blocking your ear canal:

- Soften the wax by applying a few drops of baby oil, mineral oil or glycerin with an eyedropper twice a day for no more than four to five days.
- When the wax is softened, fill a bowl with water heated to body temperature (if it's colder or hotter, it may make you feel dizzy during the procedure).
- With your head upright, grasp the top of your ear and pull upward. With your other hand, squirt the water gently into your ear canal with a 3-ounce rubber-bulb syringe. Then, turn your head and drain the water into the bowl or sink.
- You may need to repeat this several times before the extra wax falls out.
- Gently dry your outer ear with a towel or a hand-held hair dryer.
- Earwax removal kits sold in stores can be effective. If you're unsure which one is right for you, ask your doctor.

Caution

Wax removal is most safely done by a doctor. Your ear canal and eardrum are very delicate and can be damaged easily. Don't poke them with objects such as cotton swabs, paper clips or bobby pins, especially if you have had ear surgery, have a hole in your eardrum, or are having ear pain or drainage. These objects can push the wax deeper into your ear and damage the lining of the ear canal and even your eardrum.

Flushing wax out of the ears should be avoided if you've had an eardrum perforation or ear surgery, unless your doctor approves. If infection is a concern, don't flush your ears.

Some people use ear candling, a technique that involves placing a lighted, hollow, cone-shaped candle into the ear, to try to remove earwax. The theory is that the heat from the flame will create a vacuum seal and the earwax will adhere to the candle. But research has found that ear candling doesn't work, and it may cause injury, such as burns, ear canal obstructions and even perforations.

Medical help

Even if the self-care tips are followed, many people have difficulty washing wax out of their ears. Asymptomatic earwax is best left alone since it provides infection protection for your ear canal. But ask your doctor to remove earwax if you have symptomatic hearing loss. Your doctor can remove excess wax in a procedure similar to the self-care method described above.

A special instrument is used to either scoop the wax out of the ear or suction it out. If this is a recurring problem, your doctor may recommend using a wax-removal medication every four to eight weeks.

Noise-related hearing loss

Sound is measured in decibels. An average conversation is about 60 decibels. A loud conversation in a crowded building is about 70 decibels. Continual exposure to noise at 85 decibels or above can cause gradual hearing loss.

Self-care

If you're exposed to loud power tools or engines, loud music, firearms, or other equipment that produces loud noises, take the following precautions:

- **Wear protective earplugs or earmuffs.** Use commercially made protection devices that meet federal standards (cotton balls will not work, and they could get stuck in your ears). These bring most loud sounds down to acceptable levels. You can get custom-molded earplugs made of plastic or rubber to protect against excessive noise.
- **Have your hearing tested.** Early detection of hearing loss can prevent future, irreversible damage.
- **Use ear protection off the job — beware of recreational risks.** Exposure to explosive noises, such as from firearms and fireworks, can cause immediate, permanent hearing loss. Other recreational activities with dangerously high noise levels include snowmobiling, motorcycling or listening to loud music. Music played through headphones can cause lasting hearing loss if you turn the volume up high enough to mask the sound of other loud noises, such as a lawn mower. And if you can identify the music being played while your child is wearing a headset or earbuds, it's too loud. Tell your child to save his or her ears for a lifetime of music enjoyment.

Sound levels of common noises

Decibels	Noise source
	Safe range
45	Humming of a refrigerator
60	Normal conversation
	Risk range
85	Heavy city traffic
95	Motorcycle
105	MP3 player at maximum volume
	Injury range
120	Sirens
150	Firecrackers and firearms

Source: National Institute on Deafness and Other Communication Disorders, 2017

Maximal job-noise exposure allowed by law

Sound level, decibels	Duration, daily
90	8 hours
92	6 hours
95	4 hours
97	3 hours
100	2 hours
102	1.5 hours
105	1 hour
110	30 minutes
115	15 minutes or less

Source: Department of Labor's Occupational Safety and Health Administration, 2008

Age-related hearing loss

Gradual **hearing loss** that occurs as you age (presbycusis) is common. Doctors believe that heredity and long-term exposure to loud noises contribute to hearing loss over time. Age-related hearing loss can't be reversed. But a hearing aid and taking steps such as shutting off background noise to focus on the person talking may greatly improve the quality of your life. If you or a family member suspects you have serious hearing loss, see your doctor or an audiologist — a person who specializes in the diagnosis and treatment options for hearing loss.

Before you buy a hearing aid, here's sound advice

If you're thinking about trying a hearing aid for the first time or shopping for a new model, you may be happily surprised by new technology. Current models are small, simple to operate and technologically advanced.

Hearing aids come in five basic styles, shown here. Generally, the smaller the hearing aid, the less powerful and more likely it is to produce feedback (a high-pitched noise). Digital hearing aids offer greater ability to fine-tune sound, reduce feedback and reduce background noise.

Tips to keep in mind
When selecting a hearing aid:
- **Have a medical and hearing exam.** Before you buy a hearing aid, be examined by a physician, preferably an ear, nose and throat doctor (otorhinolaryngologist). It's best to have this exam within six months before you buy a hearing aid. An exam can determine whether a medical condition will prevent you from using a hearing aid.
- **Buy from a reputable audiologist.** This hearing loss specialist will evaluate hearing to determine the degree and type of hearing loss you have.

The audiologist then takes an impression of your ear, recommends and helps you choose the most appropriate aid and adjusts the device to fit appropriately. These are complex tasks, and skills of dispensers vary. Check with your state hearing aid licensing board about a dispenser's record. Be cautious of free consultations and dispensers who sell only one brand of hearing aid.
- **Be alert to misleading claims.** For years, a few manufacturers and distributors claimed their hearing aids eliminated background noise. Some newer hearing aids reduce loud sounds, making wearing a hearing aid in noisy places more comfortable. But no hearing aid can amplify the voice you want to hear and filter out other voices or noises in a crowded room.
- **Ask about a trial period.** Have the audiologist put in writing the cost of a trial and whether this amount is credited toward the final cost of the hearing aid.
- **Have the hearing aid tested.** Retest with the hearing aid in place to ensure optimal hearing.
- **Understand the warranty.** A warranty should extend for one to two years and cover both parts and labor.

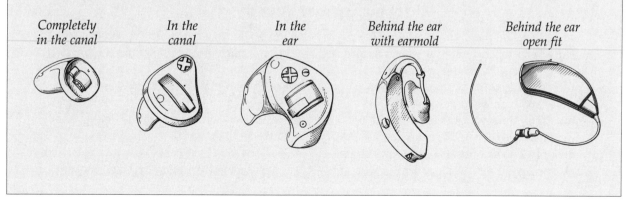

| Completely in the canal | In the canal | In the ear | Behind the ear with earmold | Behind the ear open fit |

Eyes and vision

Because your eyes are crucial in so many activities, eye problems usually demand attention. Luckily, many eye problems are more bothersome than serious.

Almost everyone has vision changes with age. Age also increases your risk of developing more-serious eye problems. Some eye problems can't be prevented, but medications or surgery can slow or stop progression. This section covers the more common eye problems and discusses some of the issues related to declining vision.

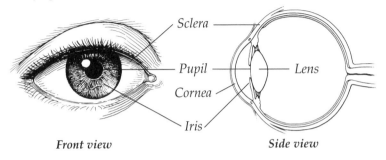

Front view　　　　　*Side view*

■ Black eye

A **black eye** is caused by bleeding beneath the skin around the eye. Sometimes a black eye indicates a more extensive injury, even a skull fracture, particularly if the area around both eyes is bruised or there has been head trauma. Although most injuries aren't serious, bleeding within the eye, called a hyphema, is serious and can reduce vision and damage the cornea. In some cases, glaucoma (see page 80) also can result.

Self-care

- Using gentle pressure, apply ice or a cold pack to the area around the eye for 10 to 15 minutes. Take care not to press on the eye itself. Apply cold as soon as possible after the injury to reduce swelling.
- Look for blood in the white and colored parts of the eye. If blood is present, contact your doctor.

Medical help

Seek medical care immediately if you experience vision problems (double vision, blurring), severe pain, or bleeding in the eye or from the nose.

Taking care of your eyes

- Have your vision checked regularly. How often you need an exam depends on several factors, such as age, health and risk of eye problems.
- Control chronic health conditions such as diabetes and high blood pressure.
- Recognize symptoms. Sudden loss of vision in one eye, sudden hazy or blurred vision, flashes of light or black spots, or halos or rainbows around lights may signal a medical problem.

- Protect your eyes against sun damage. Buy close-fitting sunglasses that block ultraviolet (UV) light.
- Eat foods containing vitamin A and beta carotene, such as carrots, yams and cantaloupe.
- Optimize your vision with the right glasses.
- Use good lighting.
- If your vision is impaired, use low vision aids, such as magnifiers and large-type books.

See back cover for online resource ⓘ

Dry eyes

Dry eyes feel hot, irritated and gritty when you blink. They may become slightly red. Tear production decreases as you age. Usually, both eyes are affected, especially in women after menopause. Some medicines (such as sleeping medications, antihistamines and some drugs for high blood pressure) can cause or worsen dry eyes. Some medical conditions may be associated with dry eyes.

Self-care

- Try over-the-counter artificial tears that don't contain a redness remover (these may worsen symptoms). If you're sensitive to preservatives, try single-use preservative-free lubricants. If your eyes are dry overnight, use a gel-type lubricant at bedtime. Ask your doctor what might work best for you.
- Don't direct hair dryers, car heaters, air conditioners or fans toward your eyes.
- Blink often to help spread your tears more evenly. Avoid rubbing your eyes.
- Wear glasses on windy days and goggles while swimming.
- Consider using a humidifier in winter to add moisture to dry indoor air.

Medical help

Seek medical care if the condition continues despite self-care efforts. Your doctor may prescribe medication for chronic dry eyes or refer you to a specialist if needed.

Excessive watering

Your eyes may actually water in response to dryness and irritation. Watery eyes also commonly occur with infections such as pink eye (see page 78). They can result from an allergic reaction to preservatives in eyedrops or contact lens solutions. Watery eyes can also result from a blockage in the ducts that drain tears to the inside of your nose. Overflowing tears can cause even more eye irritation and tearing.

Self-care

- Apply a warm compress over closed eyelids two to four times a day for 10 minutes.
- Don't rub your eyes.
- Replace mascara at least every three months. It can become contaminated with bacteria transferred by the applicator.
- Follow directions for wearing, cleaning and disinfecting contact lenses.

Floaters

The jellylike substance behind your lens (vitreous) is supported and distributed evenly within your eyeball by a framework of fine fibers (fibrils). As you age, these fibers thicken and gather in bundles, creating the appearance of specks, hairs or strings that move in and out of your vision. Floaters that appear gradually and become less noticeable over time are usually harmless and need no treatment. Floaters that appear suddenly may indicate a more serious eye disorder such as a hemorrhage or retinal detachment. The retina is the light-sensitive layer of tissue at the back of the eye that transmits visual images to the brain.

Medical help

If you see a cloud of spots or a spider web, especially if accompanied by flashes of light, see your eye doctor (ophthalmologist). These symptoms can indicate a retinal tear or retinal detachment, which requires prompt surgery to prevent vision loss.

■ Pink eye

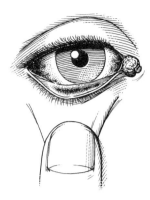

One or both eyes are pink or red in color and itchy. There may be blurred vision and sensitivity to light. You may have a gritty feeling in the eye or a discharge in the eye that forms a crust during the night.

All of these are signs and symptoms of a bacterial or viral infection commonly known as **pink eye**. The medical term is **conjunctivitis**. It's an inflammation of the membrane called the conjunctiva, which lines the inside of the eyelids and part of the eyeball.

The inflammation makes pink eye an irritating condition, but it's usually harmless to sight. However, because it can be contagious, it must be diagnosed and treated early. Occasionally, pink eye can cause eye complications.

Both viral and bacterial conjunctivitis are common among children and also affect adults — both types are very contagious. Viral conjunctivitis usually produces a watery discharge, whereas bacterial conjunctivitis often produces a good deal of thick, yellow-green matter, but sometimes it's difficult to tell the difference.

Allergic conjunctivitis usually affects both eyes and is a response to an allergen (such as pollen) rather than an infection. In addition to intense itching, tearing and inflammation of the eye, you may also experience some degree of itching, sneezing and watery discharge from the nose.

Self-care

- Apply a warm compress to the affected eye or eyes. Soak a clean, lint-free cloth in warm water, squeeze it dry and apply it over your gently closed eyelids.
- Allergic conjunctivitis is often effectively soothed with cool compresses.

Prevention

Because pink eye that's caused by infection spreads easily, good hygiene is the most useful method for control. Once the infection has been diagnosed in you or a family member, these steps may help contain it:

- Keep your hands away from your eyes.
- Wash your hands frequently.
- Change your towel and washcloth daily — don't share them.
- Wear your clothes only once before washing.
- Change your pillowcase each night.
- Discard eye cosmetics, particularly mascara, after three months.
- Don't use other people's contact lens solution, eye cosmetics, handkerchiefs or other personal items.

Medical help

If you have any symptoms of pink eye, see your health care provider. He or she may culture the eye secretions to determine which form of infection you have. A doctor may prescribe antibiotic eyedrops or ointments if the infection is bacterial. Viral conjunctivitis disappears on its own. If your doctor determines that you have allergic conjunctivitis, he or she may recommend medications to treat the allergy or your eye symptoms.

Kids' care

Because pink eye is contagious, keep your child away from other children. Many schools will send children with pink eye home to minimize the spread of infection.

■ Sensitivity to glare

Glare may result when light is scattered within the eyeball. Glare may be especially bothersome in low light when your pupils are enlarged (dilated) because light is allowed into your eyes at a wider angle. **Sensitivity to glare** may mean a developing cataract (see page 80). To evaluate your symptoms, your health care provider may measure your vision under low, medium and high levels of glare.

Self-care

- Reduce daytime glare by wearing polarized sunglasses with opaque side shields and wide frames that follow your brow.
- Have accurate correction for your distance vision to help minimize glare.

■ Other eye problems

Drooping eyelid

Your upper eyelid may droop if the muscles responsible for raising your eyelid weaken. Normal aging, trauma, or disorders of the nerves and muscles can lead to **drooping eyelid**. If your eyelid interferes with vision, your ophthalmologist may recommend surgery to strengthen supporting muscles. **Caution:** A drooping eyelid that develops suddenly needs immediate evaluation and treatment. It may be associated with stroke or other acute problems of your nervous system.

Inflamed eyelid

A chronic inflammation along the edges of your eyelids is called **blepharitis**. It may accompany dry eyes. Some people produce excess oil in glands near their eyelashes. Oil encourages growth of bacteria and causes your skin to be irritated, itchy and red. Tiny scales form along the edges of your eyelids, further irritating your skin. **Self-care:** Apply a warm compress over your gently closed eyelids two to four times a day for 10 minutes. Immediately afterward, wash away the scales with warm water or diluted baby shampoo. If the condition is caused by an infection, your health care provider may prescribe a medicated ointment or an oral antibiotic.

Twitching eyelid

Your eyelid takes on a life of its own — twitching at random, driving you crazy. The involuntary quivering of the eyelid muscle usually lasts less than a minute. The cause is unknown, but some people report that painless **eyelid twitching** is brought on by caffeine use, nervous tension or fatigue. Rarely, it can be a symptom of muscle or nerve disease. A twitching eyelid is usually harmless and needs no treatment. **Self-care:** Gentle massaging of the eyelid may help relieve twitching.

Sty

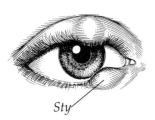

Sty

A **sty** is a red, painful lump on the edge of your eyelid. It's caused by inflammation or infection from a blocked gland in the eyelid. Sties usually fill with pus and then burst in about a week. For persistent infections, your health care provider might prescribe an antibiotic cream. **Self-care:** Apply a clean, warm compress four times a day for 10 minutes to relieve the pain and help the sty come to a point sooner. Let the sty burst on its own, and then rinse your eye thoroughly.

■ Common eye diseases

Cataract

A **cataract** is a clouding of the normally clear lens of your eye. It can develop in one or both eyes. Lens clouding blurs vision. Some degree of cataract formation is normal as you grow older, but some exposures or conditions can accelerate the process. Long-term exposure to ultraviolet (UV) light, diabetes, a previous eye injury, exposure to X-rays and prolonged use of corticosteroid drugs increase your risk. Smoking also may increase your risk of cataracts. If a cataract interferes with your daily activities, your cloudy lens can be surgically removed and replaced with a plastic lens implant. **Self-care:** Reduce glare. Prevent or slow cataracts by wearing UV-blocking sunglasses when outside in bright sun. Ensure adequate lighting.

When a cataract develops, your eye's lens becomes cloudy. The clouding scatters light passing through the lens and prevents a sharply defined image from reaching your retina. The result is blurred vision.

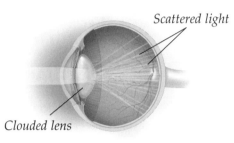

Scattered light

Clouded lens

Glaucoma

Glaucoma involves damage to the eye (optic) nerve caused by intolerance to pressure within the eyeball. Pressure increases when tiny pores that normally allow fluid to drain from inside your eye become blocked. Damage to the optic nerve causes your peripheral vision to diminish slowly. Untreated glaucoma can lead to blindness. **Caution:** Because the early symptoms can be subtle, it's important to have regular eye examinations. If diagnosed and treated early, chronic glaucoma usually can be controlled with eyedrops, oral medications or surgery. If you have symptoms such as a severe headache or pain in your eye or brow, nausea, blurred vision, or rainbows around lights at night, seek immediate evaluation. Treatment may require emergency laser surgery.

Macular degeneration

Macular degeneration (wet and dry) causes blurred central vision or a blind spot in the center of vision. It doesn't affect side vision and usually doesn't lead to total blindness. The condition occurs when tissue in the center of the retina (macula) deteriorates. When diagnosed early, treatment may help reduce or slow the loss of vision, such as injectable therapy, photodynamic therapy or laser treatment for the wet form, and specific vitamins and minerals for the dry form.

Transportation advice for those with impaired vision

- Don't drive if you fail to meet your state's vision requirements for drivers.
- Avoid stressful driving conditions — at night, in heavy traffic, in bad weather or on a freeway.
- Use public transportation or ask family members to help with night driving.
- Contact your local Area Agency on Aging about transportation options, such as shuttles, vans, volunteer drivers or ride-sharing services.
- Optimize your vision with the right glasses. Make sure to have your prescription rechecked on a regular basis.

See back cover for online resource ⓘ

Problems related to glasses and contact lenses

Many people begin to notice a change in their vision around age 40. Close-up objects that were once easy to see become blurred. The print in newspapers and books begins to seem smaller, and you instinctively hold reading material farther away from your eyes. This condition is called **presbyopia**. It refers to the difficulty with near vision that develops as the lenses in your eyes become thicker and more rigid. Another symptom is eyestrain, which may include a feeling of tired eyes and a headache.

If you're already farsighted, you may notice the changes somewhat earlier and will need to have stronger corrective lenses. Even if you're nearsighted, you'll experience the effects of presbyopia, and you may find yourself taking off your glasses to read small print. You may find that your eyes seem increasingly tired after reading.

Before trying over-the-counter reading glasses, first see an eye specialist to rule out other problems.

Medical help

If you experience frequent headaches, see your ophthalmologist or optometrist, who will test your eyes and prescribe appropriate lenses, if needed.

Respond to warnings such as blurring of vision, yellowing of colors, increased sensitivity to light or loss of side vision, which could indicate cataracts or glaucoma.

Contact lenses, laser surgery

<u>Contact lenses</u> are improving, and many people who could not use contact lenses before can now wear them comfortably. In some cases, contacts are preferable to glasses. For example, contact lenses offer markedly improved vision to people who have a malformation of the cornea.

Proper fitting of contact lenses ensures that you'll see as clearly as possible and minimizes the impact of the lenses on the surface of the eyes. If you want contact lenses, have a thorough eye exam and fitting by an experienced professional. Follow-up exams are important to monitor any changes to your vision and to update your prescription.

Laser eye surgery changes the shape of the cornea, so it focuses more precisely. Laser-assisted in-situ keratomileusis (LASIK) eye surgery involves making a thin, circular hinged cut into the cornea. The surgeon then lifts the flap and with a special laser reshapes the cornea. **LASIK eye surgery** is helpful for correcting low to moderate astigmatism in people with nearsightedness. Results aren't as good in people who are farsighted with astigmatism.

Extended-wear and disposable soft contacts

If you use extended-wear contact lenses, remove and sterilize them most nights. If you wear disposable lenses, don't wear them beyond the time recommended by your eye specialist. Wearing contact lenses too long without removing them may deprive your corneas of oxygen. Lack of oxygen can cause blurred vision, pain, tearing, redness and sensitivity to light, and may make the cornea more susceptible to infection. Remove your lenses at once if any of these signs and symptoms occur. Have regular eye exams to avoid problems that may result from extended contact lens wear.

FOR MORE INFORMATION
- National Eye Institute, 301-496-5248, *https://nei.nih.gov*
- Local services for the blind and visually impaired

Common Problems

Headache

Headaches are the most commonly reported medical complaint. They may point to a serious medical problem. But that situation is rare.

Most headaches are not linked to an underlying disease. These so-called primary headaches differ greatly. Researchers are learning more about what happens physically during a headache.

Types of headaches

There are many recognized primary headache disorders. Three well-known types are:

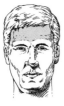

Tension
- Affects men and women nearly equally
- Gradually produces a dull pain, tightness or pressure in neck, forehead or scalp
- Is the most frequent type of headache in the general population

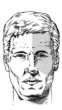

Migraine
- Produces moderate or severe and disabling pain, which is often pulsating
- Affects three times as many women as men
- May begin in childhood or teens — less common after age 40
- May be preceded by a visual change, tingling on one side of face or body, or a specific food craving
- Is often associated with nausea (with or without vomiting) and sensitivity to light and noise

Cluster
- Produces steady, boring pain in and around one eye, occurring in episodes that often begin at the same time of day or night
- Causes eye watering and redness and nasal stuffiness on one side of the face
- May occur like clockwork and be linked to light or seasonal changes
- Frequently affects men, especially heavy smokers and drinkers
- May be misdiagnosed as a sinus infection or dental problem
- Usually lasts about 15 minutes to three hours

Migraine theory

Migraines may be caused by changes in the brainstem and its interactions with the trigeminal nerve. Imbalances in brain chemicals — including serotonin, which helps regulate pain — also may be involved. Serotonin levels drop during migraine attacks. This may cause your trigeminal nerve to release substances called neuropeptides, which travel to your brain's outer covering. The result is migraine pain.

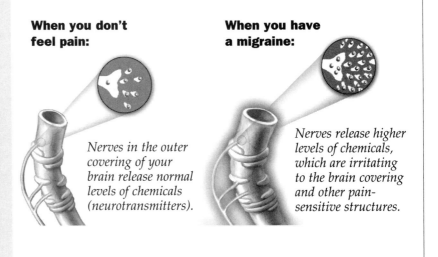

When you don't feel pain:

Nerves in the outer covering of your brain release normal levels of chemicals (neurotransmitters).

When you have a migraine:

Nerves release higher levels of chemicals, which are irritating to the brain covering and other pain-sensitive structures.

See back cover for online resource

Self-care	**For occasional tension headaches**

For occasional tension headaches

First, try massage, hot or cold packs, a warm shower, rest, or relaxation techniques. If these measures don't work, try a low dose of aspirin (adults only), acetaminophen (Tylenol, others) or ibuprofen (Advil, Motrin IB, others). Moderate exercise may help a **tension headache**.

For recurrent headaches

- Keep a headache diary. Include these factors:
  - ▸ *Severity.* Is it disabling pain or merely annoying?
  - ▸ *Frequency and duration.* When does the headache start? Does it begin gradually or strike rapidly? Does it occur at a certain time of day? In monthly or seasonal cycles? How long does it last? What makes it stop?
  - ▸ *Related symptoms.* Can you tell it's coming? Are you nauseated or dizzy? Do you see sparkling colors or blank spots?
  - ▸ *Location.* Is the pain usually on one side of your head? In your neck muscles? Around one eye?
  - ▸ *Family history.* Do other family members have similar headaches?
  - ▸ *Triggers.* Can you link your headache to any particular food, activity, weather, time frame or environmental factors? (See "Avoiding headache triggers," page 84.)
- Avoid triggers, as possible. To do so may require lifestyle changes.
- Get adequate sleep and exercise.

Special migraine self-care

Begin treatment when you feel a **migraine** coming. This approach is your best chance to stop it early. Use acetaminophen, ibuprofen or aspirin (adults only) at the recommended dosage for pain relief. Some people can abort an attack by going to sleep in a darkened room or consuming caffeine (coffee or cola).

Medical help

If self-care doesn't help after one or two days, see your health care provider. He or she will try to determine the type and cause of your headache, will try to exclude other possible sources of pain, and may do tests. Your physician may prescribe one of many pain medications. Different medications are used for different types of headaches.

For severe migraines, your physician may prescribe a medication that mimics serotonin, a nerve chemical in your body. For frequent migraine attacks, your doctor may prescribe a preventive medication to use on a daily basis.

Caution

Don't ignore unexplained headaches. Seek medical attention right away if your headache:

- Strikes suddenly and severely
- Accompanies a fever, stiff neck, rash, mental confusion, seizures, double vision, weakness, numbness or speaking difficulties
- Occurs with physical or sexual activity
- Begins or worsens after a head injury, fall or bump
- Is a new, significant problem or is worsening

Common Problems

Avoiding headache triggers

Does a specific food, drink or activity trigger your headaches? Some people can eliminate headaches by avoiding triggers. Triggers vary among individuals, but here are examples:

- Red wine or other alcohol
- Smoking
- Stress or fatigue
- Eyestrain
- Poor posture
- Changing sleeping patterns or mealtimes

- Certain foods, such as:
  ‣ Fermented, pickled or marinated food
  ‣ Caffeine
  ‣ Aged cheeses
  ‣ Chocolate
  ‣ Bananas
  ‣ Citrus fruits
  ‣ Dried fruits, such as raisins
  ‣ Food additives (sodium nitrite in hot dogs, sausages or luncheon meat, or monosodium glutamate in processed or Chinese foods) and seasonings
  ‣ Nuts or peanut butter
  ‣ Sourdough bread
- Weather, altitude or time zone changes
- Hormonal changes during your menstrual cycle or menopause, oral contraceptive use, or hormone replacement therapy
- Strong or flickering lights
- Odors, including perfumes, flowers or natural gas
- Polluted air or stuffy rooms
- Excessive noise

Kids' care

Recurrent headaches are common during late childhood and adolescence. They rarely represent a serious problem.

Headache is associated with many viral illnesses. However, if your child frequently complains of headaches, even during times when he or she is otherwise well, consult your child's health care provider.

Migraines may occur in children and may be suspected if there's a family history of migraine. In children, this type of headache often is accompanied by vomiting, light sensitivity, fatigue or sleep.

A headache may indicate stress with school, friends or family. It may be a reaction to a medication, particularly a decongestant.

If you think it's a tension headache, try the nonmedicating tips listed on page 83. If it occurs frequently, help your child keep a headache diary. Use acetaminophen (Tylenol, others) or ibuprofen (Advil, Children's Motrin, others) sparingly.

If your child's headache persists, comes on suddenly without explanation or gets steadily worse, call your health care provider. Also call about headaches that worsen and may follow recent ear infections, toothaches, strep throat or other infections. Be sure to tell your health care provider if there's any family history of migraines. That information could help lead to a diagnosis.

The link between caffeine and headaches

That morning caffeine headache can be very real, especially if you consume four or more cups of caffeinated drinks during the day. It may be a withdrawal headache after a night without caffeine.

But for some headaches, caffeine may be a cure. In fact, caffeine is a key active ingredient in many headache medications.

So for adults, if aspirin or acetaminophen (Tylenol, others) doesn't help your headache, try a medicine that includes caffeine, or a caffeinated beverage. But don't overdo. Too much caffeine can cause jitteriness, rapid heart rate, sweating and, yes, withdrawal headaches.

Limbs, muscles, bones and joints

Your body is amazingly intricate. You don't think about your body much when it's working fine. Somehow, everything holds together, and you move about easily. But you usually do notice when there's a problem.

This section focuses on problems related to your limbs. Some conditions are common to many areas of your body, such as strains, sprains, broken bones, bursitis, tendinitis, fibromyalgia and gout. These conditions are addressed on pages 87 through 92. The remainder of the chapter provides additional information about problems related to specific joints: shoulder; elbow and forearm; wrist, hand and finger; hip; leg and knee; and ankle and foot. First, here is some general information.

Anatomy

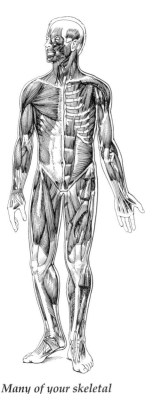

Many of your skeletal muscles are paired, enabling your body to move. Tendons connect these muscles to your bones.

Muscles and tendons

Many of your 650 muscles help you move. Each skeletal muscle is attached to bones by bands called tendons. Pairs of muscles work together to move your joints by pulling on bones. One muscle relaxes as its partner tightens.

If you're active, your muscles enable you to run, walk, swim, jump, climb stairs, bike, dance, mow the lawn or type on a computer. Your muscles let you know when you've overdone it. They become sore and stiff.

Common causes of muscle injuries include accidents, strains, sudden movements, overuse and inflammation. You can avoid many muscle and tendon aches by taking these steps:

- Exercise regularly and moderately. Build up your activity gradually. You're not ready to run a marathon if you're not regularly running more than a few miles. Even yardwork and housecleaning can cause strains if you dive into projects and work beyond a moderate pace.
- Stretch your muscles gently before and after you exercise. For some people it's also helpful to use heat and massage to loosen their muscles before activity.
- Drink plenty of water. Drinking six to eight glasses of water a day maintains good hydration. But you'll need more than that when you're active, especially in the heat of summer.
- Strengthen your muscles with resistance exercise.
- Support previously injured areas with elastic tape or a brace.
- Use appropriate ergonomic principles in the workplace.

Bones — Rigid, but alive

You can't see it, but the 206 bones in your body change constantly. Proteins form the framework. Minerals, especially calcium and phosphate, fill in to give the bones strength. Because of this need for minerals, it's a good idea to consume mineral-rich, low-fat milk and leafy green vegetables.

Common bone conditions include:

- Breaks, resulting from stress on a bone greater than it can withstand
- Bruising, usually from trauma
- Weakening, through loss of minerals (osteopenia and osteoporosis)

A child's bones are more pliable than an adult's. When under strain or pressure, they're less likely to break. As you mature, your bones become more rigid.

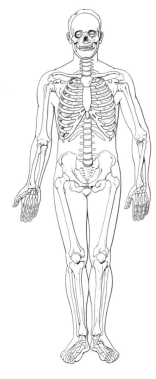

Your bones are living tissue and are always changing.

Joints — Mechanical masterpieces

Your bones come together at your joints. The end of each bone is covered by a layer of cartilage that glides smoothly and acts as a shock absorber. Tough bands of tissue (ligaments) hold your joints together.

Your body has several types of joints. This chapter discusses:

- **Hinge joints** in the ends of your fingers or your knees, for example. They allow one kind of back-and-forth movement (flexion and extension).
- **Ball-and-socket joints** in your shoulder or hip, for example. They allow a wide range of movement in many directions.

Causes of joint pain covered in this chapter include:

- Traumatic injuries or dislocation (when a joint is pushed out of place)
- Bursitis
- Gout
- Sprains

Nerves — Lines of communication

Most of this chapter focuses on bones, muscles and joints. However, all of your limbs are wired with nerves that carry messages to and from your brain. They sense pain and also help you locate its source. They direct your movement. They let you know when your muscles are tired or injured. Nerves may keep a muscle from working properly. They also help you avoid many injuries.

Muscle strains: When you've overdone it

A muscle becomes pulled (strained) — or may even tear — when it stretches unusually far or abruptly. This type of injury can also often occur when muscles suddenly and powerfully contract. A slip on the ice or lifting in an awkward position may cause a muscle strain.

Muscle **strains** vary in severity:

- **Mild.** A mild strain causes pain and stiffness when you move and lasts a few days.
- **Moderate.** A moderate strain causes small muscle tears and more extensive pain, swelling and bruising. The pain may last one to three weeks.
- **Severe.** With a severe strain, muscle becomes torn apart or ruptured. You may have significant internal bleeding, swelling and bruising around the muscle. Your muscle may not function at all. Seek medical attention immediately.

Self-care

- Follow the instructions for R.I.C.E. (see below). The earlier the treatment, the speedier and more complete your recovery.
- For extensive swelling, use cold packs several times each day throughout your recovery.
- Don't apply heat when the area is still swollen.
- Avoid the activity that caused the strain while the muscle heals.
- Use over-the-counter pain medications as needed (see page 258). Avoid using aspirin in the first few hours after the strain because aspirin may make bleeding more extensive.

Medical help

Seek medical help immediately if the area quickly becomes swollen and is intensely painful. Call your health care provider if the pain, swelling and stiffness don't improve in two to three days or if you suspect a ruptured muscle or broken bone.

R.I.C.E.: Your best tool for muscle or joint injury

You'll see R.I.C.E. mentioned often throughout this section. Here's what it means:

- **R: Rest** to promote tissue healing. Avoid activities that cause pain, swelling or discomfort.
- **I: Ice** the area immediately, even if you're seeking medical help. Use an ice pack or slush bath for about 15 minutes each time you apply the ice. Repeat every two to three hours while you're awake for the first 48 to 72 hours. Cold reduces pain, swelling and inflammation in injured muscles, joints and connecting tissues. It may also slow bleeding if a tear has occurred.
- **C: Compress** the area with an elastic bandage until the swelling stops. Don't wrap it tightly or you may hinder circulation. Begin wrapping at the end farthest from your heart. Loosen the wrap if pain increases, if the area becomes numb or if there is swelling below the wrapped area.
- **E: Elevate** the area above your heart, especially at night. Gravity helps reduce swelling by draining excess fluid.

Some additional tips:

- After 48 hours, if the swelling is gone, you may apply warmth or gentle heat. Heat can improve blood flow and speed healing.
- Apply cold to sore areas after a workout, even if you're not injured, to prevent inflammation and swelling.
- Consider taking steps to protect the area from further injury. Use an elastic wrap, sling, splint, cane, crutches or air splint.

Common Problems

■ Sprains: Damage to your ligaments

Strictly speaking, a sprain occurs when you overextend or tear a ligament. Ligaments are the tough, elastic-like bands that attach to your bones and hold your joints in place. However, the term *sprain* is commonly used to describe any instance in which a joint moves outside its normal range of movement.

Sprains frequently are caused by twisting. They occur most often in your ankles, your knees or the arches of your feet. True sprains cause rapid swelling. Generally, the greater the pain, the more severe the injury. Sprains vary in severity:

- **Mild.** Your ligament stretches excessively or tears slightly. The area is somewhat painful, especially with movement. It's tender. There is not a lot of swelling. You can put weight on the joint.
- **Moderate.** Some fibers in your ligament tear, but it doesn't rupture completely. The joint is tender, painful and difficult to move. The area may be swollen and discolored from bleeding.
- **Severe.** One or more ligaments tear completely. The area is painful. You can't move your joint normally or put weight on it. It becomes very swollen and discolored. The injury may be difficult to distinguish from a fracture or dislocation, which requires medical care. You may need a cast to hold the joint motionless, or an operation if torn ligaments cause joint instability.

Self-care

- Follow the instructions for R.I.C.E. (see page 87).
- Use over-the-counter pain medications as recommended (see page 258).
- Gradually test and use the joint after two days. Mild to moderate sprains usually improve significantly in a week, although full healing may take six weeks.
- Avoid activities that stress your joint. Repeated minor sprains will weaken it.

Medical help

Seek medical care immediately if:
- You hear a popping sound when your joint is injured and you can't use it. On the way to your health care provider, apply cold.
- You have a fever and the area is red and hot. You may have an infection.
- You have a severe sprain, as described above. Inadequate or delayed treatment may cause long-term joint instability or chronic pain.

See your doctor if you're unable to bear weight on the joint after two to three days of self-care or if you don't experience much improvement in a week.

Preventing sports injuries

- Select your sport carefully. Don't jog if you have chronic back pain or sore knees.
- Warm up for five to 10 minutes. Begin by doing the activity and movement patterns of your chosen exercise, but at a low, slow pace that gradually increases in speed and intensity.
- After exercising, cool down. Continue your workout session for five minutes or so, but at a slower pace and reduced intensity.
- Begin a new sport gradually. Increase your level of exertion over several weeks.

- Do cross-training. Alternating between a high-impact activity (such as jogging) and a low-impact activity (such as walking or swimming) can help avoid injuries from repetitive stresses.
- Stop the activity immediately if you think you may be injured, you become disoriented or dizzy, or you lose consciousness, even briefly.
- Return gradually to full activity, or switch sports until injuries heal.

■ Broken bones (fractures)

If you suspect a bone is broken, get medical care. A broken bone may or may not poke through your skin. Open fractures break through the skin. Closed fractures do not. Closed fractures are classified according to the way the bone breaks. For example, in a comminuted fracture, the bone is broken into several pieces.

| Open | Closed (simple) | Incomplete | Complete | Displaced | Comminuted (defined above) |

Emergency treatment

After serious injury or trauma, seek medical care immediately if:
- The person is unconscious or can't be moved.
- The person isn't breathing or doesn't have a pulse. Begin CPR (see page 2).
- There's heavy bleeding.
- Even gentle pressure or movement produces pain.
- The limb or joint appears deformed, or the bone has pierced the skin.
- The part farthest from the heart is numb or bluish at the tip.

Self-care

Take these precautions and seek medical care:
- Protect the area from further damage.
- If there's bleeding, try to stop it. Press directly on the wound with a sterile bandage, clean cloth or piece of clothing. If nothing else is available, use your hand. Keep pressing until the bleeding stops.
- Use a splint or sling to hold the area still. You can make a splint from wood, plastic or rolled newspaper. Place it on both sides of the bone, extending beyond the ends of the bone. Hold it firmly in place with gauze, cloth strips, tape or string, but not tight enough to stop the blood flow.
- Don't try to set the bone yourself.
- If ice is available, wrap the ice in cloth and apply it to the splinted limb.
- Try to elevate the injured area above the heart to reduce bleeding and swelling.
- If the person becomes faint or takes short breaths, he or she may be in shock. Lay the person down with the head slightly lower than the rest of the body.

Kids' care

The bones in your child's arms and legs have growth plates near the ends that allow bones to lengthen with growth. If growth plates become damaged, the bone may not grow properly. Check out any possible fractures with your health care provider.

Bursitis

Bursae

You have more than 150 bursae in your body. These tiny, fluid-filled sacs lubricate and cushion pressure points for your bones, tendons and muscles near your joints. They help you move without pain. When they become inflamed, movement or pressure is painful. This condition is called **bursitis**. Bursitis is commonly caused by overuse, trauma, repeated bumping or prolonged pressure such as kneeling for an extended period. It may even result from an infection, arthritis or gout. Most often, bursitis affects the shoulder, elbow or hip joint. But you can also have bursitis at your knee, heel and even in the base of your big toe.

Self-care

- Use over-the-counter pain medications (see page 258).
- Keep pressure off the joint. Use an elastic bandage, sling or soft foam pad to protect it until the swelling goes down.
- Apply ice for 10 to 15 minutes or until the area feels numb.
- Simple bursitis usually disappears within two weeks. Ease the area back into activity slowly.

Prevention

- Strengthen your muscles to help protect the joint. Don't start exercising a joint that has bursitis until the pain and inflammation are gone.
- Take frequent breaks from repetitive tasks. Alternate repetitive tasks with rest or other activities. Follow ergonomic principles for desk work and lifting.
- Cushion the joint before applying pressure (such as with knee or elbow pads). For bursitis in a hip, cushion a hard mattress with a foam pad or soft mattress cover.

Medical help

Seek medical care if the area becomes red and hot or doesn't improve or if you also have a fever or rash.

Tendinitis

Tendinitis produces pain and tenderness near a joint. You can usually associate it with a specific movement (grasping, for example). It usually means you have an inflammation or a small tear of the tendon. Tendinitis is usually the result of overuse or a minor injury. It's most common around the shoulders, elbows and knees.

Pain may cause you to limit movement. Rest is important, but so is maintaining a full range of movement. If you don't treat tendinitis carefully, tendons and ligaments around your joint may gradually stiffen over several weeks. Movement may become limited and difficult.

Self-care

- Follow the instructions for R.I.C.E. (see page 87).
- Gently move the joint through its full range four times a day. Otherwise rest it. A sling, elastic bandage or splint may help.
- Use an anti-inflammatory medication (see page 258).
- If soreness doesn't greatly improve in two weeks, see your health care provider.

Prevention

- Use warm-up and cool-down exercises and strengthening exercises.
- Apply heat to the area before you exercise, and apply cold afterward.
- Exercise on alternate days when starting an exercise program.

Medical help	Seek medical help immediately if you have a fever and the area is inflamed.
	Sometimes doctors inject a drug into tissue around a tendon to relieve tendinitis. Cortisone injections reduce inflammation and can give rapid relief of pain. These injections must be used with care because repeated injections may weaken the tendon or cause undesirable side effects. Other emerging treatments are available.

Fibromyalgia

Fibromyalgia is a chronic condition characterized by widespread pain in muscles, ligaments, tendons and surrounding soft tissue, as well as fatigue, sleep, memory and mood issues. The type of pain can vary but is often described as a constant dull ache. To be considered widespread, the pain must occur on both sides of your body and above and below your waist.

Women are much more likely to develop the disorder than are men. You may be more likely to develop fibromyalgia if a relative also has the condition.

Symptoms often include:

- Widespread aching, lasting more than three months
- Fatigue and nonrestful, nonrestorative sleep
- Cognitive difficulties, including the ability to focus, pay attention and concentrate on mental tasks
- Associated problems such as headaches (see page 82), irritable bowel syndrome (see page 65) and pelvic pain

Although people with fibromyalgia feel pain in their muscles, this is not a disease of the muscles. The science of fibromyalgia is still emerging, but this may eventually be found to be a disorder of sensory processing in the nervous system. Medications used for this condition affect chemical receptors in the brain and spinal cord — they don't treat your muscles.

Depressive feelings often accompany fibromyalgia and often require specific treatment. Similarly, stress usually worsens the symptoms of fibromyalgia.

Self-care

- Pace yourself. Reduce your stress and avoid long hours of repetitive activity. Develop a routine that alternates work with rest.
- Develop a regular, low-impact exercise program such as walking, biking, swimming and plenty of stretching exercises. Improve your posture by strengthening supportive muscles (see page 55).
- Improve your sleep naturally with daily physical activity. To avoid undesirable side effects, use sleep medications sparingly, if at all. (See "Self-care," page 44.)
- Find a support group that emphasizes maintaining health.
- Learn relaxation techniques. Try massage and warm baths. Yoga and tai chi have also been found helpful in controlling fibromyalgia symptoms.
- Ask your family and friends for support.

Medical help

A fibromyalgia diagnosis can be made if you've had widespread pain for more than three months — with no underlying medical condition that could cause the pain. Your doctor may prescribe medications to help reduce the pain of fibromyalgia and improve sleep, as well as specific exercises. If you think you have excessive stress or depression from trying to cope with fibromyalgia, discuss this with your doctor or mental health provider. (See "Depression," pages 200-202.)

Common Problems

■ Gout

Gout is a form of arthritis that occurs when crystals of uric acid collect in a joint. It produces a sudden pain in a single joint, usually at the base of your big toe, although it may also affect joints in your feet, ankles, knees, hands and wrists. The joint becomes tender, swollen and red. Risk factors include obesity, high blood pressure, taking blood pressure medications that cause water loss and family history.

Self-care
- Maintain a healthy weight, drink plenty of water, and limit or avoid alcohol.
- Limit or avoid organ meats (liver, brain, kidney, sweetbreads), red meats and seafood — high-protein foods that increase uric acid.
- Limit or avoid products containing high-fructose corn syrup.

Medical help
Seek medical care immediately if you have a fever and your joint is hot and inflamed. (See "Gout" on page 162.)

■ Shoulder pain

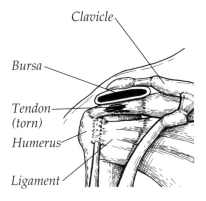

Clavicle

Bursa

Tendon (torn)

Humerus

Ligament

Treatment of shoulder pain depends on its cause. Bursitis and tendinitis are common causes of **shoulder pain** (see page 90), as are acute injury and rotator cuff tears (see page 93). Take note of how the pain began and what makes the pain worse. This can be helpful if you need medical care.

Most shoulder pain isn't life-threatening. But occasionally it may signal a heart attack. Call 911 or your local emergency number right away if your pain:
- Starts as chest pain or pressure. The pain may occur suddenly or gradually. It may radiate to your shoulder, back, arms, jaw and neck.
- Is accompanied by excessive sweating, shortness of breath, faintness, or nausea and vomiting.
- Is new and you have a known heart condition.

■ Acute shoulder pain

Acute shoulder pain centers on your upper arm and may extend to your upper back or neck. Pain may suddenly limit arm movement. Possible causes include overuse or trauma. Your shoulder may become inflamed. It may be very painful to put on a coat, extend your arm straight out from your side or reach behind you.

Self-care
- Use over-the-counter pain medications (see page 258).
- If the bone isn't broken or dislocated, it's important to move the joint through its full range four times a day to avoid stiffening or a condition called frozen shoulder.
- Once pain has resolved, exercise your arm daily.

Medical help
Seek medical care if:
- Your shoulders appear uneven or you can't raise the affected arm
- An injury causes you to wonder if a bone is broken
- You have redness, swelling or fever
- Your shoulder isn't improving after a week of self-care

See back cover for online resource ⓘ

Rotator cuff disorder

The rotator cuff is formed by the attachment of several tendons to the shoulder. Because of the shoulder's complexity, many problems are simply diagnosed as rotator cuff disorder. The tendons in your shoulder may have tiny tears, be irritated or pinched between your bones (impingement). Pain may be more severe at night. This type of disorder usually results from repetitive overhead motions, such as painting a ceiling, swimming or throwing a baseball, or from trauma, such as falling on your shoulder. In older adults, a **rotator cuff disorder** may simply stem from degeneration of the shoulder tendons from a lifetime of use.

Self-care

- Follow the instructions for R.I.C.E. (see page 87).
- Use over-the-counter pain medications (see page 258).
- Do stretching exercises and put the shoulder through its full range of motion four times daily.
- Wait until the pain is gone before gradually returning to the activity that caused the injury. You may have to wait three to six weeks.
- Alter your technique in racket sports, pitching, golf or weight training.

Medical help

Seek medical care if the area is hot and inflamed and you have a fever, if your shoulders are uneven, or if you can't move your arm at all.

If the pain hasn't diminished in one week despite the use of self-care measures, see your doctor.

Elbow and forearm pain

Bursitis and tendinitis are common sources of pain in your elbow (see page 90). Bursitis may produce a small, egg-shaped, fluid-filled sac at the tip of your elbow. Keep pressure off the elbow, for example, by using a soft foam elbow pad.

If the pain hasn't improved after a few days of treatment and the area is still very sensitive to pressure, or if it becomes red or increasingly painful, seek immediate medical care.

A **dislocated elbow**, sometimes known as nursemaid's elbow, may occur in a child if an adult suddenly pulls or jerks the child's arm. The elbow of a child — especially if younger than 6 years — cannot withstand this stress. **Dislocation** is very painful and limits movement. Seek medical treatment immediately. Your doctor will return the bones to their proper position, which usually relieves the pain. An X-ray can rule out other problems.

A **hyperextended elbow** occurs when your elbow is pushed beyond its normal range of motion, often as a result of a fall or misplay during a tennis swing. Pain and swelling occur in your elbow and in the tissues beneath your elbow. Try R.I.C.E. (see page 87) and support your elbow with a splint or sling until the pain stops. If the pain hasn't improved in a day or two, see your health care provider.

Medical help

Seek medical care immediately if:
- Your elbow seems deformed
- Your elbow is very stiff and has limited range of motion after a fall
- The pain in your arm is severe

■ Tennis elbow or golfer's elbow

The recurrent pain from **tennis elbow** or **golfer's elbow** is actually a form of tendinitis (epicondylitis). These two conditions are similar, but tennis elbow affects the outside of your elbow and golfer's elbow affects the inside. Pain may extend into your forearm and wrist. It may result from repeated tiny tears (microtears) in tendons that attach muscles of your lower arm to your elbow, or by inflammation of tissues due to overuse.

Common causes of tennis elbow or golfer's elbow include swinging a racket or club, pitching a baseball, painting, using a screwdriver or hammer, raking, weaving, typing, or any movement requiring twisting arm motions or repetitive gripping.

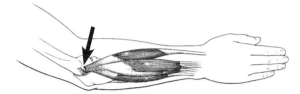

Tennis elbow produces pain on the outside of your forearm near your elbow when you exercise the joint. Tiny tears or inflammation (see arrow) causes the discomfort.

Self-care

- Follow the instructions for R.I.C.E. (see page 87).
- Take an anti-inflammatory medication (see page 258).
- It may take six to 12 weeks of treatment for the pain to disappear.

Prevention
- Use proper technique. Have a sports trainer review your technique to see if you're using the proper motion and properly sized equipment.
- Prepare for repetitive work-related tasks by participating in fitness and strengthening routines.
- Prepare for any sport season with appropriate preseason conditioning. Do strengthening exercises with a hand weight by flexing and extending the wrists.
- Wear a forearm support band just below your elbow.
- Warm up properly. Gently stretch the forearm muscles before and after use.
- Try applying a warm pack for five minutes before activity and an ice pack after heavy use.
- When lifting anything — including free weights — keep your wrist rigid and stable to reduce the force transmitted to your elbow.

Medical help

Seek medical care immediately if:
- Your elbow is hot and inflamed and you have a fever
- You can't bend your elbow at all or it looks deformed
- A fall or injury causes you to wonder if a bone is broken or a tendon is torn
  If the pain doesn't improve in a week or so, see your doctor to rule out other complications.

See back cover for online resource (i)

■ Wrist, hand and finger pain

Think of all the things you do each day with your wrists, hands and fingers. You may not consider the many nerves, blood vessels, muscles and small bones that work together as you turn a key in the door — until the movement becomes painful.

Pain and swelling in your wrists, hands and fingers can result from injury or overuse. They can begin gradually or rapidly. They may be due to:

- A strain or sprain (see pages 87 and 88)
- Fracture, bursitis, tendinitis or gout (see pages 89, 90 and 92)
- Fibromyalgia or arthritis (see pages 91 and 161).

Self-care

- Follow the instructions for R.I.C.E. (see page 87).
- Use over-the-counter pain medications (see page 258).
- If an initial X-ray doesn't show a fracture but the area is still quite painful a week later, ask your health care provider to check again. Some fractures may require special X-ray views or be invisible in the first few days.
- If pain continues, you may need more tests, a splint or cast, or physical therapy.

Prevention

- Use tools with large handles so that you don't have to grip them as hard.
- Remove your rings before manual labor. If you injure your hand, remove your rings before your fingers become swollen.
- Take frequent breaks to rest muscles you've used steadily. Vary your activities.
- Use flexibility and strengthening exercises.

Medical help

Seek medical care immediately if:

- You suspect a fracture
- A fall or accident has caused rapid swelling and moving the area is painful
- The area is hot and inflamed and you have a fever
- Your fingers suddenly become blue or white and numb

■ Other problems

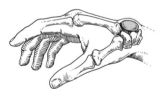

A ganglion cyst is a swelling beneath the skin. It's a fluid-filled lump lined with tissue bulging from a joint or tendon sheath.

<u>Ganglion cysts</u> are fluid-filled lumps that usually appear on the top of the wrist, but also may occur on the underside of the wrist, in the palm or over finger joints. They're filled with jellylike material leaking from a joint or tendon sheath, although they feel firm or solid. Ganglion cysts are sometimes painful and, if bothersome, may require treatment. Seek medical care immediately if the lump becomes painful and inflamed or if the cyst breaks through the skin and drains (usually at the end of the fingers).

A **jammed finger** commonly occurs during sports activities. Pain may be caused by stretched ligaments (sprain) or a fracture involving the joint surface. Follow the R.I.C.E. guidelines on page 87. To protect it during use, "buddy tape" the injured finger to an adjacent finger. Seek medical care immediately if:

- Your finger appears deformed
- You cannot straighten your finger
- The area becomes hot and inflamed and you have a fever
- Swelling and pain are significant or persistent
- The finger becomes numb or white or pale (less pink)

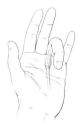

Trigger finger is a condition that causes the finger to lock or catch in a bent position. It'll straighten with a sudden "snap," but if it's severe, the finger may not fully straighten. The condition is more evident in the morning and after firmly grasping an object. The condition is caused by a binding knot in the palm that prevents smooth tendon motion. Change your habits to avoid overuse. Seek medical care immediately if your finger is hot and inflamed or you have a fever.

Carpal tunnel syndrome

A narrow tunnel through your wrist (carpal tunnel) protects your median nerve, which provides sensation to your fingers. When swelling occurs in the carpal tunnel, the median nerve can become compressed, causing numbness and pain.

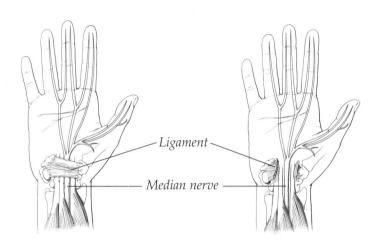

Ligament

Median nerve

The **carpal tunnel** is a passageway between your wrist and hand that protects nerves and tendons. When the tissues in the carpal tunnel become swollen or inflamed, they put pressure on a nerve that affects the sensation of your thumb and index, middle and ring fingers. Too much pressure may cause **carpal tunnel syndrome**. If left untreated, nerve and muscle damage can occur.

Risk factors for carpal tunnel syndrome include occupations, activities and hobbies that involve awkward wrist positions, pressure on the palm of the hand, and repetitive lifting or grasping actions. Pregnancy, obesity and conditions such as diabetes, thyroid disease and arthritis also are risk factors. Signs and symptoms include:

- Tingling or numbness in your thumb and index and middle fingers (but not your little finger). This sensation may occur at night, waking you up. It may also occur while you're driving or holding something, such as the phone or a newspaper.
- Pain radiating or extending from your wrist up your arm to your shoulder or down into your palm or fingers, especially after forceful or repetitive use.
- A sense of weakness in your hands and a tendency to drop objects.

Self-care

- **Take a five-minute break every hour.** Gently stretch your wrists and hands.
- **Vary your activities.** Alternate tasks when possible.
- **Watch your form.** Avoid bending your wrist all the way up or down.
- **Relax your grip.** Avoid using a hard grip when driving your car, bicycling or writing. Oversized grips on pens, pencils and tools may allow a softer grasp.
- **Use a wrist splint at night.** A wrist splint may help ease pain or numbness in your wrists and hands. The splint should be snug but not tight.
- **Consider using nonsteroidal anti-inflammatory drugs (NSAIDs).** For example, try ibuprofen or naproxen to temporarily relieve symptoms (see page 258).

See back cover for online resource ⓘ

| **Medical help** | If the symptoms continue for more than a couple of weeks, see your doctor. Splints, therapy, injection or prescription medications may be recommended. Occasionally, surgery is necessary. |

◼ Thumb pain

Pain at the base of your thumb may be the first sign of osteoarthritis in your hands (see page 161), **thumb arthritis** or tendinitis of the thumb (**de Quervain's tenosynovitis**). With any of these conditions, you may notice pain and swelling at the base of your thumb when you write, open jars, turn your key in the door or ignition, or try to hold small objects. With osteoarthritis of the hands, the pain may be limited to one joint or extend to many. It's more common in women than in men. Arthritis pain can be the result of a previous injury, repetitive activity or heredity. A common cause of de Quervain's tenosynovitis is chronic overuse of your wrist.

Self-care

- Modify behaviors and avoid activities that cause pain.
- Rest your thumb. Use a splint to stabilize the wrist and thumb. Remove the splint at least four times a day to move and stretch the joints to maintain flexibility.
- Use over-the-counter pain medications (see page 258).
- Exercise your thumb daily while your hands are warm. Move your thumb in wide circles. Bend it to touch each of the other fingers on your hand.
- Use tools specially designed for people with arthritis.

Medical help

Seek medical care immediately if pain limits activities or is too severe to tolerate most days. Cortisone injections, arthritis medicine and, occasionally, an operation are effective in alleviating pain.

◼ Hip pain

Hip pain frequently follows a fall or accident. It may also occur after vigorous speed walking or aerobics. Common causes include bursitis, tendinitis and osteoarthritis (see pages 90 and 161), or strains and sprains (see pages 87 and 88). Pain may extend to the groin or thigh, depending on the cause. Only rarely is hip pain caused by having one leg shorter than the other, since differences in leg length of up to ½ inch (1 centimeter) are common and normal.

Self-care

- Follow the instructions for R.I.C.E. (see page 87).
- Avoid activities that aggravate the pain.
- Use over-the-counter pain medications (see page 258).
- Strengthen the hip-group muscles (especially the hip abductors, which move the leg out from the body) to relieve pain and improve function in an arthritic hip.

Medical help

Seek medical care immediately if:
- You have fallen or had an accident and wonder if your hip may be broken
- You have followed the self-care instructions above after an accident or fall and your hip is more painful the following day
- You have osteoporosis and have injured your hip in a fall

Common Problems

▊ Leg pain

Leg pain and other leg problems can result from a combination of overuse, deconditioning (poor strength and flexibility), being overweight, trauma and poor circulation. Lifestyle changes may improve your legs' comfort. In some cases, the pain may radiate from the spine.

Use the following exercises to strengthen your muscles and avoid injuries:

- **Walk.** Begin with short strides. Lengthen your stride as your muscles loosen.
- **Bike.** Gradually increase your distance and speed over weeks.
- **Swim.** Stretch and tone your muscles.
- **Work paired muscles equally.** For example, be sure to exercise the muscles on the front of the thigh (quadriceps) equally with the muscles on the back of the thigh (hamstrings).

▊ Pulled hamstring muscle

Athletes often bruise or strain hamstring muscles, especially during sports such as soccer or track and field activities. You may suspect a **pulled hamstring** if you experience pain in the back of your thigh after a slip or rigorous activity.

Self-care

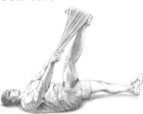

- Follow the instructions for R.I.C.E. (see page 87). If symptoms don't begin to improve after a week of R.I.C.E. treatment, see your health care provider.

Prevention

To avoid hamstring injury, try this exercise called the lying hamstring stretch:

- Lie on your back with a towel around your foot. Raise your leg and pull on the towel to keep your knee as straight as possible. Your trunk stays relaxed. Hold for 30 seconds. Repeat two to four times, reversing leg positions. Don't lock your knee.

▊ Pain, cramps and charley horses

A cramp, sometimes called a charley horse, is actually a muscle spasm. Cramps commonly occur in an athlete who's overfatigued and dehydrated during sports, especially in warm weather. However, almost everyone experiences a **muscle cramp** at some time. For most people, cramps are only an occasional inconvenience.

Self-care

- Gently stretch and massage a cramping muscle.
- For lower leg (calf) cramps, put your weight on the leg and bend your knee slightly, or do the calf stretch illustrated on page 106.
- For upper leg (hamstring) cramps, straighten your legs and lean forward at your waist. Steady yourself with a chair. Or do the hamstring stretch described above.
- Apply heat to relax tense, tight muscles.
- Apply cold to sore or tender muscles.
- Drink plenty of water. Fluid helps your muscles function normally.
- If you have troublesome leg cramps, ask your health care provider about possible medication options.

Self-care

Prevention

Stretch your leg muscles daily, using the following stretch for the Achilles tendon and calf (see the illustration on page 106):

- Stand an arm's length from a wall. Lean forward, resting your hands and forearms on the wall.
- Bend one leg at the knee and bring it toward the wall. Keep the other leg stiff. Keep both heels on the floor. Keep your back straight and move your hips toward the wall. Hold for 30 seconds.
- Repeat with the other leg. Repeat five times with each leg.
- Stretch your muscles carefully and warm up before exercising vigorously.
- Stop exercising if a cramp begins.

Shin splints

When pain occurs on the front, inside portion of the large bone of your lower leg (tibia), it may be the result of shin splints. Shin splints occur when tiny fibers of the membrane that attaches muscle to the tibia become irritated and inflamed, producing pain and sometimes swelling. Shin splints commonly occur in runners, basketball and tennis players, and army recruits.

Self-care

- Follow the instructions for R.I.C.E. (see page 87).
- Apply ice massage to the painful area.
- Try over-the-counter pain relievers (see page 258).
- Wait until the pain leaves before resuming the activity that caused it. The pain may last several weeks or even months. Meanwhile, bike or swim to maintain flexibility and strength.

Prevention

- Use stretching exercises before running to loosen the muscles in your legs and feet. Tap your foot up and down and side to side.
- A soft shoe insert may help cushion your leg.
- You may need a specially made insert (orthotic) to wear in your shoes, especially if you have flatfeet.
- A trainer can help evaluate and adjust your running style.

Medical help

Seek medical care immediately if:

- Pain in your shin follows a fall or accident and is severe
- Your shin is hot and inflamed
- You have pain in your shin at rest, at night or with walking

Special X-rays may be used to look for a stress fracture.

Swollen legs

Occasional leg swelling is a common problem and has many causes, including being overweight, sitting or standing for a long time, retaining fluids (common in women who are pregnant or menstruating), having varicose veins, having an allergic reaction, and getting too much sun exposure.

Serious and ongoing swelling can be caused by these conditions:

- **Blood clot and inflammation in a vein (phlebitis).** Phlebitis usually occurs in the lower portion of a leg. It may affect both superficial and deep veins. The leg becomes sore, red and swollen. It often follows a period of inactivity, such as a long car or plane ride or after an operation. Phlebitis that occurs in a deep vein (**deep vein thrombosis**) is a serious medical condition. See your doctor immediately.
- **Poor circulation (claudication).** A cramping pain occurs at about the same point each time you walk. It goes away when you stop and rest. It's caused by a narrowed or blocked area in your leg arteries. See your doctor.
- **Venous insufficiency.** With this condition, your legs have problems sending blood from your legs back to your heart. This is common in people who are older and overweight. See your doctor about compression stockings and other treatment.
- **Lymphedema. Lymphedema** is swelling that occurs when a blockage in your lymphatic system prevents the lymph fluid in your arm or leg from draining adequately. See your doctor about compression stockings and other treatment.
- **Heart failure.** If your heart can't keep up with the demands on it, you may retain fluid in your legs. This condition affects both legs at the same time and isn't painful, but **heart failure** is a serious condition (see page 179). See your doctor.
- **Liver or kidney disease.** These are both serious conditions. See your doctor.

Self-care

For occasional swelling
- Lose weight and limit salt intake.
- Elevate your legs to a level above your heart for 15 to 20 minutes every few hours to let gravity help move fluid toward your heart.
- For prolonged sitting and travel, walk around frequently and stretch your legs.
- Consider using compression stockings, especially when you're on your feet for long periods of time and while traveling on an airplane.

For conditions that cause swelling
Although you can't treat these conditions yourself, you can lower your risk if you:
- Stop smoking
- Control blood pressure
- Exercise moderately and regularly
- Achieve a healthy weight

Medical help

Seek medical care immediately if you have unexplained, painful swelling in your legs or if a swollen leg becomes warm, red and inflamed.

◼ Knee pain

Knee injuries are often complex. A knee bears a lot of weight and isn't designed to handle sideways stress. Many knee injuries are sports related or result from trauma. Sometimes pain is simply a matter of wear and tear. You can't always tell how severe a knee injury is by the extent of pain, swelling or both, but swelling is typically a sign of a more severe injury. It's important that your knee can bear weight, feels stable and has its full range of motion. **Knee pain** can be due to:

- **Strains and sprains.** These may occur from sudden twists or blows to your knee. A sprain will be on the opposite side of your knee from the side that took the blow. It may take days for swelling to develop fully (see pages 87 and 88).

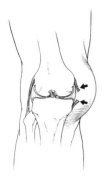

Arrows point to a torn ligament, a common form of knee injury. Swelling occurs, and the joint becomes unstable.

- **Tendinitis.** Pain may occur as a result of intense bicycling or stair climbing. Runner's knee is a form of tendinitis. This overuse injury produces pain at the front of your knee. Your tendons become inflamed, and it hurts to move your knee (see page 90).
- **Fibromyalgia.** Knee pain is a common symptom of fibromyalgia (see page 91).
- **Bursitis.** Inflamed bursae can occur near the knee (see page 90).
- **Osteoarthritis.** Arthritis often causes pain when you move or put weight on your knees (see page 161).
- **Torn cartilage or ligaments.** Tears may be caused by twisting or impact. Torn cartilage is a common injury for athletes and adults. Torn ligaments are common in skiers and basketball players, but they're not common in older adults.
- **Loose pieces of cartilage.** The pieces may become pinched in your knee joint. This is painful and can cause the joint to lock.
- **A tender, bulging cyst behind your knee.** A popliteal, or **Baker's cyst**, often indicates arthritis in your knee joint. It hurts to bend, squat or kneel.

Self-care

- Follow the instructions for R.I.C.E. (see page 87).
- Take an anti-inflammatory medication (see page 258) for a short duration. Remember that you may not feel injury-alerting pain after you take pain medication.
- Flex and straighten your leg gently every day. If it's difficult to move your knee, have someone help you at first. Try to straighten it and keep it straight.
- If you use a cane, use it on the side that's not injured to take weight off your bad knee or leg.
- Avoid strenuous activity until your knee heals. Start nonimpact exercises slowly.
- Avoid squatting, kneeling, or walking up and down hills.

Prevention

- Exercise regularly to strengthen your knee muscles. Bend your knee only to a 90-degree angle during exercise. Don't do deep knee bends.

Medical help

Seek medical care immediately if:
- The injury produces intense, immediate pain, and the knee doesn't function properly.
- Your knee is very painful, even when you're not putting weight on it.
- Pain follows an injury with a popping sound or snapping or locking feeling. Torn knee ligaments may require surgery.
- Your knee locks in one position, or your kneecap is visibly deformed (dislocated).
- Your knee seems unusually loose or unstable.
- You have rapid, unexplained swelling or a fever.

If the pain isn't improving after one week of home treatment, see your doctor.

Knee supports and braces

If your knees are unstable, try a brace or support bandage such as:
- **A rubbery, neoprene sleeve.** This slips over your knee and has a hole over your kneecap.
- **An inexpensive, nonprescription knee brace.** This may be hinged on the outer side or on both sides of your knee.

Caution: These devices appear to offer more support than they actually do. Although they don't protect your knee from injury, they may make it feel warm and secure. Use braces or supports under the direction of your doctor or therapist. Avoid tight braces that cause swelling. Don't wear a brace to bed unless it's recommended by your doctor.

■ Ankle and foot pain

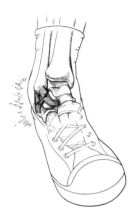

An ankle sprain occurs when ligaments that support your ankle are stretched or torn.

The ankle is one of the most commonly injured joints. The ankle, where three bones meet, allows a wide-ranging foot movement and bears your full body weight. Common causes of foot or ankle pain include the following:

- **Strains and sprains** (see pages 87 and 88).
- **Fractures** (see page 89). Repetitive or high-impact activities such as running, basketball or aerobics can cause stress fractures. Stress fractures are really hairline cracks. They're often invisible on an X-ray for 10 to 21 days after the injury.
- **Bursitis and tendinitis** (see page 90).
- **Achilles tendinitis.** This condition occurs when the tendon that links your calf muscles to the bone at the back of your heel becomes inflamed. The tiny tears in the tendon may follow strenuous exercise. You'll feel a dull ache or pain, especially when you run or jump. The tendon may also be mildly swollen or tender.
- **Bunion.** Ill-fitting footwear or hereditary factors are often the cause of this condition. Your big toe bends toward the next toe, sometimes causing overlapping or underlapping of these toes. The base of your big toe extends beyond your foot's normal profile. That bump is called a bunion. Shoe pressure over a bunion can be painful and lead to callus formation. Arthritis of the big toe joint can develop as a result of a bunion deformity.

Self-care

- Follow the instructions for R.I.C.E. (see page 87).
- Walking on an unstable joint may increase the damage, unless you stabilize it with an ankle brace, air splint or high, laced boots.

If you suspect a fracture, see your health care provider. If you have a **stress fracture:**
- Allow at least one month for healing. A cast or walking boot may be necessary, based on the location of the stress fracture.
- Avoid high-impact activities for anywhere from six weeks to several months, based on stress fracture location and advice from your health care provider.

If you have **Achilles tendinitis:**
- Wear soft-soled running shoes, and avoid running or walking up or down hills.
- Avoid any impact on your heel for several days.
- Use gentle calf stretches daily (see pages 99 and 106).

If you have **bunions:**
- Wear shoes with adequate toe width and soft leather.
- Have your shoes stretched in the area of the bunion.
- Wear sandals or lightweight shoes in the summer.

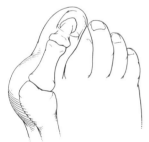

The bump of a bunion is caused when the base of the big toe extends beyond the foot's normal profile.

Prevention

- Choose well-fitting, good-quality footwear. Shoes with a wider toe box will reduce pressure on your toes. Avoid tight, thin-soled, high-heeled shoes.
- Stretch your Achilles tendon. Before exercise, follow the calf stretches outlined on pages 99 and 106.

Medical help	Seek medical care immediately if:

Medical help

Seek medical care immediately if:
- Your foot pain is severe and the area is swollen after an accident or injury
- Your foot is hot and inflamed or you have a fever
- Your foot or ankle is deformed or bent in an abnormal position
- The pain is so severe that you can't move your foot
- You can't bear weight 72 hours after any injury

◼ Flatfeet

A flat foot is normal in infants and toddlers. By the time children become teens, most have developed arched feet. Arches go both from side to side and lengthwise and help distribute weight evenly across the foot.

Some people never develop arches. Others become flat-footed after they put many miles on their feet. But that isn't necessarily a problem.

Flatfeet can be a problem when the condition:
- Places pressure on your foot's nerves and blood vessels
- Causes imbalance and joint problems in the ankles, knees, hips or lower back

Self-care
- Try arch supports. When placed in well-fitting shoes, they may give you a better weight-bearing position.
- See your health care provider if your feet are continuously painful.

Kids' care

Baby fat may make your infant's feet look flat. At about age 5 years, your child may begin to develop an arch. One in 7 children never develops well-formed arches.

There are two kinds of flatfeet:
- **Flexible flatfoot**, in which the feet look flat only when your child stands up. Arches reappear if your child stands on tiptoe or takes weight off the foot. Flexible flatfoot is painless and tends to run in families. There's usually no need to treat it. However, some health care providers recommend arch supports in firm shoes for increased comfort.
- **Fixed flatfoot**, which can be more difficult. If your child's feet are painful, stiff or extremely flat, special footwear or an operation may help.

Flatfeet occurs when little or no arch develops. Above at left (top and bottom) is a normal foot and footprint for a child age 5 or older. If your child's foot and footprint more nearly resemble the illustrations at right, then he or she may have flatfeet.

■ Burning feet

This condition involves mild or severe burning or stinging. It may be constant or temporary. See a doctor if symptoms persist. This condition is most common in people older than age 65. The cause can be difficult to pinpoint and may include the following:
- Irritating fabrics
- Poorly fitting shoes
- A fungal infection such as athlete's foot (see page 122)
- Exposure to a toxic substance such as poison ivy

Suspect a nerve or blood vessel disorder if you have:
- Burning with prickling, tingling, weakness, or a change of sensation or coordination in your legs; burning or tingling that's worse when at rest or in bed
- Burning with nausea, diarrhea, loss of urine or bowel control, or impotence
- Other family members with the problem
- A persistent condition
- Diabetes

Self-care
- Wear nonirritating cotton or cotton-synthetic blend socks and shoes of natural materials that breathe. A specially fitted insole also may help.
- Eliminate aggravating activities, such as standing for long periods.
- Bathe your feet in cool water.
- Use over-the-counter pain medications (see page 258).

■ Hammertoe and mallet toe

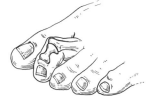

Unlike a bunion, which affects the big toe, **hammertoe** may occur in any toe (most commonly the second toe). The toe becomes bent and may be painful. Generally, both joints in a toe are affected, giving it a clawlike appearance. Hammertoe can result from wearing shoes that are too short, but the deformity also occurs in people with long-term diabetes or other diseases that cause muscle and nerve damage. A **mallet toe** is a deformity in which the very end of the toe is bent downward.

Self-care
- Special toe pads or cushions help protect the toe. Metatarsal pads may reduce pain in the ball of the foot behind the hammertoe.
- Your shoes should accommodate foot length, width and height of your toes.

Tips for proper shoe fit

You can avoid many foot, heel and ankle problems with shoes that fit properly. Here's are some tips:
- Find shoes with adequate toe room — height, width and length. Avoid shoes with pointed toes.
- Keep any heels low.
- Choose laced shoes, which are roomier and adjustable.
- Select comfortable athletic shoes, strapped sandals or soft pumps with cushioned insoles.
- Avoid vinyl and plastic shoes. They don't breathe when your feet perspire.
- Buy shoes in the afternoon and evening. Your feet are smaller in the morning and swell throughout the day. Measure both feet.
- Have your feet measured periodically. That's because as you age, your shoe size (length and width) may change.
- Have your shoe store stretch shoes in tight spots.

◼ Swelling

Most people have **swollen feet** occasionally. Causes include all of those noted under "Swollen legs," page 99.

Self-care
- Reduce your salt intake.
- Exercise your legs.
- Lie down for 30 minutes at midday with your feet elevated higher than your heart.

Prevention
- Wear support stockings. They apply constant pressure and reduce foot and ankle swelling. Poorly fitting stockings (too tight in the calf) can cause swelling.
- Maintain a regular exercise program.

Medical help
Seek medical care immediately if one foot becomes swollen rapidly, your foot is inflamed or you have a fever.

◼ Morton's neuroma

Morton's neuroma causes a sharp, burning pain in the ball of your foot. It may feel like you're walking on a stone. Your toes may sting, burn or feel numb. Soft tissue grows around a nerve in your foot (neuroma), often between your third and fourth toes. It may not hurt early in the day, but only after you stand or walk in tight shoes.

Self-care
- Wear well-fitting shoes with enough room in the toe box, or wear sandals.
- Shoe supports (orthotics) or a metatarsal pad may help.
- Reduce high-impact activities for a few weeks.

Medical help
- A cortisone injection may reduce pain.
- The growth may be surgically removed if pain is chronic and severe.

◼ Heel pain

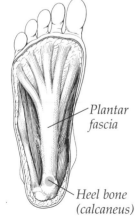

Plantar fascia

Heel bone (calcaneus)

Heel pain often results from stress on the plantar fascia.

Heel pain is irritating but rarely serious. Although it can result from a pinched nerve or a chronic condition, such as arthritis or bursitis, the most common cause is plantar fasciitis. This is an inflammation of the plantar fascia, the fibrous tissue along the bottom of your foot that connects to your heel bone (calcaneus) and toes.

The pain usually develops gradually, but it can come on suddenly and severely. It tends to be worse when you are getting out of bed in the morning, when the fascia is stiff. Although both feet can be affected, it usually occurs in only one foot.

The pain generally decreases or goes away once your foot limbers up. It can recur if you stand for a long time or get up from a sitting or lying position. Climbing stairs or standing on tiptoe also can produce pain. A bone spur (usually painless) may form from tension on your heel bone.

Plantar fasciitis can affect people of all ages. Factors increasing your risk include excess weight, improperly fitting shoes, foot abnormalities and activities that place added or prolonged pressure on your feet. Treatment involves steps to relieve the pain and inflammation. Don't expect a quick cure. Relief may take six months or longer.

Self-care

- Cut back on jogging or walking. Substitute exercises that put less weight on your heel, such as swimming or bicycling.
- Apply ice to the painful area for up to 20 minutes after activity.
- Stretching increases flexibility in your plantar fascia, Achilles tendon and calf muscles. Stretching in the morning before you get out of bed helps reverse the tightening of the plantar fascia that occurs overnight.
- Strengthening muscles in your foot can help support your arch.
- Buy shoes with good heel and arch support and shock absorbency.
- Over-the-counter medications may ease the pain (see page 258).
- If you're overweight, shed excess pounds.
- Try heel pads or cups. They help cushion and support your heel.
- Consider over-the-counter arch supports. They support your feet and help to redistribute weight on your feet.

These exercises stretch or strengthen your plantar fascia, Achilles tendon and calf muscles. Hold each for 20 or 30 seconds, and do one or two repetitions two or three times a day.

Toe curls with towel

Toe extension

Standing calf and heel stretch

Medical help

If the self-care measures aren't effective, or if you believe your condition is due to a foot abnormality, see your doctor. Treatment options include:

- Custom orthotics.
- Night splints to keep tension on the tissue so it heals in a stretched position.
- Deep heat, which increases blood flow and promotes healing.
- A cortisone injection in your heel to help relieve the inflammation when other steps aren't successful. But multiple injections aren't recommended because they can weaken and rupture your plantar fascia, as well as shrink the fat pad covering your heel bone.
- Detaching a portion of the plantar fascia from your heel bone, but this is recommended only when all other treatments have failed.

Lungs, chest and breathing

Breathing is one of the most basic reflexes. You do it thousands of times a day. When you breathe in (inhale), you draw fresh oxygen into your lungs and bloodstream. When you breathe out (exhale), you remove the air from your lungs that contains carbon dioxide, a waste product of your body's activities. Breathing is something that most people take for granted — until they have trouble with it.

■ Coughing: A natural reflex

A cough is a reflex — just like breathing. It's actually a way of protecting your lungs against irritants. When your breathing passages (bronchi) have secretions in them, you cough to clear the passages so that you can breathe more easily. A small amount of coughing is ordinary and even healthy as a way to maintain clear breathing passages.

Strong or persistent coughing can be an irritant to your breathing passages. Repeated coughing causes your bronchi to constrict. This change can irritate the interior walls of your breathing passages (membranes).

What causes coughing?

Coughing is frequently a symptom of a viral upper respiratory tract infection, which is an infection of your nose, sinuses and airways. A **cold** and **influenza** are common examples. Your voice box may become inflamed (**laryngitis**), causing hoarseness, which can affect your ability to speak. Coughing may also result from throat irritation caused by the drainage of mucus down the back of your throat, a condition called postnasal drainage.

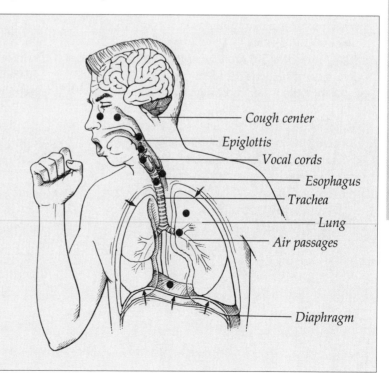

The cough

A cough begins when an irritant reaches one of the cough receptors in your nose, throat or chest (see dots). The receptor sends a message to the cough center in your brain, signaling your body to cough. After you inhale, your epiglottis and vocal cords close tightly, trapping air within your lungs. Your abdominal and chest muscles contract forcefully, pushing against your diaphragm. Finally, your vocal cords and epiglottis open suddenly, allowing trapped air to explode outward.

Cough center
Epiglottis
Vocal cords
Esophagus
Trachea
Lung
Air passages
Diaphragm

Coughing also occurs with chronic disorders. People with allergies and asthma have bouts of involuntary coughing, as do people who smoke. Irritants in the environment, such as smog, dust, secondhand smoke, and cold or dry air, can cause coughing.

Sometimes coughing is caused by stomach acid that backs up into your esophagus or, in rare cases, your lungs. This condition is called gastroesophageal reflux (see page 64). Some people also develop a "habit" cough.

Self-care

- **Drink plenty of fluids.** They help keep your throat clear. Drink water or fruit juices — not soda or coffee.
- **Use a humidifier.** The air in your home can get very dry, especially during the winter. Dry air irritates your throat when you have a cold. Using a humidifier to moisturize the air will make breathing easier (see below).
- **Honey, hard candy or medicated throat lozenges** may help to soothe a simple throat irritation and may help prevent coughing if your throat is dry or sore. Try drinking a cup of tea sweetened with honey.
- **Try sleeping with the head of your bed elevated 4 to 6 inches** if your cough is caused by a backup of stomach acids. Also avoid food and drink within two to three hours of bedtime.

Medical help

Contact a doctor if your cough lasts more than two or three weeks, or if it's accompanied by a fever, increased shortness of breath or bloody phlegm. Managing a chronic cough requires careful evaluation.

Home humidifiers — Help or hazard?

When breathing dry indoor air makes you cough, increase the humidity. But don't let the remedy to one problem create another. Dirty humidifiers can be a source of bacteria and fungi. To minimize growth, the U.S. Consumer Product Safety Commission suggests the following:

- **Change the water every day.** Don't allow film and scale to develop inside. Empty the tank, dry the inside surfaces and refill with clean water. Follow the manufacturer's instructions.
- **Use distilled or demineralized water.** Tap water contains minerals that can create bacteria-friendly deposits. When released into the air, these minerals often appear as white dust on your furniture.

- **Clean your humidifier often during use.** Unplug the device before cleaning it. If chlorine bleach or another disinfectant is used, rinse the tank well afterward to avoid breathing harmful chemicals. Clean or replace sponge filters or belts when needed.
- **Keep the humidity between 30 and 50 percent.** Levels higher than 60 percent may create a buildup of moisture. When moisture condenses on surfaces, bacteria and fungi can grow. Periodically check the humidity with a hygrometer, available at your local hardware store.
- **Clean your humidifier before you store it.** Clean it again after summer storage and remove dust on the outside of it.

Bronchitis

Bronchitis is a common condition, much like the common cold. It usually is caused by a viral infection that spreads to the bronchi, producing a deep cough that, in turn, brings up yellowish-gray matter from your lungs. The bronchi are the main air passages of your lungs. When the walls that line the bronchi become inflamed, this condition is called bronchitis.

Self-care
- Get plenty of rest. Drink lots of fluids. Use a humidifier in your room.
- Consider taking a nonprescription cold remedy (see page 259). Adults can take aspirin, another nonsteroidal anti-inflammatory drug (NSAID) or acetaminophen for a fever. Children should take only acetaminophen or ibuprofen.
- Avoid irritants to your airways, such as tobacco smoke.

Medical help

Acute bronchitis usually disappears in a matter of days. Contact a doctor if you experience shortness of breath or a fever of 101 F (38.3 C) or higher for more than three days. In addition, if your cough lasts for more than 10 days, you should seek medical attention.

Croup

Croup is caused by a virus that infects the voice box (larynx), windpipe (trachea) and bronchial tubes. Croup occurs most often in children between the ages of 3 months and 3 years. Because of a narrowing of the airway, a child with croup has a tight, brassy cough that may resemble the barking of a dog or seal. The child's voice becomes hoarse, and it's difficult for the child to breathe in. The child may become agitated and begin crying — actions that make breathing even more difficult. Croup typically lasts five or six days. During this period, it may go from mild to severe several times. The symptoms are usually worse at night.

Self-care
- Give plenty of water to soothe the throat and replace water lost by the illness.
- Since panic can worsen the symptoms, reassure and comfort the child.
- Give acetaminophen or ibuprofen in age- and weight-appropriate doses to soothe the throat and chest.
- Keep the child away from smoke (it aggravates the symptoms).
- Expose the child to humid air. Try these methods:
  - Use a cool-air humidifier in your child's bedroom and have the child put his or her face in or near the mist and breathe deeply through the mouth. Or run a hot shower with the bathroom door closed, holding the child in your lap to breathe the steamy air.
  - Weather permitting, dress the child warmly and take the child outside with you to breathe the cool, moist night air.

Medical help

If you can't calm the child and ease the cough with self-care measures, seek medical attention. The doctor may give corticosteroids by mouth or injection to break the symptoms and ease congestion in the windpipe.

Call 911 or emergency medical help if the child is in severe distress or unresponsive, or if his or her complexion is blue or dusky.

Common Problems

Wheezing

Wheezing occurs when you hear a high-pitched whistling sound coming from your chest as you breathe out. It's caused by a narrowing of the airways in the lungs and indicates breathing difficulty. In addition, your chest may feel tight.

Wheezing is a common symptom of **asthma**, **bronchitis**, smoking, allergies, **pneumonia**, **emphysema**, **lung cancer** and **congestive heart failure**. It can also stem from environmental factors, such as chemicals or air pollution. Wheezing requires medical attention. See a doctor if you have difficulty breathing or wheezing.

Shortness of breath

In general, unexpected shortness of breath is a symptom that needs medical attention. Shortness of breath can be caused by a variety of illnesses, including heart attacks to blood clots in the lung to **pneumonia**. It can also be caused by pregnancy.

In its chronic form, shortness of breath is a symptom of illnesses such as **asthma**, **emphysema**, other lung diseases, heart disease, anemia and deconditioning. All of these chronic conditions also require medical attention. Some exercises can help relieve shortness of breath if you have chronic lung disease (see below).

Simple exercises can improve your breathing

Breathing exercises may help if you have emphysema or another chronic lung disorder. They help control the emptying of your lungs and increase your lungs' efficiency. Ask your doctor about these exercises. Do them two to four times daily or as advised.

Diaphragmatic breathing
Lie on your back with your head and knees supported by pillows. Begin by breathing in and out slowly and smoothly in a rhythmic pattern. Relax.

Place your fingertips on your abdomen, just below the base of your rib cage. As you inhale slowly, you should feel your diaphragm lifting your hand.

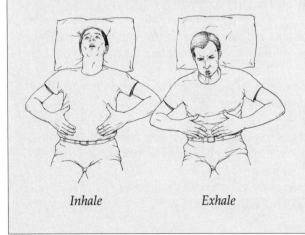

Inhale   *Exhale*

Practice pushing your abdomen against your hand as your chest becomes filled with air. Make sure your chest remains motionless. Try this while inhaling through your mouth and counting slowly to three. Then purse your lips and exhale through your mouth while counting slowly to six.

Practice this breathing on your back until you can take 10 to 15 consecutive breaths in one session without tiring. Then practice the exercise while lying first on one side and then on the other. Progress to doing the exercise while sitting erect in a chair, standing up, walking and, finally, climbing stairs.

Pursed-lip breathing
Try the diaphragmatic breathing exercises with your lips pursed as you exhale. With your lips puckered, the flow of air should make a soft "sssss" sound. Inhale deeply through your mouth and exhale. Repeat 10 times at each session.

Deep-breathing exercise
While sitting or standing, pull your elbows firmly backward as you inhale deeply. Hold the breath in, with your chest arched, for a count to five and then force the air out by contracting your abdominal muscles. Repeat the exercise 10 times.

See back cover for online resource (i)

■ Chest pain

Chest pain can be severe. It can also be difficult to interpret. The pain could be caused by something as simple as indigestion or by a serious medical situation.

Emergency care

If chest pain persists, call 911 (or your local emergency number) immediately!

Heart attack. In addition to pain or pressure in your chest, you could experience pain in your jaw, arms, neck or back. Other symptoms of a **heart attack** may include shortness of breath, sweating, dizziness, nausea and vomiting. Shortness of breath in people over the age of 65 — especially in women — is the predominant sign of a heart attack. If you think you're having a heart attack, call for emergency help. If you go to a hospital, *do not drive yourself!* **See "Heart attack," pages 5-6.**

Other causes of chest pain

Here are common forms of chest pain that don't require immediate medical attention:

Chest wall pain. This is one of the most common forms of harmless chest pain. If probing the tender area with your finger causes the pain to return, then serious conditions, such as a heart attack, are less likely. Chest wall pain usually lasts only a few days, and it can be treated with aspirin in adults. For children, treat with ibuprofen or acetaminophen. Apply low and intermittent heat to the area to help reduce the pain.

Heartburn. Symptoms are a warm or burning discomfort in the upper part of your abdomen and under your breastbone. You may also have an acid or sour taste in your mouth. **Heartburn** sometimes can be so painful that the symptoms are confused with the onset of a heart attack. Chest pain from heartburn usually can be relieved by belching or by taking an antacid.

Precordial catch. This is a condition that occurs most often in young adults. The symptom is a brief, sharp pain under the left breast that makes breathing difficult. There are no self-care measures. The condition goes away momentarily. The cause of this common condition is unknown, although it's apparently harmless.

Angina. Angina is the term used for chest pain, or pressure, associated with coronary artery disease. It's caused by a lack of oxygen reaching the heart muscle. It usually develops with physical exertion or when you're under emotional stress. If you have coronary artery disease, develop a treatment plan with your doctor.

- Don't try to "work through" an episode of angina. Stop and treat it.
- Angina usually is treated with rest and a medication such as nitroglycerin.
- If you have a change in your pattern of angina, such as increased frequency or nighttime attacks, see your doctor immediately.
- If you've tried measures to stop an angina attack but it lasts over 15 minutes, or you also have lightheadedness or palpitations, seek emergency medical care.

■ Palpitations

Heart **palpitations** are the feelings of having rapid, fluttering or pounding heart-beats. Many people experience heart palpitations from time to time. Often the cause can't be found, but palpitations can be triggered by stress, vigorous exercise, caffeine, nicotine, a fever or some medications that contain stimulants. Frequently, changes in lifestyle relieve the symptoms.

Usually palpitations are not dangerous, but check with your doctor to be sure. In some cases, palpitations are caused by a more serious heart problem.

Nose and sinuses

Your nose is the gateway to your respiratory system. Your nose filters, humidifies and warms the air you breathe as it moves from your nasal passage into your throat and lungs.

However, your nose may be affected by conditions such as a nosebleed, cold, sinus infection or hay fever. Luckily, most disorders of the nose and sinuses are temporary and easy to control.

The following pages address common disorders of the nose and sinuses. For information on respiratory allergies, see page 158.

■ Foreign objects in the nose

If a foreign object becomes lodged in your nose, follow these steps:
- Don't probe at the foreign object with a cotton swab or other tool. Don't try to inhale the object by forcefully breathing in; breathe through your mouth until the object is removed.
- Blow your nose gently to try to free the object, but don't blow hard or repeatedly.
- If the object protrudes from your nose and can be easily grasped with tweezers, gently remove it.

If these methods fail, seek emergency medical assistance.

■ Loss of sense of smell

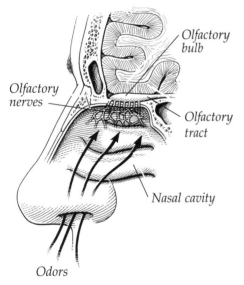

Your sense of smell begins with odors stimulating the olfactory nerve endings in the upper portion of your nose. The olfactory nerves contain very fine and sensitive fibers that transmit signals from the olfactory bulb to your brain.

Most people temporarily lose their sense of smell when they have a head cold. Usually, the sense of smell returns once the infection is gone. You may notice the loss of taste and smell together, as a large part of what people perceive as "taste" is actually the aroma associated with foods.

However, when the sense of smell is lost without an apparent cause, the condition is called anosmia. Anosmia occurs from either an obstruction in your nose or nerve damage. An obstruction prevents odors from reaching the delicate nerve fibers in your nose. Nasal polyps, infections, tumors or neurological conditions can cause obstruction. Viral infections, chronic nasal infections or allergies also can damage the nerves that transmit smell.

Medical help

If you lose your sense of smell and you don't have a cold, consult your doctor. He or she will check for polyps or tumors of the nasal passages. When the problem is caused by a viral infection, the sense of smell usually returns when the tissues of the olfactory area heal.

Nosebleeds

Nosebleeds are common. Most often they're a nuisance and not a true medical problem. But they can be both.

Among children and young adults, nosebleeds usually start from the septum, the middle partition separating your nasal chambers. Most often, this is due to dryness and nose-picking. In middle-aged and older adults, nosebleeds can begin from the septum, but may also begin deeper in the nose's interior, although the latter form is much less common. These nosebleeds begin spontaneously and are often difficult to stop.

Rarely, frequent nosebleeds may indicate a serious condition such as a bleeding disorder or tumor. See your doctor to rule out these conditions if you experience frequent nosebleeds associated with easy bruising and bleeding elsewhere in your body.

Self-care

- **Sit upright and lean forward.** By remaining upright, you reduce blood pressure in the veins of your nose. This discourages further bleeding. Sitting forward will help you avoid swallowing blood, which can irritate your stomach.
- **Pinch your nose** with your thumb and index finger and breathe through your mouth. Continue to hold pressure for five to 10 minutes. This maneuver sends pressure to the bleeding point on the nasal septum and often stops the flow of blood.
- **To prevent re-bleeding after bleeding has stopped,** don't blow your nose until one to two days after the bleeding episode. Avoid bending over. Don't pick your nose.
- **If re-bleeding occurs,** spray both sides of your nose with a decongestant nasal spray containing oxymetazoline (Afrin, Neo-Synephrine, others). Pinch your nose again for 10 minutes. If bleeding doesn't stop, seek emergency care.
- **To prevent bleeding,** increase the humidity of the air you breathe in your home. A humidifier or vaporizer can help keep your nasal membranes moist. Over-the-counter saline nasal spray may help, especially during winter months.
- **Avoid using any tissue,** cottom swabs or fingers in the nose.

Medical help

Seek medical care immediately if:

- The bleeding lasts for more than 20 minutes
- You feel weak or faint, which can result from the blood loss
- The bleeding is rapid or the amount of blood loss is great
- Bleeding begins by trickling down the back of your throat
- Other body sites are bruised or bleeding
- The nosebleed follows an accident, a fall or an injury to your head, including a punch in the face that may have broken your nose

If you have frequent nosebleeds, make an appointment with your doctor. An examination is important to rule out serious causes. Most often, though, the bleeding can be stopped by sealing the bleeding blood vessel (cautery), or it may be controlled with nasal packing.

Call your doctor if you're taking blood thinners, such as aspirin or warfarin (Coumadin, Jantoven). Your doctor may adjust the dose of your medications.

Kids' care

Frequent nosebleeds in children are common. Often, nosebleeds are due to trauma, but they can be a sign of a foreign body in the nose or of difficulty with blood clotting. Rarely, a nosebleed can be a sign of a tumor. Check with your child's health care provider if frequent nosebleeds are a problem.

Stuffy nose

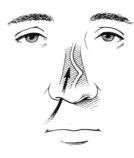

Your nasal septum separates your nasal chambers. A deviated septum may cause nasal obstruction.

A stuffy nose is a common medical complaint. A stuffy nose usually results from nasal congestion or an obstruction. In most cases, a stuffy nose is a mere nuisance, but sometimes it can severely impact sleep, speech and daily functioning. The most common causes of nasal obstruction include:

Common cold. See page 115.

Deformities of the nose and the partition (nasal septum) separating your nasal chambers are usually due to an injury. The injury may have occurred years earlier, even in childhood. Deformities of the nose such as a deviated septum are fairly common problems. For many people, a deviated septum poses few problems. But if the condition makes breathing difficult, surgery to realign your septum may help.

Allergies. Allergic rhinitis, which means nasal inflammation from allergies, is the medical term for **hay fever**, rose fever, grass fever and other allergies. The allergic reaction is an inflammatory response to specific foreign substances that enter the nose, such as pollen, mold or house dust. This can be seasonal or last year-round.

Nonallergic rhinitis. This form of inflammation is associated with triggers such as smoke, air conditioning or vigorous exercise.

Self-care

- For colds and flu, see page 115.
- Gently blow your nose if mucus or debris is present.
- Breathing steam can loosen the mucus and clear your head.
- Take a warm shower or sit in the bathroom with the shower running.
- Drink plenty of liquids.
- Use nonprescription decongestant nasal sprays or nose drops once a day for two to three days. Nonprescription oral decongestants (liquid or pills) may be helpful.
- Try saline drops or nasal saline spray. These are safe to use long term as needed.
- Try a nonprescription steroid nasal spray such as fluticasone (Flonase) and triamcinolone (Nasacort Allergy 24HR). These can also be used long term.

Medical help

If nose congestion persists for more than one to two weeks, consult your doctor, who will examine your nose for the cause of the obstruction, such as polyps or tumors.

If your doctor determines you have an allergy, he or she may prescribe a course of therapy that may include antihistamines and inhaled anti-inflammatory medications.

Runny nose

A **runny nose** commonly occurs early in a cold and in allergic irritation. Gently blowing your nose may be all the self-care you need. If the discharge is persistent and watery, an over-the-counter antihistamine may be helpful. If the discharge is thick, follow the recommendations for a stuffy nose above.

Decongestant nasal sprays

Decongestant sprays work by shrinking congested blood vessels, which allows you to breathe easier. However, after a few days of use, the blood vessels don't respond as well to the medication. Use of the medication beyond three days may result in the congestion worsening (rebound congestion). Ask your doctor or pharmacist about methods that don't cause rebound congestion.

See back cover for online resource

'Aaachoo!' Is it a cold or the flu?

Both are viral upper respiratory tract infections

	Cold	Seasonal flu (influenza)
Usual symptoms	• Runny nose, sneezing, nasal congestion • Sore throat (usually scratchy) • Cough • No fever or low fever • Mild fatigue	• Runny nose • Sore throat and headache • Cough • Fever, usually over 101 F (38.3 C), chills • Moderate to severe fatigue and weakness • Achy muscles and joints
Cause	One of more than 200 viruses typically causes two to four colds a year in adults and six to 10 a year in kids, especially preschoolers.	One of a few viruses from the influenza A or influenza B family. On average, adults have less than one infection a year.
Seriousness	Usually not serious except in people with lung disease or other serious illness.	Can be serious. A special concern in older adults and those with chronic health conditions.
Can I work?	Usually. Use care to avoid spreading a cold to others. Wash hands frequently. Cover sneezes.	No, not until fever, fatigue and all but the mild symptoms have resolved.
Preventable?	Possibly, through careful hand washing, not sharing food, towels or handkerchiefs, and getting good nutrition and enough rest.	Usually, through vaccination. You need to be immunized every fall (see pages 226-228). But the tips at left are still important.
Do antibiotics help?	No, since colds are from viral infections.	Sometimes. Antivirals may help if taken within 48 hours of the start of symptoms.
Self-care	• Drink lots of fluids. Homemade chicken soup may help clear mucus. • Increase sleep and rest. • Use cold remedies cautiously (see page 259). • Keep your room warm, but not overheated. • If air is dry, a cool-mist humidifier or vaporizer may help ease congestion.	• Drink lots of fluids. Homemade chicken soup may help clear mucus. • Increase sleep and rest. • Use over-the-counter pain relievers cautiously, as needed (see page 258).
Seek medical help	• If you have trouble breathing, faintness, change in alertness, severe sore throat, cough producing a lot of sputum or mucus, pain in the face, or a chronic health condition • If symptoms haven't resolved in 10 days Rapid flu diagnostic tests can detect if you have the flu, but this test can miss some cases.	

A word about pneumonia

Pneumonia can occur after a cold or flu or on its own. Symptoms can vary greatly, depending on the organism that caused it. Common symptoms include a cough with phlegm, fever, shortness of breath, sweating, chills, chest pain when you breathe deeply (pleurisy), headache, muscle pain or fatigue. Pneumonia can be life-threatening. See your doctor right away if you have a persistent cough, shortness of breath, chest pain, unexplained fever — especially a lasting fever of 102 F (38.9 C) or higher with chills and sweating — or if you suddenly feel worse after a cold or the flu. Vaccinations are available to prevent some types of pneumonia.

Common Problems

■ Sinusitis

Signs of __sinusitis__ include thick, yellow-green drainage with increasing stuffiness, loss of smell, and pain about your eyes or cheeks. In some cases it may be associated with a fever or tooth pain.

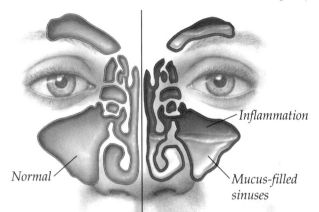

Normal

Inflammation

Mucus-filled sinuses

Sinus trouble begins when the small openings that drain into the nose and throat become blocked. The most common way this occurs is due to sinus inflammation. Inflammation causes swelling, which makes it difficult for sinuses to drain.

Your sinuses are cavities in the bones around your nose. They are connected to your nasal cavities by small openings. Normally, air passes in and out of your sinuses and mucus drains through these openings into your nose.

Sinusitis is an inflammation of the lining of one or more of these cavities. Usually, when your sinus is inflamed, the membranes of your nose also swell and cause a nasal obstruction. Swelling of the membranes of your nose may close off the opening of your sinus and thus prevent draining of pus or mucus. Pain in your sinus may result from the inflammation itself or from the pressure as secretions build up in your sinus.

Short-lived (acute) sinusitis is most often caused by the common cold. Long-term (chronic) sinusitis may be caused by an infection (viral, bacterial or fungal), allergies, nasal polyps or tumors, or other medical conditions.

Self-care

- Rinse out your nasal passages. Use a specially designed squeeze bottle (Sinus Rinse, others), bulb syringe or neti pot. This home remedy, called nasal lavage, can help clear your sinuses.
- Apply warm, damp towels around your nose, cheeks and eyes to ease pain.
- Cautiously inhale steam from a basin of boiling water or take a hot shower and breathe in the moist air.
- Drink plenty of fluids to help dilute the secretions. Don't drink alcohol, which can worsen nasal and sinus swelling.
- Gently and regularly blow your nose, then use a saline spray.
- Try over-the-counter nasal steroids such as fluticasone (Flonase) and triamcinolone (Nasacort Allergy 24HR). They can be safely used for up to two weeks.
- Refrain from bending over with your head down if this movement increases the pain.
- Ask your doctor for advice on pain relievers and over-the-counter (OTC) decongestants, such as tablets and nasal sprays. If taken too long, OTC decongestants can do more harm than good by drying out your nose too much and thickening secretions. Use them only on the recommendation of your doctor, and follow instructions carefully.

Medical help

Call your health care provider if you have an unresolving fever greater than 101.5 F, if the symptoms don't improve within 10 days, if the symptoms get worse, or if you have a history of recurrent or chronic sinusitis. CT scans and other exams may be performed to find out how serious the infection is. If sinusitis is the result of a bacterial infection, your doctor may prescribe an oral antibiotic or other medications. However, most acute sinus infections do not require antibiotics as they are either usually viral in nature or they resolve on their own.

See back cover for online resource ⓘ

Skin, hair and nails

Because your skin, hair and nails are an integral part of your appearance, changes and problems involving them are often distressing. External irritants, infections, aging and even emotional stress can affect your skin, hair and nails in many ways. Rarely, underlying medical conditions and allergies to foods or medications can trigger abnormalities.

This section explains some of the more common disorders and offers self-care tips to help you find relief. But first, here are some basic guidelines for skin care.

■ Proper skin care

Regardless of your skin color or type or your age, limiting exposure to the sun — and its ultraviolet (UV) rays — can help prevent damage and, eventually, skin cancer. Dark skin can tolerate more sun than can fair skin. However, any skin can become blotchy, leathery and wrinkled from overexposure to the sun. Protective clothing, daily use of sunscreen on sun-exposed skin, and daily lubrication or moisturizing can help.

Sun exposure enhances vitamin D production, but to avoid the risk of skin cancer, health care providers often recommend vitamin D supplements (available in daily multiple vitamins) and vitamin-D fortified foods, such as low-fat milk. If you don't get enough vitamin D, ask your health care provider for advice.

Proper cleansing is another important strategy in protecting your skin. The best procedures and cleansing ingredients vary according to your skin type — oily, dry, balanced or a combination of these.

Finally, don't smoke. It's not only bad for your heart and lungs, but nicotine affects the skin and causes it to age faster.

Self-care

- When washing your face, use comfortably cool or lukewarm (never hot) water and a washcloth or sponge to remove dead skin cells. Use a mild soap. You may need to clean oily skin two or three times each day.
- Avoid washing your body with very hot water or strong soaps. For more tips on caring for dry skin, see "Dryness," page 121.
- If you shave your beard with a blade razor, use a sharp blade. Soften your skin by applying a warm cloth for a few seconds. Then use plenty of shaving cream. Pass the blade over your beard only once, in the direction of hair growth. Reversing the stroke to get a close shave can cause skin irritation. Electric razors are less irritating to your skin. Products are available to treat skin irritation.
- Match cosmetics to your skin type: An oil base is suitable for dry skin, and a water base is suitable for oily skin.
- For women, remove eye makeup before facial cleansing. Use cotton balls to avoid damaging the delicate tissue around your eyes.
- Use a broad spectrum (protects against both UVA and UVB) sunscreen with a sun protection factor (SPF) of 30 or higher. It's important to find one that you like and are comfortable using on a daily basis. Remember to reapply every two hours and after swimming or sweating.

■ Acne

Acne is caused by plugged pores, hormonal changes and bacteria in the skin. Oil from glands combines with dead skin to plug pores (follicles), which can produce:

- **Whiteheads.** Clogged pores that have no opening
- **Blackheads.** Pores that are open and have a dark surface
- **Pimples.** Reddish lesions that signal an infection by bacteria in plugged pores
- **Cysts.** Thick lumps under the surface of the skin, from the buildup of secretions

Acne is most common in teenagers because hormonal changes stimulate certain glands to secrete a fatty oil called sebum, which lubricates hair and skin. But people of all ages can get acne. Menstruation, certain drugs or stress may aggravate acne.

Self-care

- Avoid oily or greasy cosmetics or hair-styling products or acne cover-up. Use products labeled *water-based* or *noncomedogenic*.
- Wash problem areas daily with a cleanser that gently dries your skin.
- Try over-the-counter acne lotion (containing benzoyl peroxide or salicylic acid as the active ingredient) to dry excess oil and promote peeling.
- Keep your hair clean and off your face.
- Try to get enough sleep and better manage your stress.
- Unless a food is clearly aggravating your acne, you don't need to eliminate it. Foods such as chocolate, once thought to cause acne, generally aren't the problem.
- Don't pick or squeeze blemishes. Doing so can cause an infection, skin discoloration or scarring.

Medical help

Persistent pimples, inflamed cysts or scarring may require prescription drugs. Proper evaluation and treatment can prevent the physical and psychological scarring associated with acne. In rare cases, a sudden onset of severe acne in an older adult may signal an underlying disease requiring medical attention.

Cosmetic surgery can decrease acne scars. The main procedures are laser resurfacing, scar revision, or peeling of the skin by freezing or chemicals.

■ Boils

Boils are tender bumps under the skin with overlying redness that occur when bacteria infect hair follicles. The bumps are usually larger than $1/2$ inch wide. They grow rapidly, fill with pus and then burst, drain and heal, usually within about two weeks.

Boils can occur anywhere on your skin, but most often occur on the face, neck, underarms, buttocks or thighs. Poor health, clothing that binds or chafes, and disorders such as acne, dermatitis, diabetes and anemia can increase your risk of infection.

Self-care

To avoid spreading this infection and to minimize discomfort, follow these measures:

- Soak the area with a warm washcloth or compress for at least 10 minutes every few hours. Use warm salt water. (Add 1 teaspoon of salt to 1 quart of boiling water and let it cool.) Doing so may help the boil burst and drain much sooner. Prevent the drained matter from contacting other skin areas.
- Gently wash the boil two to three times a day with antibacterial soap. Then apply an over-the-counter antibiotic ointment and cover with a bandage.
- Never squeeze or lance a boil because you might spread the infection.
- Wash your hands thoroughly after treating a boil. Also, launder towels, compresses and clothing that have touched the infected area.

Medical help	Contact your doctor if the boil is located on your spine, groin or face, worsens rapidly or causes severe pain, isn't gone within two weeks, or if you have a fever or reddish lines radiating from the boil. Antibiotics or surgical drainage may be needed to clear the infection. MRSA (see below) can be a cause, so ask if a culture is needed.

◼ Cellulitis

<u>Cellulitis</u> may appear gradually over a couple of days or rapidly over a few hours. It begins as a localized area of red, painful, warm skin. You may also have a fever and swelling. This common and potentially serious infection occurs when bacteria or a fungus enters your body through a break in the skin and infects the deeper layers of skin.

Good hygiene and proper wound care can help prevent cellulitis. However, bacteria can enter your skin through even tiny cuts or abrasions, such as a sore inside your nostril. The incidence of MRSA (below) as a cause is on the rise.

Self-care	To prevent cellulitis and other wound infections: • Keep wounds clean. Cover the area with a bandage to help keep it clean and keep harmful bacteria out. Keep draining blisters covered until a scab forms. • Change the bandage daily or whenever it becomes wet or dirty.
Medical help	Contact your doctor right away if you have a red, swollen, tender rash or a rash that's changing rapidly, especially if accompanied by a fever. Antibiotics can prevent the infection from spreading. Left untreated, cellulitis can spread rapidly through your body and turn into a life-threatening condition.

◼ MRSA infection

Methicillin-resistant *Staphylococcus aureus* (MRSA) is a potentially dangerous type of staph bacteria that's resistant to certain antibiotics. Most infections occur in health care facilities in older adults and people with serious health problems.

But community-associated <u>MRSA</u> can occur among otherwise healthy people. This type of MRSA is spread by direct contact with an infected person or by sharing personal items, such as towels or razors that have touched infected skin.

Staph skin infections, including MRSA, generally start as small red bumps. These bumps can quickly become painful, warm to the touch, fill with pus or other drainage, and be accompanied by a fever. The bacteria may remain confined to the skin. But they can also spread into the body, causing potentially life-threatening infections.

Self-care	To protect yourself from MRSA: • In the hospital, ask staff to wash their hands or use an alcohol-based hand sanitizer before touching you — every time. And wash your own hands often. • In the community, wash your hands often; carry hand sanitizer that has at least 60 percent alcohol; don't share personal items, such as towels and athletic equipment; keep wounds covered; and shower after athletic games or practices.
Medical help	Contact your doctor right away if you suspect MRSA infection. Treatment may include draining the infection, and in some cases, taking certain antibiotics. Don't try to drain the infection yourself — you may worsen it and spread it to others.

Corns and calluses

These thickened, hardened layers of skin typically appear on your hands and feet. Corns often appear as raised bumps of hardened skin less than ¼ inch long. Calluses vary in size and shape. **Corns and calluses** are your skin's attempt to protect itself. Although they can be unsightly, treatment may be necessary only if they cause discomfort. For most people, eliminating the source of friction or pressure will help corns and calluses disappear.

Self-care

- Wear properly fitted shoes, with adequate toe room. Have your shoe shop stretch your shoes at any point that rubs or pinches. Place pads under your heels if your shoes rub. Try to cushion or soften the corn while wearing shoes.
- Wear padded gloves when using hand tools, or try padding your tool handles with cloth tape or covers.
- Rub your corn or callus with a pumice stone or washcloth during or after bathing to gradually thin some of the thickened skin. This advice isn't recommended if you have diabetes or poor circulation.
- Try over-the-counter corn dissolvers containing salicylic acid. These are available in plaster-pad disks or solutions containing a thickener called collodion.
- Don't cut or shave corns or calluses.
- Apply a moisturizer to your hands and feet to keep them soft.

Medical help

If a corn or callus becomes very painful or inflamed, contact your health care provider. Since they can look similar to a wart, contact your health care provider if you're unsure.

Dandruff

Dandruff is a common chronic scalp condition, which is marked by itching and flaking of the skin on your scalp. Causes include dry skin, irritated and oily skin (seborrheic dermatitis), not shampooing enough, psoriasis, eczema, sensitivity to hair care products (contact dermatitis), or a yeast-like fungus (malassezia).

Self-care

- Shampoo regularly. Start with a mild, nonmedicated shampoo. Gently massage your scalp to loosen flakes. Rinse thoroughly.
- Use medicated shampoo for stubborn cases. Look for shampoos containing zinc pyrithione, salicylic acid, coal tar or selenium sulfide in brands such as Head & Shoulders, Neutrogena T/Sal or T/Gel, Denorex or Selsun Blue. Use a dandruff shampoo each time you shampoo, if necessary, to control flaking. Rotate shampoos every month or so.
- Kill dandruff-causing fungi that live on your scalp by using the antifungal shampoo Nizoral 1%. This shampoo is available over-the-counter or by prescription.
- If you use tar-based shampoos, use them carefully. They can leave a brownish stain on light-colored or gray hair and make the scalp more sensitive to sunlight.
- Use a conditioner regularly. For mild dandruff, alternate dandruff shampoo with your regular shampoo.

Medical help

If dandruff persists or your scalp becomes irritated or severely itchy, you may need a prescription shampoo. If your dandruff persists, you may have some other skin condition. See your doctor.

See back cover for online resource ⓘ

Dryness

This is by far the most common cause of itching, flaking skin. Although dryness can be a problem any time of the year, cold air and low humidity can be especially tough on your skin. **Dry skin** due to the weather depends on where you live (for example, the Minnesota "winter itch" and the Arizona "summer itch").

Self-care

- Take fewer baths or showers. Keep them short and use lukewarm water and minimal amounts of soap. Soap is only needed for the face, underarms, genital areas, hands and feet. Mild superfatted soaps (Cetaphil, Dove, Vanicream, others) will dry skin less. Consider adding bath oils to the bath.
- Pat (rather than wipe) your skin dry after bathing, then immediately moisturize your skin with an oil or cream. Use a heavy, water-in-oil moisturizer rather than a light "disappearing" cream that contains mostly water.
- Avoid creams or lotions containing alcohol.
- Use a humidifier and keep room temperatures cool.

Eczema (dermatitis)

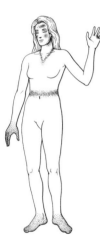

Frequent locations of irritation from contact dermatitis, the most common form of dermatitis

The terms *eczema* and **dermatitis** are both used to describe irritated and swollen or reddened (inflamed) skin. Patches of dry, reddened and itchy skin are the major symptoms. Patches can thicken and develop blisters or weeping sores in severe cases.

Contact dermatitis results from direct contact with one of many irritants that can trigger this reaction. Common culprits include poison ivy (see "Poisonous plants," page 29), rubber, metals, jewelry, perfume and cosmetics.

Neurodermatitis can occur when something such as a tight garment rubs or scratches (or causes you to rub or scratch) your skin, resulting in a chronic itch cycle.

Seborrheic dermatitis (cradle cap in infants) can appear as a stubborn, itchy dandruff. You may notice greasy, scaling areas at the sides of your nose, between your eyebrows, behind your ears or over your breastbone. This version tends to be chronic.

Stasis dermatitis may cause the skin at your ankles to become discolored (red or brown), thickened and itchy. It can occur when fluid accumulates in the tissues just beneath your skin. This condition can lead to infection.

Atopic dermatitis causes itchy, thickened, fissured skin, most often in the folds of the elbows or backs of the knees. It frequently runs in families and is often associated with seasonal allergies and sometimes asthma.

Self-care

- Try to identify and avoid direct contact with irritants.
- Follow the self-care tips to prevent dry skin (see above).
- Soak in cool to warm water for 20 to 30 minutes a day.
- Apply a moisturizing cream and an over-the-counter hydrocortisone cream.
- Avoid scratching whenever possible. Cover the itchy area with a dressing if you can't keep from scratching it. Trim nails and wear cotton gloves when you sleep.
- Shampoo with an anti-dandruff product if your scalp is affected.
- Support hose may help relieve swelling (edema) with stasis dermatitis.
- Dress appropriate to weather conditions to help avoid excessive sweating.
- Wear smooth-textured cotton clothing.
- Avoid wool bedding and clothes and harsh soaps and detergents.
- Occasional use of over-the-counter antihistamines can reduce itching.

Common Problems

◼ Fungal infections

Fungal infections are caused by microscopic organisms that become parasites on your body. Mold-like fungi called dermatophytes cause athlete's foot, jock itch, and ringworm of the skin or scalp. These fungi live on dead tissues of your hair, nails and the outer layer of your skin. Poor hygiene, moist skin, minor skin or nail injuries, and health conditions such as diabetes increase your susceptibility to fungal infections.

Athlete's foot usually begins between your toes, causing your skin to itch, burn and crack. Sometimes the sole and sides of the foot are affected, becoming thickened and leathery in texture. Although locker rooms and public showers are often blamed for spreading athlete's foot, the environment inside your shoes is probably more important. Athlete's foot becomes more common with age.

Jock itch causes an itching or burning sensation around your groin. In addition to the itching, you'll usually notice a red rash that may spread to the inner thighs, anal area and buttocks. This infection is mildly contagious. It can be spread by contact or sharing towels.

Ringworm affects children and adults, but it has nothing to do with worms. Symptoms are itchy, red, scaly, slightly raised, expanding rings on the trunk, face, or groin and thigh fold. The rings grow outward as the infection spreads, and the central area begins to look like normal skin. This infection is passed from shared clothing, combs and barber tools. Pets also can transmit the fungus to humans.

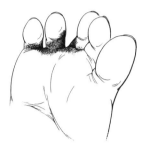

Typical pattern of athlete's foot

Self-care

General
- Practice good personal hygiene to prevent all forms of fungal infections.
- The appropriate treatment depends on the type of fungal infection. For athlete's foot or jock itch, for example, try over-the-counter antifungal creams or drying powder two or three times a day until the rash disappears — consider topical agents such as terbinafine (Lamisil AT) or clotrimazole (Lotrimin AF).

For athlete's foot
- Keep your feet dry, particularly the area between your toes.
- Wear well-ventilated shoes. Avoid shoes made of synthetic materials.
- Don't wear the same shoes every day, and don't store them in plastic.
- Change socks (cotton or polypropylene) twice a day if your feet sweat a lot.
- Wear waterproof sandals or shoes around public pools, showers and locker rooms.

For jock itch
- Keep your groin clean and dry.
- Shower and change clothes after exercise and dry your skin thoroughly.
- Avoid clothes that chafe, and launder athletic supporters frequently.

For ringworm
- Thoroughly clean brushes, combs or headgear that may have been infected.
- Wash hands before and after examining your child.
- Keep your child's linens separate from the rest of the family's.

Medical help

See your doctor if symptoms last longer than four weeks or if you notice increased redness, drainage or fever. You may need prescription oral medications, but some oral medications can have significant side effects, so discuss this with your doctor.

See back cover for online resource ⓘ

■ Hives

Hives are raised, red, often itchy welts of various sizes that appear and disappear on the skin. They're more common on areas of the body where clothes rub your skin. Hives tend to occur in batches and last anywhere from a few minutes to several days.

Angioedema, a similar swelling, causes large welts below your skin, especially near your eyes and lips, but also on your hands and feet and inside your throat. **Hives and angioedema** result when your body releases a natural chemical called histamine in your skin. Allergies to foods, drugs, pollen, insect bites, infections, illness, cold and heat, and emotional distress can trigger a reaction. In most cases, hives and angioedema are harmless and leave no lasting marks. However, serious angioedema can cause your throat or tongue to block your airway and can be life-threatening.

Self-care

- Avoid substances that have triggered past attacks.
- Take cool showers. Apply cool compresses. Wear lightweight clothing. Minimize vigorous activity.
- Use a lubricating cream or over-the-counter antihistamines such as loratadine (Claritin), cetirizine (Zyrtec) or fexofenadine (Allegra) to help relieve the itching.
- If you suspect that food may be causing the problem, keep a food diary.
- If hives persist and there is difficulty breathing, seek emergency care.

Medical help

Seek emergency care if you feel lightheaded or have difficulty breathing or if hives continue to appear for more than a couple of days.

■ Impetigo

Impetigo is a common skin infection that usually appears on the face. The infection begins when staphylococcus or streptococcus bacteria penetrate your skin through a cut, scratch or insect bite. Impetigo is highly contagious and easily spread by contact.

The infection starts as a red sore that blisters briefly, oozes for a few days and forms a sticky, yellow crust. Scratching or touching the sores can spread this contagious infection to other people and other parts of your body.

Impetigo is more common among young children. In adults, it appears mostly as a complication of other skin problems such as dermatitis and breaks in the skin.

Self-care

Good hygiene is essential for preventing impetigo and limiting its spread. For limited or minor infections that haven't spread to other areas, try the following:

- Keep the sores and skin surrounding them clean.
- Apply an antibiotic ointment three or four times daily. Wash the skin with an antibacterial soap before each application, and pat the skin dry.
- Avoid scratching or touching the sores unnecessarily until they heal. Wash your hands after any contact with them. Children's fingernails should be trimmed.
- Don't share towels, clothing or razors with others. Replace linens often.

Medical help

If the infection spreads, your health care provider may prescribe oral antibiotics such as penicillin or erythromycin or an ointment of mupirocin (Bactroban).

Itching and rashes

Finding the source of itching and rashes can be difficult. For information on problems that cause itching and rashes, see: "Allergic reactions," page 12; "Lice," page 126; "Insect bites and stings," page 15; "Baby rashes," below; "Childhood rashes," page 125; "Hives," page 123; "Dryness," page 121; and "Eczema," page 121.

Baby rashes

Cradle cap. Crusty, scaly skin on your baby's scalp. You may apply baby oil to the crusty areas and gently scrape off the scales with a soft brush after bathing. Use a gentle "no tears" shampoo. Make a lather in your hand (not on the child's scalp) to wash the scalp nightly until the condition is under control and then weekly to keep it under control. If the rash is red and irritated, apply a 1 percent hydrocortisone cream twice a day for seven days. You must wait seven days between courses before reapplying. Seek medical care if the cradle cap is severe.

Heat rash. Fine red spots or bumps, usually on the neck or the upper back, chest or arms. This rash often develops during hot, humid weather, especially if your baby is dressed too warmly. It can also occur if your baby has a fever. Remove layers of clothing and avoid overheating the child.

Milia. Tiny (pinpoint) white spots on the nose and cheeks. It's usually present at birth. The spots will disappear without treatment.

Infant acne. Red bumps progressing to acne-like pimples that can appear during the first few months after birth. If few in number, you need not treat. If these progress, seek medical attention. Do not use adolescent acne medications without approval and instructions from a doctor.

Drool rash. A red rash on the cheeks and chin that comes and goes, caused by contact with food, saliva and other liquids. Clean and dry the skin after feeding or spitting up to help clear this rash. An unperfumed, uncolored emollient can serve as a barrier before feeding and after washing to aid in treatment and prevention.

Diaper rash. Reddish, puffy skin in the diaper area. This usually is caused by moisture, the acid in urine or stool, and chafing of diapers. Some babies also get a rash from detergent used to wash cloth diapers, plastic pants, elastic, or certain types of disposable diapers and wipes. Sometimes a yeast infection is the cause.

Self-care for recurrent diaper rash	• Change your baby's diapers frequently to minimize exposure to urine and stool. • If using cloth diapers, use softened water for washing and rinsing and make sure that all the detergent is rinsed out. • Wash and pat dry the area at each diaper change, using plain water or a mild soap and water. • Apply a thin barrier of cream or ointment such as zinc oxide. • Try switching to a different brand of diapers if you use disposable diapers. • Avoid diaper wipes because many contain perfume and alcohol. Use a washcloth with plain water instead. • Persistent diaper rash may require corticosteroids or anti-yeast treatments.
Medical help	See your health care provider if the above tips don't help; if the rash is purple or bruised-looking, crusty, blistered or weepy; or if your baby has a fever.

See back cover for online resource

Childhood rashes

Symptoms	Self-care	Seek medical help

Chickenpox

Itchy, red spots on the face or chest that spread to the arms and legs. Spots fill with a clear fluid to form blisters, rupture and turn crusty. New spots generally continue appearing over four to five days. Fever, a runny nose or cough often accompanies chickenpox. Chickenpox seldom lasts for more than two weeks after the first spot appears. Symptoms usually appear 14 to 21 days after exposure. The child is contagious until the rash heals.	• Give child cool baths every three or four hours to reduce the itching. Sprinkle baking soda in the bath water for added relief. • Apply a lubricating cream to the rash. • Switch to a bland diet of soft foods, and avoid citrus fruits if blisters are present in the mouth. • Trim fingernails. Put gloves on the child at night to prevent scratching.	• If the rash involves the eyes, or if a cough or shortness of breath develops. • If you're an older adult, have an impaired immune system, or are pregnant and have not been previously exposed. • An antiviral medication can shorten duration of the infection. In severe cases, a doctor may prescribe an antibiotic. A vaccine is recommended for children 12 months or older.

Roseola

Often begins with a high fever lasting about three days. When it subsides, a rash appears on the trunk and neck, lasting a few hours to a few days. The virus typically affects children, most often between 6 months and 3 years.	The rash causes little discomfort and disappears on its own without treatment. Acetaminophen may help relieve the discomfort caused by the fever.	• If the rash lasts longer than three days. • If the child has a convulsion triggered by the fever.

Measles

Typically begins with a fever, often as high as 104 to 105 F, and a cough, sneezing, sore throat and inflamed, watery eyes. Two to four days later, a rash appears. It often begins as fine red spots on the face and spreads to the trunk, arms and legs. Spots may become larger and usually last about a week. Small white spots may appear on inside lining of the cheeks.	• Bed rest, acetaminophen (Tylenol, others) and an over-the-counter cough medication may help relieve the discomfort. • Lukewarm baths, lubricant creams and antihistamines may relieve itching.	• If you suspect that you or a family member has measles. Measles has uncommon but potentially serious complications, such as pneumonia, encephalitis or a bacterial infection. • Anyone 12 months or older who has not had measles should receive the vaccine.

Fifth disease (parvovirus infection)

Bright red, raised patches appear on both cheeks. During the next few days, a pink, lacy, slightly raised rash develops on the arms, trunk, thighs and buttocks. The rash may come and go for up to three weeks. Often, there are no symptoms, or only mild, cold-like symptoms.	No specific treatment. You may use acetaminophen to relieve discomfort from the fever.	• If you aren't sure whether a rash is fifth disease. • If you're pregnant and suspect you've been exposed.

Common Problems

■ Lice

Louse

Lice are tiny parasitic insects. Head lice often are spread among children by contact, shared hats and clothing, combs, or hairbrushes. Body lice are generally spread through clothing or bedding. Pubic lice — commonly called crabs — can be spread by sexual contact, clothing, bedding or even toilet seats.

The first sign of lice is intense itching. With body lice, some people have hives and others have abrasions from scratching. Head lice are found on the scalp and are easiest to see at the nape of the neck and behind the ears. Small eggs (nits) that resemble tiny pussy willow buds can be found on the hair shafts. Body lice are difficult to find because they burrow into the skin, but they usually can be detected in the seams of underwear. Pubic lice are found on the skin and hair of the pubic areas. Lice live only one to two days off the body. Eggs hatch in a little over a week.

Self-care

- Several lotions and shampoos, both prescription and over-the-counter, are available. Apply the product to all infected and hairy parts of the body. Any remaining nits can be removed with tweezers or a fine nit comb used on wet hair. Repeat treatment with the lotion or shampoo in seven to 10 days.
- Treat all infected household members at the same time, and consider preventively treating others. Keep infected children home until you complete the first treatment.
- Wash sheets, clothing and hats with hot, soapy water and dry them at high heat. Soak combs and brushes in very hot, soapy water for at least five minutes.
- Vacuum carpets, mattresses, pillows, upholstered furniture and car seats.

Medical help

Consult your doctor before using products on a child younger than 2 months or if you're pregnant. The Food and Drug Administration (FDA) cautions that products containing lindane can cause serious side effects, even when used as directed.

■ Scabies

Almost impossible to see without a magnifying glass, **scabies** mites cause itching by burrowing under the skin. Itching is usually worse at night. The burrowing leaves tiny bumps and thin, snake-like tracks just under your skin. They appear most often in the following areas: between your fingers, in your armpits, around your waist, along the insides of your wrists, on the back of your elbows, on your ankles and the soles of your feet, around your breasts and genitals, and on your buttocks. Almost any part of the skin may be involved.

Close physical contact and, less often, sharing clothing or bedding with an infected person can spread these tiny mites. Often an entire family, members of a child care group or school class will experience scabies.

Self-care

Bathing and over-the-counter products won't get rid of scabies. Talk to your doctor if you have symptoms or believe you had contact with someone who has scabies.

Medical help

Your doctor may prescribe a medicated cream or lotion that you must apply all over your body and leave on overnight. All family members and sexual partners may require treatment. Sometimes oral prescription medications may be needed. In addition, all clothing and bedding that you used before treatment must be washed with hot, soapy water and dried with high heat or sealed in plastic bags for three days.

See back cover for online resource ⓘ

■ Psoriasis

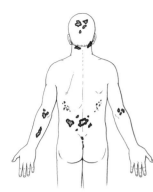

Some of the most common locations of psoriasis

For some people, **psoriasis** brings little more than recurrent bouts of mild itching, but for others, it's a lifetime of discomfort and unsightly skin changes. There are several types, including the type associated with arthritis, called psoriatic arthritis.

Most often, psoriasis causes dry, red patches covered with thick, silvery scales. You may see a few spots of scaling or large areas of damaged skin. The knees, elbows, trunk and scalp are the most common locations. Patches on your scalp can shed large quantities of silvery-white scales resembling severe dandruff.

In more-severe cases, pustules, cracked skin, itching, minor bleeding or aching joints also may develop. In addition, your fingernails and toenails may lose their normal luster and develop pits or ridges.

Many people inherit a tendency toward psoriasis. Dry skin, skin injuries, infections, certain drugs, obesity, stress and lack of sunlight can all aggravate your symptoms. This condition isn't contagious — you can't spread it to other parts of your own body, or to other people, simply by touching it. Psoriasis typically goes through cycles. The symptoms can persist for weeks or months, followed by a break.

Self-care

- Maintain good general health: a balanced diet, adequate rest and exercise.
- Maintain a normal weight. Psoriasis occurs often in skin creases or folds.
- Avoid scratching, rubbing or picking at the patches of psoriasis. Trauma worsens psoriasis.
- Bathe daily to soak off the scales. Avoid hot water or harsh soap.
- Keep your skin moist (see "Dryness," page 121).
- Use soaps, shampoos, cleansers or ointments containing coal tar or salicylic acid.
- Expose your skin to moderate sunlight, but avoid sunburn.
- Apply over-the-counter cortisone creams, 0.5 or 1 percent, for a few weeks when symptoms are especially bad.

Medical help

If self-care remedies don't help, stronger cortisone-type creams or phototherapy may be prescribed. Phototherapy involves a combination of medications and ultraviolet light. Skin ointments containing a form of vitamin D (Dovonex) also may offer some relief. In severe cases, the anti-inflammatory medication methotrexate or other oral drugs may be prescribed. Biologics may be given by infusion or injection. Discuss benefits and risks of medications for severe cases — some side effects can be serious.

■ Moles

Sometimes called beauty marks, **moles** (nevi) are usually harmless collections of pigment cells. They may contain hairs, stay smooth, become raised or wrinkled, and even fall off in old age.

In rare cases, a mole can become cancerous melanoma. Talk to your health care provider if pain, bleeding or inflammation occurs or if you notice a change in a mole (see "Signs of skin cancer," page 129). Keep an eye on moles located around your nails, hands, feet or genitals, and those present since birth. Giant moles, present at birth, may need to be removed to avoid the risk of cancer.

Self-care

Healthy moles usually don't require special care unless they become cut or irritated. Normal skin care is sufficient.

■ Shingles

Shingles (also known as herpes zoster) emerges when the virus that causes chicken-pox (varicella zoster) reactivates after lying dormant in your nerve cells for years.

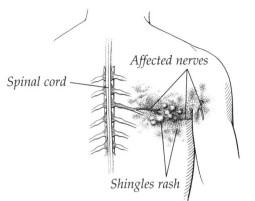

Spinal cord

Affected nerves

Shingles rash

The shingles rash is associated with an inflammation of nerves beneath the skin.

As this virus reactivates, you may notice pain, burning, numbness or tingling in a limited area, usually on one side of your body or face. These symptoms occur as the virus spreads along one of the nerves and can continue for several days or longer.

Then a rash with blisters typically appears and may continue to spread over the next few days. Typically the shingles rash develops as a band of blisters that wraps around one side of your back from your spine to your breastbone, abdomen or groin. Sometimes the rash occurs around one eye or on one side of the neck or face.

The blisters usually dry up in a few days, forming crusts that fall off over the next few weeks. The blisters contain a contagious virus, so avoid contact with others, especially people with weak immunity, pregnant women and newborns. Chickenpox in a newborn can be deadly.

Self-care

The shingles vaccine is recommended for all adults age 60 and older, whether or not they have had shingles previously. The vaccine is for prevention, not treatment. If you have shingles, you can relieve some discomfort by doing the following:

- Take a cool bath or soak your blisters with cool, wet compresses.
- Apply a lubricating cream or ointment.
- Take over-the-counter pain relievers to alleviate pain.
- Over-the-counter analgesic creams also may alleviate your pain.
- Shingles is only contagious after the rash appears and until it crusts (forms scabs).

Medical help

Contact your doctor if you suspect shingles, especially in the following situations:

- The pain and rash occur near your eyes. If left untreated, this infection can lead to permanent eye damage.
- You or someone in your family has a weakened immune system (due to cancer, medications or a chronic medical condition).
- The rash is widespread and painful.

Within the first three days, treatment with acyclovir (Zovirax), famciclovir or valacyclovir (Valtrex) may speed healing and reduce the severity of complications.

When the pain persists after shingles

Pain persisting for months or even years after a bout with shingles is called **postherpetic neuralgia** (PHN). PHN is as individual as you are, and effective treatment for you may be useless for someone else. But new treatments show promise, and new findings support the benefit of early treatment of the acute viral infection that precedes PHN.

Because the pain of PHN tends to lessen as time passes, it's difficult to tell whether a medication is effective or the pain is subsiding on its own.

Several treatments may provide relief, including analgesic medications, antidepressants, certain anti-convulsant medications and steroid injections. It may take a combination of treatments to reduce the pain.

    See back cover for online resource ⓘ

■ Signs of skin cancer

Each year, nonmelanoma **skin cancer** is diagnosed in millions of people in the United States. An additional 87,000 people are diagnosed each year with melanoma, and about 10,000 people die of their cancer each year. Most skin cancers are sun-related or from tanning lights. Other risk factors include a genetic tendency, chemical pollution and X-ray radiation.

Here are the signs of the three most common types of skin cancer:

Basal cell cancer, by far the most common skin cancer, usually appears as a smooth, waxy or pearly bump that grows slowly and rarely spreads or causes death.

Squamous cell cancer causes a firm, nodular or flat growth with a crusted, ulcerated or scaly surface on the face, ears, neck, hands or arms.

Melanoma is the most serious but least common skin cancer.

The **ABCD** guideline below can help you tell a normal mole from one that could be cancer. **Also remember "E" for evolving.** Changes over time, such as fast growth, changes in color or shape, bleeding, or nonhealing sores could be signs of cancer.

A

B

C

D

Asymmetrical in shape: Half of the lesion is unlike the other half.

Border is irregular (ragged, notched or blurred).

Color varies from one area to another. It may have many colors or an uneven distribution of color.

Diameter is larger than the head of a pencil eraser (¼ inch, or 6 millimeters).

Self-care

- Avoid a sunburn or a suntan. Both result in skin damage, which accumulates over time. Minimize your time in the sun and wear tightly woven clothing and a broad-brimmed hat. Snow, water, ice and concrete reflect the sun's harmful rays, and you can get sunburned on a cloudy day.
- Use sunscreen regularly and year-round. Apply a broad-spectrum sunscreen (protects against UVA and UVB rays) with a sun protection factor (SPF) of at least 30. Apply 20 to 30 minutes before sun exposure. Reapply every two hours and after swimming or sweating.
- Use 1 ounce of sunscreen per application — about 2 tablespoons.
- Avoid tanning salons.
- Check your skin monthly for the development of new skin growths or changes in existing moles, freckles, bumps and birthmarks.

Medical help

If you notice a new growth, change in skin or sore that doesn't heal in two weeks, see your doctor. You may need a skin biopsy. Skin cancers usually are not painful. The cure rate is high if you get treated early. Typically, treatment is outpatient surgery, and a local anesthetic is given. If you have a family history of melanoma or many moles, get regular exams by a dermatologist.

Kids' care

Severe, blistering sunburns as a child increase the risk of melanoma as an adult. Set time limits when at the pool or beach. Ultraviolet rays are strongest between 10 a.m. and 4 p.m. For babies under 6 months, limit sun exposure, and dress them appropriately to prevent sunburn. If necessary, apply sunscreen (at least SPF 30) containing zinc oxide or titanium dioxide and reapply every two hours. Don't use products that mix sunscreens with insect repellents.

 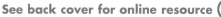

Warts

Warts are skin growths caused by a common virus, but they can be painful and disfiguring and can spread to other individuals.

There are more than 200 types of warts. They can appear on any part of your body, but they are most common on the hands or feet. Warts found on the feet, called plantar warts, can be painful because they press inward as you stand on them.

You can acquire warts through direct contact with an infected person or surface, such as a shower floor. The virus that causes them stimulates the rapid growth of cells on the outer layer of your skin.

Each person's immune system responds to warts differently. Most warts aren't a serious health hazard and disappear without treatment. Warts are more common among children than adults, likely because many adults develop immunity to them. In adults, warts generally disappear within two years.

Certain warts trigger or signal more-serious medical problems. Genital warts require treatment to avoid spreading them through sexual contact. Some strains of human papillomavirus increase cancer risk, including cancers of the cervix, throat and anus. Women also can pass this virus to their babies during birth, causing complications.

Self-care

- Over-the-counter topical medications may remove warts of the hands and feet. Look for products containing salicylic acid, which peels off the infected skin. They require daily use, often for a few weeks. **Caution:** The acid can irritate or damage normal skin.
- To avoid spreading warts to other parts of your body, avoid touching, brushing, combing or shaving areas with warts.

Medical help

You may want to see your health care provider if your warts are a cosmetic nuisance or interfere with your activities. Common treatments for warts include freezing with liquid nitrogen or dry ice, electrical burning, laser surgery, or various topical treatments.

Wrinkled skin

Skin wrinkles

Wrinkles are an inevitable part of aging. As you grow older, your skin gets thinner, drier and less elastic. Sagging and wrinkling begin because connective tissue in your skin deteriorates. Some people don't seem to age as quickly as others. This difference is typically due to heredity and avoiding extensive sun exposure. Cosmetic products that promise youthful skin are often expensive and fail to deliver improvements.

Self-care

There's no cure for wrinkled skin. These measures may help slow the process:
- Maintain good general health.
- Don't smoke cigarettes.
- Avoid prolonged exposure to the sun. Use sunscreen daily and year-round.
- Avoid harsh soaps and hot water when bathing.

Medical help

Prescription medical treatments such as retinoic acid creams may be helpful for treating fine lines. Injection of botulinum toxin type A (Botox) or various soft tissue fillers are also used to reduce the appearance of wrinkles. Cosmetic procedures such as chemical peels, dermabrasion or lasers are sometimes used. Ask your doctor about the benefits and risks of the different options.

■ Hair loss

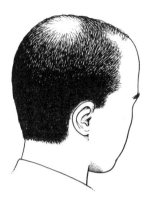

Male-pattern baldness typically appears first at the hairline or crown.

Healthy, lustrous hair has long been a symbol of youth and beauty. As a result, many people cringe at the first signs of hair thinning or baldness.

If your hair seems to be thinning, take comfort in the fact that it's normal to lose between 50 and 100 strands a day. Like your nails and skin, your hair goes through a cycle of growth and rest. Gradual thinning occurs as a normal part of the aging process.

Common **baldness**, which is largely hereditary, affects both men and women. Male-pattern baldness usually begins with thinning at the hairline, followed by moderate to extensive hair loss on the crown of the head. In contrast, bald patches rarely develop in women with common baldness. Instead, the hair thins all over the head, especially on top. Hormones and age also play roles in common baldness.

Gradual hair loss can also occur any time your hair's delicate growth cycle is upset. Diet, medications, hormones, pregnancy, improper hair care, poor nutrition, underlying diseases and other factors can cause too many follicles to rest at once, producing diffuse thinning.

Sudden patches of hair loss are usually due to a condition called alopecia areata. This fairly rare condition causes smooth, circular bald patches that may overlap. Stress and heredity may play a role in this disorder. Alopecia areata generally resolves without treatment over a period of weeks to years.

Self-care

There's no magic bullet to prevent hair loss or encourage new growth, but the following tips can help keep your hair healthy:

- Eat a nutritionally balanced diet.
- Handle your hair gently. Whenever possible, allow your hair to air-dry naturally and avoid styling with heat.
- Avoid tight hairstyles such as braids, buns or ponytails.
- Avoid compulsively twisting, rubbing or pulling your hair.
- Check with hair care experts about hairpieces or styling techniques that help minimize the effects of common baldness.
- An over-the-counter medication called minoxidil (Rogaine) can promote new hair growth in a small percentage of people. Other over-the-counter hair growth products are of no proven benefit.

Medical help

Although there's no cure for common baldness, you may want to ask your health care provider about medical treatments or hair replacement surgery. Because sudden hair loss can signal an underlying medical condition that may require treatment, contact your physician for evaluation.

Kids' care

If your child has patches of broken hairs on the scalp or eyebrows, he or she may be rubbing or pulling out the hair. This signals a behavioral disorder called trichotillomania. Bald patches in children can also be a sign of a fungal infection or ringworm. Contact your health care provider for evaluation.

Common Problems

Nail fungal infections

Typical fungal infection

This stubborn, but harmless, problem often begins as a tiny white or yellow spot on your nail. Fungal infections can develop on your nails or under their outer edges if you continually expose them to a warm, moist environment. Depending on the type of fungus, your nails may discolor, thicken and develop crumbling edges or cracks.

Fungal infections usually affect your toenails more frequently than your fingernails and are more common among older adults. Your risk of a toenail fungal infection is greater if your feet perspire heavily, and if you wear socks and shoes that hinder ventilation and don't absorb perspiration. You can also contract this infection by walking barefoot in public places and as a complication of other infections.

Fingernail fungal infections often result from overexposure to water and detergents. Moisture caught under artificial nails also can encourage fungus growth.

Self-care

To help prevent **nail fungal infections**, try the following:
- Keep your nails dry and clean. Dry your feet thoroughly after bathing.
- Change your socks often and wear leather-soled shoes.
- Use an antifungal spray or powder on your feet and inside your shoes.
- Don't pick at or trim the skin around your nails.
- Avoid walking barefoot around public pools, showers and locker rooms.

Medical help

Self-care measures usually fail to prevent the infection. Oral antifungal medications such as griseofulvin, itraconazole, terbinafine and fluconazole are more effective than topical drugs, but they can cause side effects. Their use requires careful monitoring. In severe cases, surgical removal of the nail may be necessary.

Ingrown toenails

Pain and tenderness in your toe often signal an **ingrown toenail**. This common condition occurs when the sharp end or side of your toenail grows into the flesh of your toe. It affects your big toe most often, especially if you have curved toenails, if your shoes fit poorly or if you cut your nails improperly.

Self-care

- Trim your toenails straight across and not too short.
- Wear socks and shoes that fit properly, and don't place excessive pressure on your toes. Wear open-toe shoes, if necessary, or try sandals.
- Soak your feet in warm salt water (1 teaspoon salt per pint of water) for 15 to 20 minutes twice a day to reduce swelling and relieve tenderness.
- After soaking, put tiny bits of sterile cotton or dental floss under the ingrown edge. This will help the nail eventually grow above the skin edge. Change daily until the pain and redness subside.
- Apply an antibiotic ointment to the tender area.
- If there's severe pain, take a nonprescription pain reliever and make an appointment to see your doctor.

Medical help

If you experience severe discomfort or pus or redness that seems to be spreading, seek medical attention. Your doctor may need to remove the ingrown portion of the nail and prescribe antibiotics.

See back cover for online resource (i)

Throat and mouth

■ Sore throat

The tight, scratchy feeling in your throat may be a familiar sign that a **cold** or the flu (**influenza**) is on the way. Most sore throats run their course in a few days, sometimes needing over-the-counter lozenges or gargles.

Most sore throats are caused by two types of infections — viral and bacterial — but they can also be caused by allergies, dry air and problems with acid reflux. When a sore throat involves enlarged, tender tonsils, it's sometimes called tonsillitis.

Viral infections usually are the source of common colds and the flu and the sore throat that accompanies them. Colds usually go away on their own in about a week, once your system has built up antibodies that destroy the virus. Antibiotic medications are *not* effective in treating viral infections. Common signs and symptoms include:

- Sore or scratchy, dry feeling
- Coughing and sneezing
- Mild fever or no fever
- Hoarseness
- Runny nose and postnasal dripping

Bacterial infections aren't as common as viral infections, but they can be more serious. **Strep throat** is the most common bacterial infection. Often a person with strep was exposed to someone else with strep throat in the past two to seven days. Generally it's spread by nose or throat secretions. Strep throat requires medical treatment. Common signs and symptoms are:

- Swollen tonsils and lymph nodes
- Back of throat is bright red with white patches
- Fever, often more than 101 F, and often accompanied by chills
- Pain when swallowing

Most sore throat germs are passed by direct contact. Mucus and saliva from one person's hands are transferred to objects, doorknobs and other surfaces, then to your hands, and eventually to your mouth or nose.

Mononucleosis: A tiresome illness

Infectious **mononucleosis** is sometimes called the kissing disease. It's also known as mono, and it can be spread by kissing or, more commonly, through exposure resulting from coughing, sneezing, or sharing a glass or cup.

Mono is caused by the Epstein-Barr virus. It's believed that most adults between ages 35 and 40 have been exposed to the Epstein-Barr virus and have built up antibodies. Full-blown mono is most common during adolescence and young adulthood. Children infected with the virus before age 15 may have only a mild flu-like illness.

Most people with mono experience fatigue and weakness. Other signs and symptoms include a sore throat, fever, swollen lymph nodes in the neck and underarms, swollen tonsils, headache, rash, and loss of appetite. Most symptoms abate within 10 days, but you shouldn't expect to return to your normal activities or contact sports for three weeks or longer (your liver or spleen may be enlarged and at risk of injury). It may be two to three months before you feel completely normal.

Rest and a healthy diet are the primary treatments for mono. Review with your doctor if other treatments are recommended. If symptoms linger more than a week or two or if they recur, see your doctor.

Self-care

- **Double your fluid intake.** Fluids help keep your mucus thin and easy to clear.
- **Gargle with warm salt water.** Mix about ½ teaspoon of salt with a glass of warm water to gargle and spit. This will soothe and help clear your throat of mucus.
- **Suck on a lozenge or hard candy, or chew sugarless gum.** Chewing and sucking stimulate saliva production, which bathes and cleanses your throat.
- **Take pain relievers.** Over-the-counter medications, such as acetaminophen (Tylenol, others), ibuprofen (Advil, Motrin IB, others) and aspirin, relieve sore throat pain for four to six hours (see page 258).
- **Rest your voice.** If your sore throat has affected your voice box (larynx), talking may lead to more irritation and temporary loss of your voice, called laryngitis.
- **Humidify the air.** Adding moisture to the air prevents your mucous membranes from drying out. This can reduce irritation and make it easier to sleep. Saline nasal sprays also are helpful.
- **Avoid smoke and other air pollutants.** Smoke irritates a sore throat. Stop smoking, and avoid all smoke and fumes from household cleaners or paint. Keep children away from secondhand smoke exposure.

Prevention

- Wash your hands frequently, especially during the cold and flu season.
- Keep your hands away from your face to avoid getting bacteria and viruses into your mouth or nose.

Medical help

Serious throat infections, such as epiglottitis, can cause swelling that closes your airway. Seek emergency care if your sore throat is accompanied by any of the following signs and symptoms:

- Drooling or difficulty swallowing or breathing
- A stiff, rigid neck and severe headache
- A temperature higher than 101 F in babies under age 6 months and 103 F in older children
- A rash
- Persistent hoarseness or mouth ulcers lasting two weeks or more
- Recent exposure to strep throat

If your doctor suspects strep throat, a throat swab may be ordered. For this test a cotton swab is rubbed against the back of your throat, and secretions on the swab are analyzed in a laboratory. A rapid strep test can give an initial result within an hour. However, it misses up to 30 percent of strep cases. So it's often necessary to do a traditional throat culture, which takes one to two days for a confirmed result. There is a DNA strep test that provides a final, confirmed result in about eight hours. If the test is positive, an antibiotic is typically prescribed.

Generally only in cases of recurrent infection that cause serious problems will removal of the tonsils (tonsillectomy) be considered.

Caution

If your doctor does prescribe a medication, take it for the full time indicated. Stopping use of the medication early could lead to recurrence and the development of resistant organisms, as well as complications such as rheumatic fever or a blood infection.

If your child has been taking antibiotics for at least 24 hours, has no fever and feels better, it's usually OK for him or her to return to school or child care.

■ Bad breath

Everyone would like to have breath that's always fresh. Because fresh breath is important to people, makers of mints and mouthwashes sell millions of dollars' worth of products every year. These products are only temporarily helpful for controlling **bad breath**. They actually may be less effective than simply rinsing your mouth with water, brushing and flossing your teeth, and increasing hydration.

There are many causes of bad breath. First, your mouth itself may be the source. Bacterial breakdown of food particles and other debris in and around your teeth can cause a foul odor. A dry mouth, such as occurs during sleep or as the result of some drugs or smoking, enables dead cells to accumulate on your tongue, gums and cheeks. As a result, they decompose and cause odor.

Eating foods containing oils with a strong odor causes bad breath. Onions and garlic are the best examples, but other vegetables and spices also may cause bad breath.

Lung disease can cause bad breath. Chronic infections in the lungs can produce very foul-smelling breath. Usually, much of the mucus you cough up (sputum) is produced by these conditions. Several illnesses can cause a distinctive breath odor. Kidney failure can cause a urine-like odor, and liver failure may cause a musty sweet breath odor. People with diabetes often have a fruity breath odor. This smell is also common in ill children who have eaten poorly for a few days. Bad breath in these situations can be corrected by treatment of the underlying condition.

Self-care

For most people, bad breath can be improved by following a few simple steps:
- Brush your teeth after every meal.
- Brush or scrape your tongue to remove dead cells.
- Floss once a day to remove food particles from between your teeth.
- Drink plenty of water (not coffee, pop or alcohol) to keep your mouth moist.
- Avoid strong foods that cause bad breath. Tooth paste and mouthwash only partially disguise odors of garlic or onion that come from your lungs.
- Change your toothbrush every two to three months.
- Rinse your mouth after using inhaler medications.
- If after trying these approaches your breath is still bad, talk to your dentist.

■ Hoarseness or loss of voice

Hoarseness or loss of voice (**laryngitis**) occurs when your vocal cords become swollen or inflamed and no longer vibrate normally. They produce an unnatural sound, or they may not produce any sound at all.

Your speaking voice is formed when the muscle above your stomach (diaphragm) pushes air from your lungs through your vocal cords. The controlled escape of air vibrates the vocal cords, producing the sound that's your voice.

In addition to hoarseness, you may feel pain when speaking or have a raw and scratchy throat. Sometimes, your voice sounds higher or lower than normal.

Common causes of hoarseness or loss of voice are infections (as a result, you may lose your voice when you have a cold or flu), allergies, talking too loudly for too long or yelling (vocal strain), smoking, not rinsing a steroid inhaler after use, and chronic esophageal reflux. Reflux — the backwash of acidic stomach contents into the food pipe — can sometimes spill into the voice box.

Common Problems

| **Self-care** | • Limit your talking and whispering. Whispering strains your vocal cords as much as talking.
• Drink lots of warm, noncaffeinated fluids to keep your throat moist.
• Avoid clearing your throat.
• Stop smoking and avoid exposure to smoke. Smoke dries your throat and irritates your vocal cords.
• Stop drinking alcohol, which also dries your throat and irritates your vocal cords.
• Use a humidifier to moisturize the air you breathe. Follow the manufacturer's instructions to clean the humidifier and prevent bacterial buildup. |
|---|---|
| **Medical help** | If hoarseness lasts for more than two to four weeks, seek medical help. Your doctor may prescribe medications for infection or allergy. |

◼ Mouth sores

Irritating, painful and repetitive. That's how many people describe canker sores and cold sores. But the terminology can be confusing. Cold sores have nothing to do with the common cold. What's more, the cause, appearance, symptoms and treatments of canker sores and cold sores are very different. Other mouth sores and conditions are often mistaken for canker sores and cold sores.

◼ Canker sores

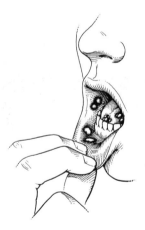

A **canker sore** is an ulcer on the soft tissue inside your mouth — on the tongue, soft palate, inside part of the lips or inside the cheeks. Typically, you notice a burning sensation and a round whitish spot with a red edge or halo. Pain usually lessens in a few days.

Despite a great deal of research into the problem, the cause of canker sores remains a mystery. Current thinking suggests that stress or tissue injury may cause the eruption of common canker sores. Some researchers believe certain nutritional deficiencies or food sensitivities may complicate the problem. In addition, some gastrointestinal and immune deficiency disorders have been linked to canker sores, as well as some medications, including nonsteroidal anti-inflammatory drugs and beta blockers.

The two most common types of canker sores are major and minor. Minor canker sores are the more common of the two and are usually small and oval shaped with a red edge. This type of canker sore heals without scarring in one to two weeks.

Major canker sores are larger and deeper than minor canker sores. They are usually round with defined borders, but may have irregular edges when very large. These canker sores can be extremely painful. They may take up to six weeks to heal and can leave extensive scarring.

Self-care

Treatment usually isn't necessary for minor canker sores, which tend to clear on their own in a week or two. But large, persistent or painful sores often need care. The following suggestions may provide temporary relief:

- Avoid abrasive, acidic or spicy foods, which may increase the pain.
- Brush your teeth carefully to avoid irritating the sore.
- Try an over-the-counter topical product that contains a numbing agent, such as Orabase, Anbesol and Orajel.
- Rinse your mouth with over-the-counter preparations.
- Use an over-the-counter pain reliever.

Medical help

For severe attacks of canker sores, your dentist or doctor may recommend a prescription mouthwash, a corticosteroid salve or an anesthetic solution called viscous lidocaine.

Contact your doctor in any of the following situations:

- High fever with canker sores
- Spreading sores or signs of spreading infection
- Pain that's not controlled with the measures listed above
- Sores that don't heal completely within a week

See your dentist if you have sharp tooth surfaces or dental appliances that are causing sores.

■ Cold sores (fever blisters)

Also known as fever blisters, cold sores are very common. They may appear on your mouth, lips, nose, cheeks or fingers.

The herpes simplex virus causes **cold sores**. Herpes simplex virus type 1 usually causes cold sores. Herpes simplex virus type 2 is usually responsible for genital herpes. However, either form of the virus can cause sores in the facial area or on the genitals. You can get cold sores from another person who has an active condition. Eating utensils, razors, towels and direct skin contact are common means of spreading this infection.

Symptoms may not start for as long as 20 days after you were exposed to the virus. Small, fluid-filled blisters develop on a raised, red, painful area of skin. Pain or tingling (prodromal stage) often precedes blisters by one to two days. Cold sores typically clear up in seven to 10 days.

After the first infection, the virus periodically re-emerges. Fever, menstruation, stress, oral trauma and exposure to the sun may trigger a recurrence.

The herpes simplex virus can be transmitted even when blisters aren't present. But the greatest risk of infection is from the time the blister appears until it has completely crusted over. Cold sores occur most often in adolescents and young adults, but they can occur at any age. Outbreaks decrease after age 35.

Self-care

Cold sores generally clear up without treatment. These steps may provide relief:

- Rest, take over-the-counter (OTC) pain relievers (if you have a fever) or use OTC creams for comfort (they won't speed healing).
- Don't squeeze, pinch or pick at any blister.
- Avoid kissing and skin contact with people while blisters are present.
- Wash your hands carefully before touching another person.
- Use sunblock on your lips and face before prolonged exposure to the sun — during both the winter and the summer — to prevent cold sores.

Medical help	If you have frequent bouts of cold sores, an antiviral medication may help. These medications inhibit the growth of the herpes virus. The topical antiviral medication penciclovir (Denavir), available as a cream, also has shown some benefit in treating cold sores. Talk with your health care provider to learn more about treatment options if you have multiple episodes during a year. You may feel a tingling sensation before the outbreak of a cold sore. Many doctors recommend using medication as soon as the tingling begins.
Caution	• If you have a cold sore, take special care to avoid contact with infants or anyone who has a skin condition known as eczema (see page 121). They're more susceptible to infection. Also, avoid people who are taking medications for cancer and organ transplantation because they have decreased immunity. The virus can cause a life-threatening condition in them. • Pregnant women and nursing mothers should avoid using antivirals, such as acyclovir (Zovirax) or penciclovir (Denavir), for treatment of cold sores unless specifically advised by their doctors to use it. • Herpes simplex virus infections have potentially serious complications. The virus can spread to your eye. This is the most frequent cause of corneal blindness in the United States. If you have a burning pain in the eye or a rash near the eye or on the tip of your nose, see your doctor immediately.

■ Other oral infections and disorders

Oral thrush. **Oral thrush** (candidiasis) is an infection that's caused by a fungus. Symptoms may include creamy-white soft patches in your mouth or throat, lesions with a cottage cheese-like appearance, pain, slight bleeding if the lesions are rubbed or scraped, cracking at the corners of your mouth, a cottony feeling in your mouth, or loss of taste. It often occurs when your body is weakened by illness or when your mouth's natural balance of microbes has been upset by medications.

Oral thrush is most common among babies, young children and older adults. In addition, risk is increased if you smoke, have lowered immunity, wear dentures, have other health conditions (such as diabetes or anemia), take certain medications (such as antibiotics or oral or inhaled corticosteroids), are having chemotherapy or radiation treatment for cancer, or have conditions that cause dry mouth.

Although painful, oral thrush isn't a serious disorder. It can, however, interfere with eating. There's no self-care for this condition, but a dentist or physician can prescribe an oral medication that is taken for seven to 10 days. Thrush tends to recur.

Leukoplakia. Thickened, white patches on a cheek or the tongue are often signs of **leukoplakia**. Leukoplakia is the mouth's reaction to chronic irritation. It may be caused by ill-fitting dentures or a rough tooth rubbing against the cheek or gum. When white patches develop in the mouths of smokers, the condition is called smoker's keratosis. Snuff and chewing tobacco also produce chronic irritation. Tobacco use can lead to oral cancer.

You can have leukoplakia at any age, but it's most common among older adults. Treatment involves removing the source of irritation. Once that's done, the patch may clear up. A doctor or dentist should evaluate white patches in the mouth. If the white patches don't clear up, a biopsy may be needed — in some instances leukoplakia may be precancerous or early signs of cancer.

See back cover for online resource ⓘ

Oral cancer. Oral cancer includes cancer of the lips, mouth, tongue, gums and tonsils. The tumors often are painless at first and frequently are visible or can be felt with a finger. The standard oral cancer screening is a visual inspection of all areas inside the mouth. A screening should be done every time you see a dentist or periodontist, who looks for abnormal white or red patches that could become cancerous.

Other signs and symptoms of oral cancer include:

- Bleeding in the mouth or a sore that doesn't heal
- Lump or thickening of the skin in your jaw, neck or lining of your mouth
- Loose teeth
- Problems wearing dentures
- Tongue pain
- Jaw pain or stiffness
- Difficult or painful chewing
- Difficult or painful swallowing
- Sore throat

Many people have abnormal sores in their mouths, with the great majority being noncancerous. While the incidence is smaller than many other cancers, it's often a deadly disease.

Tobacco use and heavy alcohol use are risk factors for oral cancer. Age is a factor, too. Most oral cancers occur in people age 45 or older. Sun exposure is a risk factor for oral cancer that occurs on the lips.

Increasingly, younger adults who aren't smokers or heavy drinkers are developing oral cancer. This group has a high incidence of the sexually transmitted human papillomavirus (HPV), which has been linked to an increased risk of oral cancer.

Every time you see your dental care provider, make sure he or she looks for signs of oral cancer. An oral lesion that persists for more than two weeks should be evaluated. Like all cancers, oral cancer is most successfully treated when it's caught early.

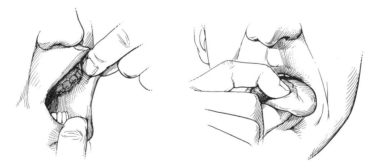

Routine self-examination of your mouth and tongue may enable you to see or feel an oral cancer when it's small and treatment may be most effective.

Men's health

■ Testicular pain

Any sharp and sudden pain in your testicles should be treated carefully because it can be a symptom of a serious medical condition. Seek medical help if you have sudden pain in your testicles that doesn't go away in 10 or 15 minutes or if you have pain that recurs. Some causes of sudden testicular pain are discussed below.

Testicular torsion is caused when the spermatic cord, which carries blood to and from the testicle, gets twisted. This twisting cuts off the blood supply to the testicle, causing sharp and sudden pain. Testicular torsion sometimes occurs after strenuous physical activity, but it can happen with no apparent cause, even during sleep. This condition can occur at any age, but it usually occurs in boys. Symptoms include sudden and severe pain, which can cause fever, nausea and vomiting. You may also notice the elevation of one testicle within the scrotum. Testicular torsion is serious and requires immediate medical attention.

Epididymitis occurs when the epididymis, a coiled tube that carries sperm from the testicles to the spermatic cord, becomes inflamed, usually by a bacterial infection. Symptoms include aching to moderately severe pain in the scrotum, which develops over several hours or days. Fever and swelling also may occur. Epididymitis is occasionally caused by chlamydia or gonorrhea (see page 185). In these cases, your sexual partner may be infected and also should receive a medical exam.

Orchitis is an inflammation of the testicle, usually due to an infection. Orchitis frequently occurs with epididymitis (see above). Orchitis may occur when you have the mumps, or it may develop if you have a prostate infection. Orchitis is rare, but it may cause infertility if left untreated. Signs and symptoms include pain in the scrotum, swelling (usually on one side of the scrotum) and a feeling of weight in the scrotum.

Screening for cancer of the testicle

Testicular cancer accounts for less than 1 percent of cancers in men, occurring most often in young men between the ages of 20 and 39. Signs and symptom include a lump, swelling or heavy feeling in a testicle.

A simple two-minute self-examination each month can help detect early signs of testicular cancer. Perform the examination after a shower or warm bath, when the skin of your scrotum is loose and relaxed. Examine one testicle at a time. Roll it gently between your thumbs and forefingers, feeling for any lump on the surface of the testicle. Also pay attention if the testicle is enlarged, hardened or otherwise in a different condition from the last examination. If you notice anything unusual, it may not necessarily mean cancer, but you should contact your doctor.

Don't be alarmed if you feel a small, firm area near the rear of the testicle and a tube leading up from the testicle. This is normal. These are the epididymis and the spermatic cord, which store and transport sperm.

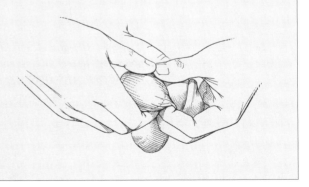

■ Enlarged prostate

The prostate is a walnut-sized gland in males, beneath the bladder, that produces semen. Testosterone, the male sex hormone, causes the prostate to slowly enlarge with age. As the prostate enlarges, some men develop bothersome symptoms.

Signs and symptoms of **prostate gland enlargement** (benign prostatic hyperplasia, or BPH) may include a weak or slow urine stream, trouble starting urination, stopping and starting while urinating, dribbling at the end of urination, frequent and sometimes urgent need to urinate, frequent nighttime voiding, dribbling after voiding, or voiding twice in a row within minutes.

Prostate gland enlargement rarely causes problems before age 40. More than half the men in their 60s and as many as 90 percent in their 70s and 80s experience symptoms of BPH. Some men with BPH may need treatment for the condition.

An enlarged prostate can produce difficulty with urination because the flow of urine is restricted.

Bladder — Rectum — Normal prostate

Bladder — Rectum — Enlarged prostate

Medical help

Your health care provider may ask you detailed questions about your symptoms and may do tests on urine and blood samples. Using a gloved, lubricated finger, your health care provider may examine your prostate for enlargement and lumps. Called the digital rectal examination, this procedure causes only mild discomfort.

Initial treatment for an enlarged prostate may be medications that reduce the size of the prostate gland or improve urine flow by relaxing the tissues in the prostate gland. Various types of surgery can reduce the size of the prostate.

Screening for prostate cancer

Cancer of the prostate is the third-leading cause of cancer death in American men. The risk of **prostate cancer** increases with age.

Prostate cancer is the most treatable when it's detected early. Symptoms are sometimes similar to those of prostate enlargement, such as trouble urinating, starting and stopping while urinating, or decreased force in the urine stream. Other signs include blood in your urine or semen. However, many men may have no noticeable early symptoms. Warning signs that prostate cancer has spread may include swelling in your legs, discomfort in the pelvic area, bone pain that doesn't go away, bone fractures or compression of the spine.

Screening for prostate cancer typically involves digital rectal examination and a blood test for prostate-specific antigen (PSA). Professional organizations vary in their recommendations about the PSA screening test. The American Cancer Society and Mayo Clinic urologists recommend that men at average risk discuss prostate screening with their doctors beginning at age 50.

If you're at increased risk of prostate cancer — you're black or you have a family history of the disease or of genes that increase your risk of breast cancer (BRCA1 or BRCA2) — it's recommended that screening begin earlier. A transrectal ultrasound may be needed if other tests raise concerns.

Common Problems

■ Prostatitis

Prostatitis, a disease of the prostate gland, can cause pain in the groin, painful urination, difficulty urinating and related symptoms. Prostatitis is an inflammation of the prostate gland, due to an infection or another factor that's irritating the gland. Although many things are unclear about the disease, an accurate diagnosis is crucial to successful treatment. There are four categories of prostatitis:

Acute bacterial prostatitis. This severe form of prostatitis results from an infection in the prostate gland that produces severe and often sudden signs and symptoms, such as high fever, chills, nausea, vomiting and a general feeling of being unwell. Bacteria found in the urinary tract or large intestine are often the cause.

Chronic bacterial prostatitis. This form also results from bacterial infection, but symptoms typically develop slower and are often less severe. The cause often isn't clear, but it may result from bacteria in your urinary tract, a bladder infection or a blood infection. It may also follow trauma to your urinary tract or insertion of an instrument such as a catheter or cystoscope.

Chronic prostatitis/chronic pelvic pain syndrome. The most common form of prostatitis, it's also the most difficult to diagnose and treat. The symptoms may be similar to chronic bacterial prostatitis, but there's no evidence of bacteria, and white blood cells identified in urine specimens may signal the presence of inflammation. Possible causes include other infectious agents, heavy lifting, occupations or hobbies that irritate the gland, structural abnormalities of the urinary tract, or other reasons.

Asymptomatic inflammatory prostatitis. This form is usually found during an examination that's done for another reason. It often doesn't require treatment.

Medical help

If you have signs or symptoms of prostatitis, see your doctor, who can determine whether you need to see a urologist. Bacterial prostatitis is treated with antibiotics. Left untreated, acute bacterial prostatitis can cause serious problems, including an inability to urinate. Without treatment, chronic bacterial prostatitis can lead to a serious infection. Chronic prostatitis tends to be frustrating and efforts may focus on therapies to help manage symptoms, including medications.

■ Erectile dysfunction (ED)

Occasional episodes of **erectile dysfunction** (ED) are common in men. Formerly called impotence, ED is the inability to obtain or maintain a firm erection long enough to have sex. When ED is a recurring problem, it may affect self-image and relationships. Fortunately, it can be treated successfully.

ED is more often caused by physical problems than by psychological ones. Clogged blood vessels (atherosclerosis) may cause ED. If you have ED, you may be at increased risk of heart disease, especially if you have risk factors, such as high blood pressure. ED can also be a side effect of excessive alcohol use and some medications (such as some drugs used to treat high blood pressure). ED can be caused by obesity and diseases such as diabetes or multiple sclerosis or other chronic diseases. Surgeries or injuries that affect the pelvic area or spinal cord may result in ED. There are numerous other possible physical causes. Also, stress, anxiety or depression can lead to ED or worsen it. If ED is recurrent or persistent, discuss it with your doctor.

See back cover for online resource ⓘ

Self-care	If you can still get an erection at certain times of the day, such as the morning, you may benefit from the following advice:
	• Limit alcohol consumption, especially before sexual activity.
	• Quit smoking.
	• Exercise regularly.
	• Reduce stress.
	• Work with your partner to create an atmosphere conducive to sexual relations.

Medical help	**Medications.** Pills, such as sildenafil (Viagra), tadalafil (Cialis) or vardenafil (Levitra), or testosterone injections or topical cream may be prescribed by your doctor.
	Penile injections. If ED is caused by decreased blood supply to the penis, medications that increase blood flow may be prescribed. They're injected into the penis. The injections can be performed at home after training by your doctor.
	Intraurethral medication. A small suppository — half the size of a grain of rice — is slid into the opening of the penis to help achieve an erection.
	Vacuum constriction device. A tube is placed over the penis, and air is withdrawn, creating a vacuum. As a result, blood flows to the penis and causes an erection. A rubber constricting band is placed around the base of the penis to prolong the erection. This low-cost device is available at most drugstores with a doctor's prescription.
	Surgery. Surgery can be performed to increase blood flow to the penis or to implant devices to help in achieving an erection.
	Psychological treatment. If stress, anxiety or depression is the cause of ED, you may want to seek counseling with a mental health professional or a sex therapist, either alone or with your partner.

■ Male birth control

Vasectomy involves cutting and sealing the vas deferens, the tube that carries sperm. The procedure doesn't interfere with your ability to maintain an erection or reach orgasm, nor does it stop the production of male hormones or of sperm in the testicles. The only change is that the sperm's link to the outside is severed permanently. After a vasectomy, you continue to ejaculate about the same amount of semen because sperm account for only a small part of the ejaculate.

A vasectomy is usually done in an outpatient setting while you're awake. Before the procedure, you'll be given an injection of anesthetic in the scrotum to numb the area so that you won't feel pain. A pair of small cuts are made in the skin of the scrotum. Each of the tubes that carry semen (vas deferens) is then pulled through the opening until it forms a loop. A very small section is cut out of each vas deferens and removed. The two ends of each vas deferens are closed by stitches or cauterization (or both) and are placed back in the scrotum. The incisions are closed with stitches.

The surgery usually takes about 20 to 30 minutes. After a vasectomy, avoid strenuous activity, including intercourse, for at least two weeks. The stitches often are the type that dissolve in three to four weeks. You may notice swelling and minor discomfort in the scrotum for several weeks. If the pain is severe or if fever develops, call your doctor.

The failure rate for a vasectomy is less than 1 percent. Until your doctor has determined that your ejaculate doesn't contain sperm, continue to use another form of birth control. This typically takes several months and more than 10 ejaculations.

Women's health

■ Lump in your breast

Most breast lumps aren't cancerous. Even so, all lumps should be carefully assessed because of the risk of cancer. Many breast lumps are fluid-filled cysts that enlarge near the end of your monthly cycle. The lumps may or may not be painful. Many doctors encourage breast self-awareness and advise evaluation of any new breast symptoms as one means of early cancer detection.

Self-care

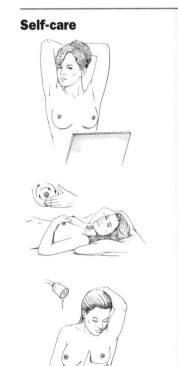

- Consider checking your breasts about once a month for lumps or any other changes.
- If you're still menstruating, the best time to examine your breasts is seven days after your last period started. If you take oral contraceptives, examine your breasts each time you open a new package of pills. Notify your health care provider of any changes.
- Breast self-awareness is to become familiar with the texture of your breasts and nodules within them, and to watch carefully for any changes.
  - **Start by looking into a mirror with your arms at your sides.** Raise your arms and examine your breasts for puckering, dimples or changes in their size or shape. Look for changes in the natural symmetry of both breasts. Check to see whether your nipples are pulled in (inverted). Note any unusual discharge from your nipples. Check for the same signs while resting your hands on your hips and again with your hands behind your head.
  - **Examine your breasts while lying on your back or standing in the shower.** Hold one hand behind your head and use a circular massaging motion with the other hand to check the tissue over the entire opposite breast, including the nipple and the tissue under your armpit. Repeat the procedure on the other side.
  - **Check for lumps that don't disappear.** Abnormal lumps may seem to appear suddenly and remain. They vary in size and firmness and often feel hard with irregular edges. Sometimes they just feel like thickened areas without distinct outlines. Cancerous lumps usually aren't painful.

Medical help

See your doctor if a breast lump doesn't go away after your menstrual cycle. A painful or enlarging fluid-filled cyst may be drained with a needle after an injection of a local anesthetic. If you have a breast infection, an antibiotic is typically prescribed. Lumps that aren't filled with fluid may require a needle biopsy to see if they're cancerous. Women should see their doctors if a lump lasts more than a week or becomes reddened, painful or enlarged.

A word on breast density

Breast density is an important risk factor for breast cancer. Your risk of cancer is four to six times higher if you have dense breasts.

Dense breasts also pose a screening challenge, as they contain less fatty tissue and more fibroglandular tissue. On a mammogram image, fatty tissue appears dark and transparent. Dense tissue, on the other hand, appears as patchy white areas. Because cancers also look white on a mammogram, having dense breast tissue makes it more difficult to identify breast cancer through standard mammography. Because of this, your doctor may suggest supplemental screening.

Mammograms: Who should have them?

A mammogram is a breast X-ray that can detect very small tumors. Mammography saves lives by identifying breast cancer at a stage when it's potentially curable. However, the test isn't perfect. Occasionally it fails to show a tumor — such as for women with dense breasts — or indicates a problem when there isn't one, leading to unnecessary testing.

Screening standards continue to change. However, Mayo Clinic supports the stance that women should have the opportunity to begin annual screening at age 40, and should continue as long as their overall health is good and their life expectancy is 10 years or longer. Women who are considered at high risk of breast cancer may need to start mammograms at an earlier age or may need additional imaging. Discuss your situation with your doctor and make a decision that's best for you.

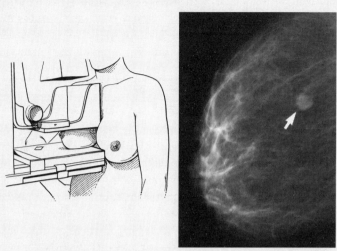

Mammograms are produced by a special X-ray device that can often detect tumors before you or your doctor can feel them. If your mammogram is digital, images are electronic and are displayed on a video monitor.

■ Breast cancer

After nonmelanoma skin cancer, **breast cancer** is the most common cancer diagnosed in women in the United States.

Warning signs. Signs and symptoms of breast cancer may include:
- A breast lump or thickening that feels different from the surrounding tissue
- Bloody discharge from the nipple
- Change in the size or shape of a breast
- Changes to the skin over the breast, such as dimpling
- New onset of an inverted nipple; or peeling, flaking or rash on the nipple skin
- Redness or pitting of the skin over your breast, like the skin of an orange

Risk factors. A number of factors may increase your risk:
- Being older than age 50
- Personal or family history of premenopausal breast cancer, multiple family members with breast or ovarian cancer, cancer in both breasts, or ovarian cancer
- Inherited genes that increase cancer risk
- Dense breast tissue
- Radiation treatments to your chest as a child or young adult
- Being overweight or obese
- Starting your period before age 12 or starting menopause after age 55
- Having never given birth or breast-fed, or having your first child after age 30
- Using combination hormone therapy for more than five years after menopause
- Drinking alcohol (more than one drink a day)

Checkups and screening. See page 144 on breast self-awareness and above on mammography. For some women, other screening methods, such as ultrasound, magnetic resonance imaging (MRI) or molecular breast imaging (MBI), are appropriate.

Medical help	Breast cancer treatment options are based on type of breast cancer, stage, whether the cancer cells are sensitive to hormones, your overall health and your own preferences. Most women have surgery and may also receive additional treatment, such as chemotherapy, hormone therapy or radiation. If you find a lump or other change in your breast, even if a recent mammogram was normal, see your doctor right away.

■ Pain in your breast

Generalized tenderness in both breasts is common, especially during the week before a menstrual period, and it's also a symptom of premenstrual syndrome (see page 147). Vigorous exercise can cause breast tenderness, or it may be caused by an inflamed cyst. If fever and redness occur, infection is a concern. Mastitis, caused by an infection or inflammation, usually occurs in only one breast. Infections can occur with breast-feeding.

Self-care	• Wear a comfortable and supportive bra. • Take an over-the-counter pain reliever (see page 258). • Reduce the salt in your diet before your period and avoid caffeine. • If pain is due to high-impact exercises, switch to a low-impact workout, such as biking, walking or swimming, and use an athletic bra. • See other tips in the section on premenstrual syndrome (page 147).
Medical help	If you have fever or redness with the pain, see your doctor. You may need an antibiotic. Also see your doctor if pain is associated with a lump or change in breast texture. Rarely, inflammatory breast cancer can be confused with mastitis.

■ Menstrual cramps

Chances are you've dealt with menstrual cramps — dull, throbbing or cramping pains in your lower abdomen that may extend to the lower back and thighs. Some women also have nausea, vomiting, diarrhea, sweating or dizziness. The discomfort may be merely annoying, or severe pain may interfere with everyday activities.

If there's no underlying gynecological disorder, the pain is called primary dysmenorrhea. It's caused by high levels of a substance that makes the muscles of the uterus contract and shed its lining. Although painful, this isn't harmful. Pain caused by an underlying gynecological disorder is called secondary dysmenorrhea. It may be due to a benign tumor in the wall of your uterus, a sexually transmitted infection, endometriosis, pelvic inflammatory disease, or an ovarian cyst or tumor.

Self-care	• Take a nonprescription pain reliever. Nonsteroidal anti-inflammatory drugs (see page 257) taken as directed from the start of cramps until the cramps go away relieves pain in most women. • Try soaking in a warm tub or exercising.
Medical help	Treating the underlying cause should relieve the pain. If no cause for the pain is found, birth control pills may relieve the discomfort. Talk to your doctor if the pain is severe or is associated with fever; if you have unusual nausea, vomiting or abdominal pain, vaginal discharge or odor; or if the pain lasts several days a month.

Irregular periods

It's common for women to experience unexplained irregularities in their periods. Irregular periods are due to changes in hormone levels, which can be affected by stress or other emotional experiences, significant changes in the amount of aerobic exercise or dramatic changes in weight. Among women with excessively lean bodies who exercise extensively, their periods may stop altogether.

Self-care

- Keep a menstrual calendar for at least three cycles. Record the first day of flow, the day of maximum flow, the day that flow stops and times of intercourse, to help evaluate menstrual changes.
- If your periods are irregular for more than three cycles, talk with your doctor.
- If you miss a period and have had intercourse, look for symptoms of pregnancy and contact your health care provider.

Bleeding between periods

Occasional bleeding between menstrual periods is common. It may occur spontaneously or with sexual intercourse. Usually it isn't serious, and is caused by a variation of your usual hormone cycles. Stress, new contraceptive pills, benign growths of tissue (polyps) and many other conditions can affect your menstruation. Because abnormal bleeding can also be the first warning sign of cancer, or a sign of ectopic (tubal) pregnancy, it needs prompt evaluation by your health care provider.

Premenstrual syndrome

If you experience a predictable pattern of physical and emotional changes in the days before your period, you may have **premenstrual syndrome** (PMS). This condition is related to normal hormone cycles and occurs with normal hormone levels. One clue to its cause may lie in your response to serotonin. Serotonin is a substance in the brain that has been associated with clinical depression and other emotional disorders. Sometimes an underlying psychological condition such as depression is aggravated by the hormonal changes before a period.

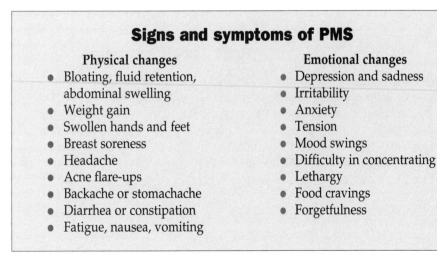

Signs and symptoms of PMS

Physical changes	Emotional changes
• Bloating, fluid retention, abdominal swelling	• Depression and sadness
• Weight gain	• Irritability
• Swollen hands and feet	• Anxiety
• Breast soreness	• Tension
• Headache	• Mood swings
• Acne flare-ups	• Difficulty in concentrating
• Backache or stomachache	• Lethargy
• Diarrhea or constipation	• Food cravings
• Fatigue, nausea, vomiting	• Forgetfulness

Self-care

You can usually manage PMS with a combination of education and lifestyle changes.

- Maintain a healthy weight.
- Eat smaller, more-frequent meals. Don't skip meals. Eat at the same time every day if possible.
- Limit salt and salty foods for one to two weeks before your period to reduce bloating and fluid retention.
- Avoid caffeine to reduce irritability, tension and breast soreness.
- Avoid alcohol before your period to minimize depression and mood swings.
- Eat a balanced diet (see page 210). Eat plenty of fruits, vegetables and whole grains.
- Get enough calcium. Drink fat-free or low-fat milk daily and choose other calcium-rich foods (see page 149). If you can't tolerate foods with calcium or you're unsure about the adequacy of calcium in your diet, a daily calcium supplement may help. Ask your health care provider what dose is best.
- Reduce stress (see page 221). Stress can aggravate PMS.
- Plan ahead for PMS. Don't overbook yourself the week you're expecting symptoms.
- Walk, jog, bike, swim or perform some other aerobic activity at least three times a week.
- Record your symptoms for a few months. You may find that PMS is more tolerable if you see that your symptoms are predictable and short-lived.

Medical help

There are no physical findings or lab tests for diagnosing PMS. Instead, doctors rely on careful evaluation of your medical history. As part of the diagnostic process, women are asked to record the onset, duration, nature and severity of symptoms for at least two menstrual cycles.

If your PMS symptoms seriously affect your life and the suggestions listed above don't help, your doctor may recommend the following medications:

- Nonsteroidal anti-inflammatory drugs (NSAIDs) can ease cramps and breast discomfort (see page 257).
- Birth control pills often relieve symptoms by stopping ovulation.
- Antidepressants are often effective in reducing severe emotional symptoms of PMS. Examples include citalopram (Celexa), escitalopram (Lexapro), fluoxetine (Prozac), sertraline (Zoloft), paroxetine (Paxil) and venlafaxine (Effexor). These drugs can be used in doses lower than those usually prescribed for depression and may be effective when taken only during the week or two before menstruation.

Toxic shock syndrome

Toxic shock syndrome (TSS) is a rare, life-threatening complication of a bacterial infection that is often associated with the use of tampons. It's also occasionally occurs with use of contraceptive sponges, after surgical procedures or with wounds.

Warning signs may include a sudden high fever, low blood pressure, vomiting, diarrhea, confusion, muscle aches, redness of eyes, mouth and throat, a rash resembling a sunburn (particularly on palms of hands and soles of feet), headaches, and seizures.

TSS requires immediate medical attention.

If you use tampons, avoid superabsorbent brands. Change tampons at least every eight hours. If you've ever had TSS, don't wear tampons at all.

■ Menopause

Menopause is the permanent end of menstruation and fertility, defined as occurring 12 months after your last menstrual period. Some women reach **menopause** in their 30s or 40s, others in their 50s or 60s. The average age in the United States is 51.

During menopause, the ovaries gradually stop producing estrogen. Your periods become irregular. Eventually, your menstrual periods stop, and you can no longer become pregnant.

As your ovaries produce fewer hormones, various changes occur, although they vary a great deal from person to person. Your uterus shrinks, and the lining of your vagina becomes thin. Your vagina may also become dry, making intercourse painful. Hot flashes cause flushing or sweating that may last from several minutes to more than an hour and may interrupt sleep and produce night sweats.

During and after menopause, your body fat typically is redistributed as your metabolism changes. Your bones lose density and strength. Osteoporosis may occur.

Mood changes are not uncommon during menopause. They may be related to sleep disruption due to hot flashes, other hormonal changes or the normal midlife issues that affect both men and women.

Self-care

- Remember that menopause is normal and healthy.
- Eat a balanced diet. Get regular physical activity. Dress in layers (if needed).
- Use a water-soluble lubricating jelly if intercourse is painful.

Medical help

Your doctor may prescribe hormone therapy (HT) in the lowest dose needed to relieve postmenopausal symptoms, such as hot flashes. The disadvantage of HT is that it may slightly increase the risk of breast cancer, as well as vascular diseases, including blood clots and stroke. While HT can be very effective for menopausal symptoms, its risks, especially at an older age, lead many women to seek other treatments.

Other treatments include medications that may affect temperature regulation in the brain, such as low-dose antidepressants, other types of medications and vaginal estrogen. Talk with your doctor about the benefits and risks of treatment options.

Vaginal bleeding after menopause is not normal and should be promptly evaluated by your doctor. The cause of bleeding may be entirely harmless, but postmenopausal bleeding has a number of serious causes, including cancer.

How to prevent osteoporosis

Loss of estrogen after menopause increases the likelihood of **osteoporosis**, a disorder in which your bones become porous and brittle. The most effective way to manage osteoporosis is to prevent it by maximizing your bone density when you're young.

- Get enough calcium: 1,000 milligrams (mg) a day for women ages 19 to 50 and for men ages 19 to 70, 1,200 mg for women over age 50 and men over age 70. Foods rich in calcium include milk, yogurt, fish with bones that are eaten, broccoli and calcium-fortified foods. One 8-ounce glass of milk has about 300 mg of calcium.

- If you're at an increased risk, your doctor may suggest calcium supplements. Keep the amount within your doctor's recommendations, since too much calcium may be harmful for certain conditions.
- Get enough vitamin D to help absorb the calcium. Food sources include vitamin D-fortified milk, vitamin D-fortified foods and fatty fish such as salmon. Take a daily supplement of 600 international units (IU) — or 800 IU for adults over age 70 — if needed.
- Regularly do weight-bearing exercises (such as walking or jogging) and strength training.

Urination problems

Urinary tract infections (UTIs) are common among women. With the beginning of sexual activity, women have a marked increase in the number of infections. Sexual intercourse, pregnancy and urinary obstruction all contribute to the likelihood of such an infection. Symptoms of UTI include pain or a burning sensation during urination, increased frequency of urination, and a feeling of urgency every time you need to urinate. If you have an infection, your doctor will prescribe an antibiotic.

Urinary incontinence is involuntary loss of urine, which can be urge or stress incontinence. If leakage occurs when you feel the need to void, it's called urge incontinence. It's often caused by a mild UTI or by excessive use of bladder stimulants such as caffeine. Stress incontinence is loss of urine when pressure is put on your bladder by coughing, laughing, jumping or lifting something heavy. It's usually caused by weakening of the muscles that support your bladder. These muscles can weaken because of childbirth, being overweight, having a chronic cough or aging.

Self-care for urine leakage

- Try Kegel exercises. Imagine that you're trying to stop the flow of urine. If you're using the right muscles, you'll feel a pulling sensation. Pull in your pelvic muscles and hold for a count of three. Relax for a count of three. Work up to 10 to 15 repetitions each time you exercise. Do Kegel exercises at least three times a day. It may take up to 12 weeks before you notice an improvement in bladder control.
- Empty your bladder more often.
- Lean forward when urinating to empty your bladder more completely.
- Decrease your intake of caffeine-containing foods and beverages.
- Use tampons while exercising to support the urethra.

Vaginal discharge

Vaginal discharge is one sign of **vaginitis**. Vaginitis is an inflammation of your vagina. It usually is caused by an infection or an alteration in the normal vaginal bacteria. In addition to vaginal discharge, you may have itching, irritation, pain during intercourse, pain in your lower abdomen, vaginal bleeding and odor.

Common types of vaginitis include yeast infections, bacterial vaginosis and trichomoniasis. Yeast infections are caused by a fungus. You're more susceptible to a yeast infection if you are pregnant or have diabetes; if you're taking antibiotics, cortisone or birth control pills; or if you have an iron deficiency. The main symptom is itching. A white discharge also may occur. Bacterial vaginosis usually produces a gray discharge. This can be treated with metronidazole (Flagyl, MetroGel) or clindamycin (Cleocin). Trichomoniasis is caused by a parasite and is often sexually transmitted. It may cause a smelly, greenish-yellow, sometimes frothy discharge. Your doctor may prescribe metronidazole (Flagyl) or tinidazole (Tindamax) tablets. Your partner also should be treated.

Self-care for yeast infection

- Use a nonprescription antifungal cream or suppository for suspected yeast infections.
- Abstain from intercourse or have your partner use a condom for a week after beginning treatment.
- See your health care provider if symptoms persist still after one week.

See back cover for online resource

■ Cancer screening

See page 145 for breast cancer screening recommendations. Screening tests for **cervical cancer** include a Pap test and a pelvic exam. The Pap test can detect cervical cancer at an early and curable stage.

Cervical cancer is linked to forms of the human papillomavirus (**HPV**), which can be passed on through sexual contact. A male or female condom usually prevents infection.

Most cervical cancers develop slowly, beginning with changes in cells on the surface of the cervix. These abnormal cells, called precancerous cells, may become cancerous over time. Early precancerous changes in surface cells are called dysplasia. Some of these abnormalities go away on their own, but others progress. Precancerous conditions generally don't cause any symptoms, including pain.

American Cancer Society guidelines recommend that:

- All women should have an initial Pap test at age 21, with subsequent Pap tests every three years until age 30.
- Beyond age 30, women should have a Pap test combined with HPV testing (co-testing) every five years, or a Pap test alone every three years.
- Women who have had their uterus and cervix removed (complete hysterectomy) can stop having Pap tests unless they had the surgery to treat cervical cancer or precancerous changes.
- Women over age 65 who have had regular screening in the previous 10 years with no serious pre-cancers found in the last 20 years may discontinue the test.

Women at high risk should have more frequent testing. You're at high risk if:

- You've had prior cervical cancer and your cervix was not removed
- You have HIV or a weakened immune system
- Your mother took diethylstilbestrol (DES) while she was pregnant with you
- You've had an organ transplant

Ovarian cancer

Until recently, ovarian cancer was known as a silent killer because it usually wasn't found until it had spread to other areas of your body. But new evidence shows that awareness of symptoms may lead to earlier detection.

Signs and symptoms often include:

- Abdominal pressure, fullness, swelling or bloating
- Urinary urgency
- Pelvic discomfort or pain

Signs and symptoms may also include:

- Persistent indigestion, gas or nausea
- Unexplained changes in bowel habits, such as constipation
- Changes in bladder habits, including a frequent need to urinate
- Loss of appetite or quickly feeling full
- Increased abdominal girth or clothes fitting tighter around your waist
- Pain during intercourse
- A persistent lack of energy
- Low back pain
- Changes in menstruation

Treatment usually involves a combination of surgery and chemotherapy. Women who are at very high risk of developing ovarian cancer may elect to have their ovaries removed to prevent the disease.

Cervical cancer vaccine

The vaccine Gardasil is approved by the Food and Drug Administration (FDA) to prevent four types of human papillomavirus (HPV) that are known to cause cervical cancer. Another vaccine, Cervarix, protects against two HPV strands.

These vaccines are recommended for girls ages 11 to 12, but they may be used in girls as young as age 9 or for females ages 13 to 26 who haven't been vaccinated (Gardasil is also recommended for boys ages 11 to 12). This results in high antibody levels and greater protection before the person is likely to encounter HPV. This vaccine is part of the routine childhood immunization schedule (see page 228).

It's important to note that these vaccines don't guard against all HPV strains, nor do they prevent all cervical abnormalities. While they're valuable for prevention, they shouldn't replace periodic cervical cancer screening.

◼ Other common medical conditions

Endometriosis

Endometriosis is a disorder of the reproductive system in which some of the lining of the uterus (endometrium) migrates out of the uterus through the fallopian tubes. Most often, this growth is on your fallopian tubes, ovaries or the tissue lining your pelvis. During menstruation, blood from this tissue is absorbed by the surrounding organs, causing inflammation. This can create scar tissue that causes organs to stick together (adhesions), which can prevent pregnancy. Symptoms include severe cramping during periods, pelvic pain during intercourse, and pain during bowel movements or urination. Some women have severe pain, but others have few or no symptoms. Various hormone therapies may relieve symptoms, stop progression and prevent infertility. Sometimes surgery, traditional or laparoscopic, is needed.

Uterine fibroids

Uterine fibroids are noncancerous growths of the uterus that often appear during childbearing years. Fibroids often go undetected because many women don't have symptoms. When they occur, signs and symptoms may include heavy or prolonged menstrual bleeding, pelvic pressure or pain, frequent urination, difficulty emptying your bladder, constipation, backache or leg pains. See your doctor if you have pelvic pain that doesn't go away, overly heavy or painful periods, pain during intercourse, bleeding between periods, or difficulty with urination or bowel movements. Uterine fibroids seldom require treatment. If needed, treatment may include medications, surgery, or other procedures to shrink or destroy the fibroids.

Uterine polyps

Overgrowth of cells in the lining of the uterus leads to the formation of **uterine polyps**. Uterine polyps can range from tiny to golf ball sized or larger. They most commonly occur in women in their 40s and 50s. It's possible to have uterine polyps without signs or symptoms. Signs include irregular menstrual bleeding, bleeding between menstrual periods, excessively heavy menstrual periods, vaginal bleeding after menopause or infertility. Possible treatments include watchful waiting, medication, surgical removal or hysterectomy (if the polyp contains cancerous cells).

Hysterectomy

A hysterectomy is a procedure in which your uterus is removed. A **vaginal hysterectomy** is removal of the uterus through an incision in the vagina. An **abdominal hysterectomy** is removal of the uterus through an incision in the abdomen. Abdominal hysterectomy is performed if you have suspected or confirmed uterine or ovarian cancer, extensive endometriosis or scarring in the pelvis, a history of pelvic infection, or a uterus that's too large to remove vaginally.

Sometimes one or both ovaries are removed along with the uterus. This is called an **oophorectomy**, which may be done with one large abdominal incision or less invasively (laparoscopically or robotically), using multiple small incisions. Women who haven't reached menopause will experience premature menopause if both ovaries are removed.

Ask your doctor about the benefits and risks of surgery, including physical and emotional aftereffects. Also ask if there are alternatives to surgery.

Birth control methods

Method	How it works	Effectiveness*	Cautions
Implantable rod	Hormone released from rod placed under skin; up to 3 years.	99%	Irregular bleeding; uncommonly, acne and headache.
Intrauterine devices (IUD): copper IUD; IUD with progestin	Inserted into the uterus; inhibit sperm migration and fertilization.	99%	Copper IUD may increase menstrual blood flow; progestin decreases flow; must ensure that IUD stays in place.
Surgical sterilization†	Fallopian tubes are tied and cut or cauterized.	99%	Requires outpatient surgery, not readily reversible.
Injection	Hormone shot in the arm, buttock or under the skin every 3 months that blocks ovulation.	94%	May cause headache, menstrual irregularities, acne and weight gain. Prolonged use may raise risk of (reversible) bone loss.
Birth control pills (oral contraceptives)	Synthetic hormones prevent ovulation and impair implantation.	91%	Don't smoke, especially after age 35.
Patch	Skin patch that releases hormones into bloodstream.	91%	Less effective in women who weigh more than 198 pounds.
Hormonal vaginal contraceptive ring	Ring placed inside vagina that releases hormones.	91%	Side effects can include headache, nausea, breast tenderness, vaginal irritation and discharge.
Diaphragm	Fitted silicone or latex cap inserted into the vagina to cover the cervix. Inserted before intercourse and left in for 6 to 30 hours afterward.	88%	May cause cervical irritation and increased risk of urinary tract infections.
Male condom	Latex sheath placed over penis.	82%	Avoid natural or lambskin (does not protect against STIs); avoid if you have an allergy to latex.
Female condom	Polyurethane or nitrile membrane inserted into the vagina.	79%	Must be inserted before intercourse. Insertion cumbersome for some.
Sponge	Foam barrier that contains spermicide. Can be put in 24 hours before intercourse.	76-88%	Should not be worn for more than 30 hours. Less effective in women who have given birth.
Natural family planning	Intercourse determined by menstrual cycle.	76%	Works best in stable relationships and with regular cycles. Requires training.
Emergency contraception	High-dose hormones in morning-after pill or copper IUD insertion.	75%	Must be started within 5 days of having unprotected sex.
Spermicide alone	A chemical that inactivates sperm. Can be used alone or with a barrier method.	72%	May cause vaginal burning and irritation.

*Effectiveness is defined as preventing pregnancy during the first year of typical use.
†For information on male sterilization (vasectomy), see page 143.

Based on *Managing Contraception 2017-2018*; American College of Obstetricians and Gynecologists, 2014-2016.

■ Pregnancy

Before and during **pregnancy**, you want to take especially good care of your health to help ensure that your baby will have the best possible start in life. It's a good idea to see your health care provider for a complete physical exam before you become pregnant. You may be checked for conditions that may not cause symptoms but can complicate pregnancy. These include diabetes, high blood pressure, anemia and others. If you have a health problem, your health care provider will want to control the condition, ideally before you become pregnant. Your health care provider will also review your immunizations to be sure you're immune to German measles (rubella), a viral infection, and tell you what medications to avoid, such as antibiotics.

Self-care

To prepare for pregnancy

- If you're overweight, reduce your weight before you become pregnant. Don't begin a diet if you're pregnant unless advised by your doctor.
- If you smoke, stop. And, if possible, avoid secondhand smoke (see page 195).
- Don't drink alcohol if you're trying to become pregnant.
- Take a multivitamin daily. Make sure it contains folic acid, which decreases the risk of birth defects of the spinal column (neural tube defects).
- Check with your health care provider about taking over-the-counter or prescription medicines.

During pregnancy

Once you're pregnant, the best ways to ensure a healthy baby are to:
- Eat a healthy diet. Allow for appropriate weight gain.
- Make regular visits to your health care provider.
- Take a prenatal vitamin with folic acid, as prescribed by your physician.
- Obtain a book on pregnancy. Understand the changes your body is experiencing.
- Avoid harmful substances such as cigarettes, alcohol, and some medications and chemicals.
- **Caution:** Bleeding from your vagina during pregnancy may indicate that something is wrong. Call your health care provider immediately. Although some harmless spotting and bleeding occur in many women during early pregnancy, your health care provider will want to rule out miscarriage, tubal (ectopic) pregnancy or other conditions.

Home pregnancy tests

Home pregnancy tests provide a private way to find out whether you're pregnant. Most tests use a wand or stick placed into a urine stream or a collected urine specimen to detect the hormone human chorionic gonadotropin (HCG). The placenta begins to produce this hormone soon after conception. When performed correctly, the tests are 97 to 99 percent accurate around the time of a missed period.

Home pregnancy tests can help you get off to a good nutritional start by using prenatal vitamin supplements early. An early pregnancy test also helps you avoid things that could harm the fetus such as alcohol, smoking, some medications or chemicals at home or work. For women who are at risk of a tubal pregnancy or early miscarriage, home tests alert them early in their pregnancy so they can see their health care provider promptly.

See back cover for online resource ⓘ

■ Common problems during pregnancy

Common but bothersome concerns you may have during pregnancy are morning sickness, heartburn, backache and other problems. These may make you uncomfortable, but usually they don't threaten your health or the health of your developing baby. If they're severe or persist despite self-care measures, see your doctor.

Morning sickness

During the first 12 weeks of pregnancy, the majority of women experience nausea and many experience vomiting. Commonly referred to as morning sickness, this condition doesn't always happen during the morning, and it's usually harmless. If you have problems with morning sickness:

- Munch a few crackers before arising in the morning.
- Eat several small meals a day so that your stomach is never empty.
- Avoid smelling or eating foods that trigger the nausea, and avoid spicy, rich and fried foods if you are nauseated.
- Drink plenty of liquids, especially if you're vomiting. Try crushed ice, fruit juice or frozen ice pops if water upsets your stomach.
- Try using acupressure or motion sickness bands to combat nausea.
- Take vitamin B-6 supplements, if recommended by your health care provider.

Anemia

Some pregnant women develop an inadequate level of hemoglobin in the blood (**anemia**) because of an iron deficiency or not having enough folic acid. Symptoms of anemia include fatigue, breathlessness, fainting, palpitations and pale skin. This condition can be risky for both you and your baby. It's easily diagnosed with a blood test. If you're anemic:

- Eat a diet rich in iron (including meat, liver, eggs, dried fruit, whole grains and iron-fortified cereals)
- Eat plenty of leafy green vegetables, liver, lentils, black-eyed peas, kidney beans and other cooked dried beans, oranges and grapefruit
- Follow your health care provider's recommendations about other steps to take

Swelling (edema)

When you're pregnant, your body tissues accumulate more fluid, and swelling is common. Warm weather may aggravate the condition. If you have problems with edema:

- Use cold-water compresses to help relieve swelling
- Eat a low-salt diet
- Lie down and elevate your legs for an hour in the middle of the day

If your face or hands become swollen, or if you gain weight very rapidly, it may be a sign of a serious condition called preeclampsia. See your doctor right away.

Varicose veins

Pregnancy increases the volume of blood in your body and may impair the flow of blood from your legs to your pelvis. Such impairment can cause the veins in your legs to become swollen and sometimes painful, a condition called **varicose veins**. If you have problems with varicose veins:

- Stay off your feet as much as possible, and elevate them as often as you can
- Wear loose clothing around your legs and waist
- Wear support stockings from the time you awaken until you go to bed

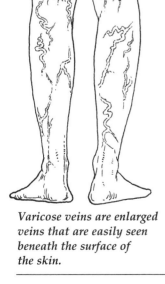

Varicose veins are enlarged veins that are easily seen beneath the surface of the skin.

Constipation

Constipation may worsen during pregnancy. Bowel activity may be slowed because of the increased pressure on the bowels from the growing baby inside the uterus.

- Drink plenty of liquids — at least eight to 10 glasses a day.
- Exercise moderately every day.
- Eat several servings of fresh fruits, vegetables and whole grains.
- Try a nonprescription bulking agent that contains psyllium or a stool softener.
- Don't take a laxative without discussing it with your health care provider.

Heartburn

Heartburn is a burning sensation in the middle of your chest, often with a bad taste in your mouth. It's caused by reflux — stomach acid flowing up into your food pipe (esophagus). It has nothing to do with your heart. During the later part of pregnancy, your expanding uterus pushes the stomach out of position, which slows the rate that food empties from the stomach.

- Eat smaller meals more often, but eat slowly.
- Avoid greasy foods.
- Don't drink coffee. Both regular and decaffeinated coffee may worsen heartburn.
- Don't eat for two to three hours before you go to bed, and raise the head of your bed four to six inches. Reflux is worse when you lie flat.
- If these steps don't work, consult your health care provider, who may recommend an antacid. (See page 64.)

Backache

Backache is common in pregnancy and may worsen if you bend, lift, walk too much or are fatigued. Pain may be in the lower back, or it may radiate down your legs. Your abdomen also may hurt because of the stretching of ligaments. During pregnancy your ligaments are more elastic, and so your joints are more prone to strain and injury. Your center of balance also changes during pregnancy. This puts more strain on your back.

- Don't gain more weight than your health care provider recommends.
- Eliminate as much strain as possible. Try wearing a maternity support belt.
- Follow medical advice for exercises to relieve pain and strengthen back muscles.

Hemorrhoids

Hemorrhoids are enlarged veins at the anal opening. They become enlarged from increased pressure. They're often worse during pregnancy and accompany constipation.

- Avoid becoming constipated.
- Don't strain during bowel movements.
- Take frequent warm-water baths.
- Apply a cotton pad soaked with cold witch hazel or a hemorrhoidal cream.
- Lie down during pregnancy to help relieve pressure in the anal area.

Sleeping problems

Your sleep may be disturbed during the later stages of pregnancy because of the frequent need to urinate, the movements of your baby or the many things on your mind.

- Avoid caffeine.
- Don't eat a large meal right before bedtime; take a warm bath before going to bed.
- Exercise more during the day.
- If you can't sleep, get out of bed and do something else.
- Don't take any medicines unless recommended by your health care provider.

See back cover for online resource

Specific Conditions

- **Respiratory allergies**
- **Thyroid disorders**
- **Arthritis**
- **Asthma**
- **Cancer**
- **Diabetes**
- **Heart disease**
- **Hepatitis**
- **High blood pressure**
- **Sexually transmitted infections**

Many of the diseases and medical conditions discussed in this section are common. But they warrant examination and follow-up by a doctor for correct diagnosis and treatment.

In this section, you'll find general guidelines on the prevention and management of these diseases. In some cases, new treatments are included. Talk with your doctor about what's right for you.

Respiratory allergies

Do you develop itchy, watery eyes or a stuffy, runny nose during the same season every year? Do you sneeze frequently when you're around animals or at work? If you answered yes to either of these questions, you may be one of millions of Americans with an allergy (see "Allergic reactions," page 12, and "Hives," page 123).

Allergic reactions and immune response

An allergy is an overreaction by your immune system to an otherwise harmless substance, such as pollen or pet dander. Contact with this substance, called an allergen, triggers production of the antibody immunoglobulin E (IgE). IgE causes immune cells in the lining of your eyes and airways to release inflammatory substances, including histamine.

When these substances are released, they produce the familiar signs and symptoms of allergy — itchy, red and swollen eyes, a stuffy or runny nose, frequent sneezing or cough, and hives or bumps on the skin. This allergic reaction causes or aggravates some forms of asthma (see page 165).

Substances found outdoors and indoors can cause allergic reactions. The most common allergens, listed below, are inhaled:

- **Pollen.** Spring, summer and fall are the pollen-producing seasons in many climates, with exposure to airborne pollen from trees, grasses and weeds.
- **Dust mites.** House dust harbors many allergens, including pollen and molds. But the main allergy trigger is the dust mite. Thousands of these microscopic insects are in a pinch of house dust. House dust can cause year-round allergy symptoms.
- **Pet dander.** Dogs and especially cats are the most common animals to cause allergic reactions. An animal's skin flakes (dander), saliva, urine and sometimes hair are the main culprits.
- **Molds.** Many people are sensitive to airborne mold spores. Outdoor molds produce spores mostly in the summer and early fall in northern climates and year-round in subtropical and tropical climates. Indoor molds shed spores all year long.

Discovering causes

It's not clear why some people become sensitive to allergens. But doctors know the tendency to develop **allergies** is inherited. Yet, you and your relatives won't necessarily be sensitive to the same allergens.

If your symptoms are mild, over-the-counter (OTC) allergy medications may be all you need. But if your symptoms are persistent or bothersome, see your doctor. To diagnose allergies accurately, your doctor will need to know about your:

- Symptoms
- Past medical problems
- Past and current living conditions
- Work environment
- Possible exposure to allergens
- Family's medical history
- Diet, lifestyle and recreational habits

The next steps are typically a physical exam and skin tests. During a skin test, tiny, diluted drops of suspected allergens are applied to your skin. Then small pricks are made through the drops. If your response to an allergen is positive, a skin reaction similar to a mosquito bite or small hive appears within 20 minutes. A positive result of a skin test means only that you might be allergic to a particular substance.

The difference between colds and allergies

Many people mistake allergies for colds. But with a cold, symptoms usually go away in a few days. If you have allergies, symptoms may flare under certain conditions or may seem never-ending.

<u>Hay fever</u> (seasonal allergic rhinitis) is a common allergy. The symptoms often appear during pollen season — spring, summer or fall. Signs and symptoms include:

- Stuffy or runny nose
- Itchy eyes, nose, throat or roof of your mouth
- Frequent sneezing
- Cough

Self-care

The best approach for managing allergies is to know and avoid your triggers.

Pollen

- Shower and change clothes upon entering your home after outdoor exposure.
- Use an air conditioner with a good filter. Change filters monthly.
- Wear a pollen mask when outdoors and for yardwork.
- Vacation out of the region during the height of the pollen season.

Dust or molds

- Limit your exposure by cleaning your home at least once a week. Wear a mask while cleaning, or have someone else clean for you.
- Encase mattresses and pillows in dustproof or allergen-blocking covers.
- Consider replacing upholstered furniture with leather or vinyl, and replacing carpeting with wood, vinyl or tile (particularly in the bedroom).
- Maintain indoor humidity between 30 and 50 percent. Use kitchen and bathroom exhaust fans and a dehumidifier in the basement.
- Change furnace filters monthly. Also, consider installing a high-efficiency particulate air (HEPA) filter in your heating system.
- Clean humidifiers and dehumidifiers often to prevent mold and bacterial growth.

Pets

- Avoid pets with fur or feathers. If you choose to keep a furry pet, keep it out of the bedroom and in an area of the home that's easily cleaned. Keep your pet outside as much as possible.

Medical help

Discuss medications with your doctor. **Antihistamines** are used to control sneezing, runny nose, and itchy eyes or throat. Caution: Some types can cause drowsiness.

Decongestants may reduce congestion, allowing you to breathe easier. Decongestants may cause heart palpitations or increase blood pressure.

Nasal spray options include:

- *Corticosteroids.* Available by prescription and over-the-counter (OTC), they relieve congestion when used daily but may take at least a week to become fully effective.
- *Saline.* OTC nasal sprays with a saltwater solution relieve mild congestion and loosen mucus.
- *Decongestants.* These sprays aren't intended for relief of chronic allergy symptoms. Avoid them or use sparingly for no more than two or three days.

Allergy shots (immunotherapy) involve injecting tiny amounts of allergens into your body to desensitize your immune system to allergens, usually over three to five years.

Thyroid disorders

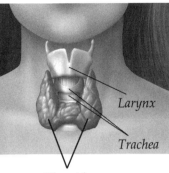

Larynx

Trachea

Thyroid

Abnormal hormone production in the butterfly-shaped thyroid gland can cause hyperthyroidism or hypothyroidism.

Your thyroid is a gland located at the base of your neck. Thyroid hormones control metabolic rate and have a major impact on health. Thyroid disorders are common in the United States, affecting women much more often than men, but children also can have thyroid problems. Two of the more common thyroid disorders are noted below.

Hyperthyroidism

With overactive thyroid (**hyperthyroidism**), your thyroid gland produces too much of the hormone thyroxine, accelerating metabolism. Symptoms vary widely, and older adults are more likely to have no symptoms or subtle ones. Signs and symptoms may include:

- Weight loss despite normal or increased appetite
- Rapid heartbeat, irregular heartbeat or pounding of your heart (palpitations)
- Nervousness, anxiety or anxiety attacks, and irritability
- Tremor — usually a fine trembling in your hands and fingers
- Sweating and increased sensitivity to heat
- In women, changes in menstrual patterns
- More-frequent bowel movements and sometimes diarrhea
- Enlarged thyroid gland (goiter) that looks like swelling at the base of your neck
- Fatigue and muscle weakness
- Difficulty sleeping

Hypothyroidism

With underactive thyroid (**hypothyroidism**), your thyroid gland doesn't produce enough of the hormone thyroxine, slowing your metabolism. The condition may develop slowly over years. Signs and symptoms vary widely but may include:

- Fatigue and sluggishness
- Slow heart rate
- Increased sensitivity to cold
- Unexplained weight gain
- Constipation
- Dry skin and hair
- Puffy face
- Hoarse voice
- High cholesterol
- Muscle aches and weakness
- In women, heavier than normal menstrual periods
- Depression

Medical help

Untreated hyperthyroidism or hypothyroidism can lead to serious complications, including heart problems. Treatment for hyperthyroidism depends on the underlying cause and severity. Radioactive iodine is the most common treatment. Treatment for hypothyroidism involves daily use of the synthetic hormone levothyroxine (Synthroid, Levoxyl, others). This oral medication restores adequate hormone levels.

Thyroid cancer

Although thyroid cancer isn't common in the United States, rates seem to be increasing. It occurs more often in women than in men. Typically there are no signs or symptoms in the early stages. As thyroid cancer grows, it may cause a lump that you can feel on your neck, voice changes (including hoarseness),

trouble swallowing, neck or throat pain, or swollen lymph nodes in your neck.

Risk increases with exposure to high levels of radiation, personal or family history of goiter, or hereditary disorders. If you think you're at increased risk or you have symptoms, talk with your doctor.

See back cover for online resource ⓘ

Arthritis

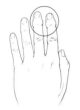

Rheumatoid arthritis can lead to swelling and deformities in the large and middle knuckles.

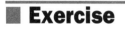

Heberden's nodes are lumps of bone and cartilage at the ends of fingers. They are a sign of osteoarthritis.

Arthritis is one of the most common medical problems in the United States. There are more than 100 forms of arthritis, and they have varying causes, symptoms and treatments. See the chart on page 162 for a summary of signs and symptoms of some forms of arthritis.

The signs and symptoms of inflammatory arthritis include the following:

- Swelling in one or more joints
- Prolonged early-morning stiffness
- Recurring pain or tenderness in any joint
- Inability to move a joint normally
- Obvious redness and warmth in a joint
- Unexplained fevers, weight loss or weakness associated with joint pain

Any of these warning signs, when new, that last for more than two weeks require prompt medical evaluation. Distinguishing arthritis from simple aches and pains is important for treating the problem correctly.

Arthritis has many causes. It may result from degeneration of cartilage in your joints (osteoarthritis) or from genetics, injury, inflammation, infection or any number of unknown causes. Most joint problems caused by inflammation are termed arthritis, from the Greek words *arthron,* for "joint," and *itis,* for "inflammation."

The remainder of this section focuses on the management of **osteoarthritis**, which is the most common form of arthritis. Some of the self-care tips may apply to the other forms. Consult your doctor regarding management of other forms of arthritis.

■ Exercise

Over time, exercise is probably the one therapy that will do the most good for managing your arthritis. Exercise must be done regularly to produce and sustain improvements. That's why you should check with your health care provider and begin a regular exercise program for your specific needs.

Overall, you want to be in good physical condition. This means maintaining flexibility, strength and endurance. Doing so will help protect your joints against further damage, keep them aligned, reduce stiffness and minimize pain.

Different types of exercise achieve different goals. For flexibility, range-of-motion exercises (gentle stretching) move the joint from one end position to the other (bending and straightening your knee, for example). In severe arthritis, range-of-motion exercises may cause pain. Don't continue an exercise beyond the point that's painful without the advice of your doctor or physical therapist.

Moving large muscle groups for 15 to 20 minutes is the primary way of exercising aerobically to strengthen muscles and build endurance. Walking, bicycling, swimming and dancing are good examples of aerobic-type exercises with low to moderate stress on the joints.

If you're carrying a lot of extra weight, moving around is more difficult. You're putting stress on your back, hips, knees and feet — all common places to have osteoarthritis. Obesity clearly worsens arthritis symptoms, as does deconditioning from lack of physical activity. This makes low-impact activities, such as swimming, a effective tool for helping manage your symptoms

Common forms of arthritis

About the condition	Key symptoms	How serious is it?

Osteoarthritis

Osteoarthritis is often associated with wear and tear on some joints. Obesity, aging, injury or genetics can increase risk. It's common in people older than 50; uncommon in young people unless a joint is injured or a metabolic abnormality exists.

- Pain in a joint after use.
- Swelling and a loss of flexibility in a joint.
- Bony lumps at finger joints.
- Aching is common. Redness and warmth are less common.

Seriousness may depend on age and joints affected. Osteoarthritis doesn't go away, although the pain may come and go. The effects may be disabling in some cases. Joints such as the hip and knee may deteriorate to the point of needing surgical replacement.

Rheumatoid arthritis

Rheumatoid arthritis is the most common form of inflammatory arthritis.* It most often develops in middle age, but it can occur in any age group. The cause is unknown but it's an autoimmune disease. The immune system triggers inflammation in the linings of joints and in other areas.

- Pain and swelling in the small joints of hands and feet. Joints may become deformed.
- Overall severe aching or stiffness, especially first thing in the morning or after periods of rest.
- Affected joints are swollen, painful and warm during initial attack and flare-ups.

Rheumatoid arthritis is one of the most debilitating forms of arthritis. It tends to affect smaller joints first. As the disease progresses, it affects larger joints. It frequently causes deformed joints. In some people, it can affect other parts of the body, such as the lungs or heart.

Infectious arthritis

Infectious agents include bacteria, fungi and viruses. Infectious arthritis can be a complication of sexually transmitted infections. It can occur in anyone.

- Pain and stiffness in one joint, typically the knee, shoulder, hip, ankle, elbow, finger or wrist.
- Surrounding tissues are warm and red.
- Chills, fever and weakness.
- May be associated with a rash.

Prompt diagnosis and treatment of a joint infection usually result in a rapid and complete recovery. However, major long-term complications are possible.

Gout

With gout, urate crystals form in a joint. Gout most commonly affects men older than age 40, but women can be affected.

- Severe pain that strikes suddenly in a single joint, often at the base of the big toe. But gout can affect other areas, such as joints in your feet, knees, ankles, hands and wrists.
- Swelling and redness.

An acute gout attack can be treated effectively. After an attack has run its course, the affected joint usually returns to normal. Attacks can recur and may require preventive treatment to lower uric acid levels in the blood. (See "Gout" on page 92.)

*Other types of inflammatory arthritis include psoriatic arthritis, which occurs in people with psoriasis, especially in the finger and foot joints; post-infectious arthritis, which often is transmitted by sexual contact and is characterized by pain in the joints, penile discharge, painful inflammation of the eye and a rash; ankylosing spondylitis, which affects the joints of the spine and sometimes the limbs and, in advanced cases, causes a very stiff, inflexible backbone.

See back cover for online resource

Medications control discomfort

Common over-the-counter (OTC) and prescription drugs used for **osteoarthritis** are described below. (See pages 257-258 for more on the use of OTC medications.)

- **Nonprescription pain creams and gels.** These may provide temporary pain relief for joints close to the skin surface (fingers, knees). Read the labels carefully.
- **Acetaminophen.** This nonprescription product is less likely to upset your stomach, but excessive use can damage your liver. Acetaminophen (Tylenol, others) doesn't reduce inflammation, but it can be effective for mild to moderate pain.
- **NSAIDs.** Nonsteroidal anti-inflammatory drugs (NSAIDs) include ibuprofen, naproxen, nabumetone and diclofenac. Dosage makes a difference. Your doctor should specify the amount that's right for you. NSAIDs vary in side effects and costs. Some are only available by prescription.
- **COX-2 inhibitor.** This type of drug blocks production of an enzyme that triggers inflammation and pain. But because COX-2 inhibitors appear to be linked with a higher risk of heart attack and stroke, only the drug celecoxib (Celebrex) remains on the market. Ask an arthritis specialist about the benefits and risks of this drug.
- **Corticosteroids.** These drugs decrease inflammation. A number of corticosteroids are available, but the most common is prednisone. Doctors don't prescribe oral corticosteroids for osteoarthritis, but they may occasionally inject a cortisone drug into a painful joint. If used too often, cortisone injections can cause soft tissue damage, tendon weakness, and, rarely, rupture of tendons or ligaments.

Caution

Many over-the-counter pain relievers and anti-inflammatory drugs can irritate the lining of your stomach and intestines and cause ulcers and even severe bleeding with long-term use. Stomach and intestinal perforation (without bleeding), high blood pressure, or leg swelling can occur. Some NSAIDs may increase your risk of heart attack or stroke. **Talk with your doctor if you're using NSAIDs regularly for more than two weeks to treat joint pain.**

Other methods to relieve pain

Ask your health care provider about these therapies:

- **Heat** soothes and helps relax muscles around a painful joint. You can apply heat with warm water, a paraffin bath, electric pad, hot pack or heat lamp, but take care to avoid a burn. For deep penetration, a physical therapist has other options.
- **Cold** acts as a local anesthetic. It also decreases muscle spasms. Cold packs may help when you ache from holding muscles in the same position to avoid pain.
- **Splints** support and protect painful joints during activity and provide proper positioning at night, which promotes restful sleep. Constant splinting, however, can weaken muscles and decrease flexibility.
- **Relaxation** techniques, including hypnosis, visualization, deep breathing, muscle relaxation, yoga and other techniques may decrease pain.
- **Glucosamine and chondroitin supplements** are popular for joint pain, but data is conflicting. Use caution when selecting one. The products are not regulated by the Food and Drug Administration. (See page 263.)
- **Other techniques,** such as low-impact exercise, shoe inserts (orthotics), and canes and walking sticks (gait aids), help strengthen muscles, reduce joint pressure and decrease pain. See a physical therapist for proper instruction.

Joint protection

Correct body mechanics help you move with minimal strain. A physical or occupational therapist can suggest techniques and equipment that protect your joints by decreasing stress and conserving energy.

Modifications you can make include the following:

- Avoid grasping actions that strain your finger joints. For example, instead of a clutch-style purse or briefcase, select one with a shoulder strap. Use hot water to loosen a jar lid and pressure from your palm to open it, or use a jar opener. Don't twist or use your joints forcefully.
- Spread the weight of an object over several joints. Use both hands, for example, to lift a heavy pan or large book. Try using a walking stick or cane.
- Take a break periodically to relax and stretch and avoid muscle fatigue.
- Maintain good posture to help promote even weight distribution and to help avoid strain on ligaments and muscles.
- Throughout the day, use your strongest muscles, and try to favor nonarthritic joints. Don't push open a heavy glass door. Lean into it. To pick up an object, bend your knees and squat while keeping your back straight. But if your knees hurt, get advice from your health care provider for the preferred technique.
- Utilize special tools that make gripping easier, such as those available for buttoning shirts and kitchen use. Look for them at grocery, hardware or discount stores, or contact your pharmacy or doctor for information on ordering these items.

Surgery for severe osteoarthritis

Surgery is generally reserved for severe osteoarthritis that isn't relieved by other treatments. You may consider surgery if your osteoarthritis makes it difficult to go about your daily tasks. Surgical treatments include:

- **Joint replacement.** Your surgeon removes your damaged joint surfaces and replaces them with plastic and metal devices called prostheses. The hip and knee joints are the most commonly replaced joints.
- **Cleaning up the area around the joint (debridement).** This involves removing loose pieces of cartilage and bone from around your joint to relieve pain. Debridement is most useful if you're experiencing a locking sensation from a torn cartilage or loose debris in your knee joint.
- **Realigning bones.** Surgery to realign bones may relieve pain. This is typically used when joint replacement surgery isn't an option.
- **Fusing bones.** Surgeons can permanently fuse bones in a joint to increase stability and reduce pain. The fused joint, such as an ankle, can bear weight without pain, but it has no flexibility.

Discuss options with your doctor, and weigh the benefits and risks carefully. See page 252 for advice on choosing a surgeon and questions to ask.

FOR MORE INFORMATION

- Arthritis Foundation, 800-283-7800, *www.arthritis.org*
- National Institute of Arthritis and Musculoskeletal and Skin Diseases, National Institutes of Health, 877-226-4267, *www.niams.nih.gov*
- American College of Rheumatology, 404-633-3777, *www.rheumatology.org*

Asthma

<u>Asthma</u> occurs when the main air passages of your lungs, called bronchial tubes, become inflamed and constricted. The muscles of the bronchial walls tighten, and your airways produce extra mucus. Airflow is diminished, often causing wheezing.

Asthma is a serious medical condition, but with proper care and treatment you usually can control symptoms and lead a healthy, active life.

Common signs and symptoms are wheezing, difficulty breathing, chest tightness and coughing. In emergencies, you may have extreme difficulty in breathing and the signs and symptoms shown in the box below. Asthma attacks can vary from mild to severe and can last for a few minutes, a few hours or even days.

Millions of Americans, adults and children, have asthma. It isn't clear why some people get asthma and others don't, but it's probably due to a combination of environmental and genetic (inherited) factors. Causes and asthma triggers differ among people. But these factors can increase your risk: a family history of asthma, frequent respiratory infections as a child, gastroesophageal reflux disease (GERD), exposure to secondhand smoke, living in an urban area (especially an area with lots of air pollution), exposure to occupational chemicals, low birth weight and being overweight.

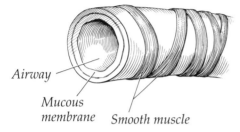

The image above shows normal airways in your lungs

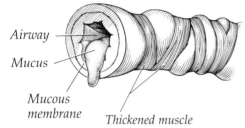

In asthma, airways in your lungs are inflamed and swollen.

Common asthma triggers

There are many triggers of asthma attacks, including:

- Air pollutants such as smoke or fumes
- Chemical smells
- Cockroaches
- Cold air or air conditioning
- Colds or flu (influenza)
- Dust or dust mites
- Exercise, physical activity or sports
- Foods, such as peanuts or shellfish
- Heartburn
- Medications, such as aspirin or beta blockers
- Menstrual cycle
- Mold and mildew
- Perfume and deodorants
- Pet allergy
- Pollen
- Stress or strong emotional reactions, such as crying
- Sulfites — preservatives in some foods and beverages
- Tobacco smoke
- Weather, such as high humidity

Recognizing a life-threatening attack

Prevent fatal attacks by treating signs and symptoms early. Don't wait for wheezing as a sign of severity. Wheezing may disappear when airflow is severely restricted. Get emergency care if:

- Breathing becomes difficult and your neck, chest or ribs pull in with each breath
- Pulse rate increases and sweating and severe cough occur
- Nostrils flare

- Fingernails or lips turn blue
- Walking or talking becomes difficult
- Peak airflow (measured with a hand-held meter you can use at home) reading decreases 50 percent below your normal level or keeps decreasing even after you take your medication

---

See back cover for online resource ⓘ

Specific Conditions

Your doctor can work with you to identify triggers. Together, you can devise a strategy to limit your exposure to these triggers, help control your signs and symptoms and make sure that your breathing is not severely obstructed.

Self-care

Educate yourself about asthma. The more you know, the easier it is to control. These tips can help control symptoms by trigger-proofing your environment:

- Avoid allergens that might trigger your symptoms. If you're allergic to cats or dogs, consider removing them from your home, and avoid contact with other people's pets. Avoid buying clothing, furniture or rugs made from animal hair.
- If you're allergic to airborne pollens and molds, use air conditioning at home, at work and in your car. Keep doors and windows closed to limit exposure to airborne pollens and molds.
- Avoid activities that might contribute to your symptoms. For example, home improvement projects might expose you to triggers that lead to an asthma attack, such as paint vapors, wood dust or similar irritants.
- Check your furnace. If you have a forced-air heating system and you're allergic to dust, use a filter for dust control. Change or clean filters on heating and cooling units monthly. The best filter is a high-efficiency particulate air (HEPA) filter. Wear a mask when you remove dirty filters.
- Use a vacuum cleaner with a small-particle filter.
- Avoid projects that raise dust. If you can't do so, then use a dust mask. Dust masks are available at drugstores and hardware stores.
- Review exercise habits and consider adjusting your routine (see below). Consider exercising indoors, which may limit your exposure to asthma triggers.
- Don't smoke and avoid secondhand smoke. Avoid all types of smoke, even from a fireplace or burning leaves. Smoke irritates the eyes, nose and bronchial tubes.
- Reduce stress and fatigue.
- Read labels carefully. If you're sensitive to aspirin, you may need to avoid other nonprescription pain relievers, including ibuprofen (Advil, Motrin IB, others) and naproxen sodium (Aleve, others).

Staying active with well-planned workouts

Well-planned regular workouts are beneficial with asthma, especially if you have mild to moderate forms of the disease. If you're fit, your heart and lungs don't have to work as hard to expel air.

However, because vigorous exercise can asthma trigger an attack, discuss a safe exercise program with your doctor before you begin. In addition, follow these guidelines:

- **Know when not to exercise.** Avoid exercise when you have a viral infection or in below zero or extremely hot and humid conditions. If it's cold, wear a face mask to warm the air you breathe.

- **Medicate first.** Use your inhaled short-acting beta agonist 15 to 60 minutes before exercise.
- **Start slowly.** Five to 10 minutes of warm-up exercises may relax your chest muscles and widen your airways to ease breathing. Gradually work up to your desired pace.
- **Choose the type of exercise wisely.** Cold-weather activities such as skiing and long-distance, nonstop activities such as running often cause wheezing. Exercise that requires short bursts of energy, such as walking, golf and leisure bicycling, may be better tolerated.

Medical help

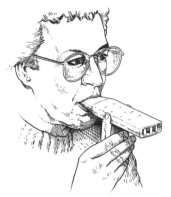

A peak flow meter is a device used to evaluate lung function.

Testing for allergies. Your health care provider may perform some tests to try to determine the triggers of your asthma attacks. A skin test or blood test may be performed. The blood test is more expensive and is less sensitive than a skin test, but a blood test is sometimes preferable when you have a skin disease or you're taking medications that might affect the test results.

Medications. Your doctor may prescribe some of the medications listed below to prevent or treat your asthma attacks. Take all the medications as prescribed, even if you aren't experiencing any symptoms. Don't take more than the prescribed amount because excessive use of medications can be dangerous. These medications can be taken using an inhaler, or they may come in liquid, capsule or tablet form.

Long-term control medications reduce the inflammation in your airways and also help reduce the production of mucus. The result is a reduction of the spasms in your breathing passages. Take the daily dose of these medications as prescribed to prevent asthma attacks from occurring. Medications include inhaled corticosteroids, long-acting inhaled bronchodilators (for use with an inhaled corticosteroid regimen but not for use alone or for quick relief), leukotriene modifiers and others.

Quick-relief medications are taken when you're experiencing an asthma attack. These medications help open narrow airways to allow you to breathe easier during an attack. They include short-acting inhaled bronchodilators, and oral and intravenous corticosteroids.

There are also medications for allergy-induced asthma and combination therapies.

Self-monitoring with peak flow meter. You may be trained to use a device that measures how well you are breathing (peak flow meter). The flow meter acts like a gauge for your lungs, giving you a number that helps evaluate lung function. A low reading means your air passages are narrow and is an early warning that you may experience an asthma attack.

Inhalers: Risks of misuse

Inhaling a **bronchodilator** helps you breathe better immediately during an attack. But the drug doesn't help with inflammation.

Maximal daily use of a bronchodilator is two puffs every four to six hours. If you're using one more frequently to control symptoms, you need a more effective program of preventive medications.

Fast relief may make it difficult to recognize worsening symptoms. Once the medication wears off, asthma returns with more severe wheezing. You're then tempted to take another dose of the medication, delaying adequate treatment with anti-inflammatory medications.

Overuse of a bronchodilator can be dangerous. If you're not getting relief from using a bronchodilator more than the recommended maximum use, talk to your doctor. If your asthma symptoms keep getting worse even after you take medication as your doctor directed, you may need emergency care. Your doctor can help you learn to recognize an asthma emergency so that you'll know when to get help.

FOR MORE INFORMATION
- Asthma and Allergy Foundation of America, 800-727-8462, *www.aafa.org*
- American Lung Association, 800-586-4872, *www.lung.org*
- National Institute of Allergy and Infectious Diseases, National Institutes of Health, 866-284-4107, *www.niaid.nih.gov*

 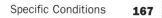

Specific Conditions

Cancer

One of the best approaches to fighting **cancer** is an early diagnosis. In most cases, the earlier a cancer is detected, the greater the chances it can be treated before it spreads to other tissues or organs. With the cancer-screening procedures available today, many cancers can be detected early. You can help in early detection by learning the warning signs and getting proper screenings.

Estimated new cases of cancer in the United States, 2017

This shows the 10 leading types of new cancer cases by sex. Estimates are rounded to the nearest 10 and cases exclude basal cell and squamous cell skin cancers and carcinoma in situ *except urinary bladder.*

Based on Siegel RL, et al., "Cancer Statistics, 2017," in CA: A Cancer Journal for Clinicians, 2017; 67:7

Men

Prostate
161,360 (19%)
Lung & bronchus
116,990 (14%)
Colon & rectum
71,420 (9%)
Urinary bladder
60,490 (7%)
Melanoma of the skin
52,170 (6%)
Kidney & renal pelvis
40,610 (5%)
Non-Hodgkin's lymphoma
40,080 (5%)
Leukemia
36,290 (4%)
Oral cavity & pharynx
35,720 (4%)
Liver & intrahepatic bile duct
29,200 (3%)

All sites
836,150 (100%)

Women

Breast
252,710 (30%)
Lung & bronchus
105,510 (12%)
Colon & rectum
64,010 (8%)
Uterine corpus
61,380 (7%)
Thyroid
42,470 (5%)
Melanoma of the skin
34,940 (4%)
Non-Hodgkin's lymphoma
32,160 (4%)
Leukemia
25,840 (3%)
Pancreas
25,700 (3%)
Kidney & renal pelvis
23,380 (3%)

All sites
852,630 (100%)

■ Signs, symptoms and screening

This section gives examples of signs and symptoms of some common cancers. Talk to your doctor about your cancer risks and what types of cancer screening would be best for your individual needs.

Prostate cancer

While some types of **prostate cancer** grow slowly and may need minimal or no treatment, other types are aggressive and can spread quickly.

Warning signs. There are often no warning signs in the early stages. With more advanced cancer, warning signs include trouble urinating; decreased force in the stream of urine; blood in the semen; discomfort in the pelvic area; bone pain; and erectile dysfunction.

Risk factors. Risk is increased if you:
- Are over age 50
- Are black
- Have a family history of prostate cancer or breast cancer
- Eat a high-fat diet and are obese

Checkups and screening. See "Screening for prostate cancer," page 141.

Breast cancer

Breast cancer can occur in both men and women, but it's far more common in women. See page 145 for information on warning signs, risk factors and screening.

Lung cancer

Most **lung cancer** deaths can be prevented. That's because smoking accounts for most cases. However, it's possible for nonsmokers to get lung cancer.

Warning signs. Lung cancer typically doesn't cause signs and symptoms in its earliest stage. Later warning signs include new cough that doesn't go away; changes in chronic cough or "smoker's cough;" coughing up blood; chest pain; shortness of breath; wheezing or hoarseness; and repeated problems with pneumonia or bronchitis.

Risk factors. Lung cancer is associated with:

- Smoking
- Exposure to secondhand smoke
- Exposure to radon gas
- Exposure to environmental carcinogens such as asbestos, arsenic and chromium
- Family history of lung cancer

Checkups and screening. Several organizations recommend that people with an increased risk of lung cancer consider annual computerized tomography (CT) scans to look for lung cancer. If you're age 55 or older and smoke or used to smoke, talk with your doctor about the benefits and risks of lung cancer screening. At any age, talk with your doctor if you're concerned about your risk of lung cancer. Together, you can determine strategies to reduce your risk and decide whether screening tests are appropriate for you.

Colorectal cancer

Colon cancer is cancer of the large intestine (colon), the lower part of your digestive system. Rectal cancer is cancer of the last several inches of the colon. Together, they're often referred to as colorectal cancer.

Warning signs. Colorectal cancer may cause rectal bleeding or blood in your stool; a change in bowel habits, including diarrhea or constipation, or a change in consistency of your stool for more than a couple of weeks; persistent abdominal discomfort, such as cramps, gas or pain; a feeling that your bowel doesn't empty completely; weakness or fatigue; and unexplained weight loss.

Risk factors. Colorectal cancer is associated with:

- Older age — typically over age 50
- History of colorectal cancer or polyps
- Family history of colorectal cancer or polyps
- Inflammatory diseases of the colon, such as ulcerative colitis or Crohn's disease
- Inherited syndromes such as hereditary nonpolyposis colorectal cancer (HNPCC), also called Lynch syndrome, or familial adenomatous polyposis
- Tobacco use
- High-fat or low-fiber diet or both
- Diet low in fruits and vegetables
- Heavy use of alcohol
- A sedentary lifestyle
- Obesity
- Diabetes
- Abdominal radiation therapy for previous cancers

Checkups and screening. If you're age 50 or older, get a screening for colorectal cancer. There are many screening options, but some are more thorough and more liable to detect cancer than others. Screening options include:

- Colonoscopy, every 10 years
- Virtual colonoscopy (CT colonography), every five years (not always covered by insurance)
- Fecal occult blood test or fecal immunochemical test, annually
- Flexible sigmoidoscopy, every five years
- Stool DNA test, every three years

Colonoscopy is generally considered the gold standard for colorectal cancer screening. Discuss the benefits and risks of each screening option with your doctor. If you're at increased risk of colorectal cancer, you may need more-frequent screening.

Bladder cancer

Most cases of **bladder cancer** are diagnosed at an early stage, when bladder cancer is highly treatable. However, even early-stage bladder cancer is likely to recur. So cancer survivors often need follow-up screening tests for years after treatment.

Warning signs. Bladder cancer may cause blood in urine (may appear cola colored or bright red, or appear on a microscopic exam of urine); frequent or painful urination; abdominal pain or back pain; loss of weight and appetite; persistent fever; and anemia.

Risk factors. A number of factors may increase your risk:

- Being male and age 50 or older (the majority of people are over 65)
- Family history of bladder cancer
- Tobacco use
- History of chronic urinary tract infections or inflammation (cystitis)
- Working around industrial chemicals, such as chemicals used in the dye or petrochemical industries or in the production of of rubber, leather, textile or paint products
- Family history of hereditary nonpolyposis colorectal cancer (HNPCC)

Checkups and screening. A routine urinalysis during an annual physical exam may reveal blood in your urine, the most common warning sign. Additional procedures may include using a scope to see inside your bladder (cystoscopy), removing suspicious cells for testing and doing imaging tests.

Uterine cancer (endometrial cancer)

Endometrial cancer, sometimes called uterine cancer, is often detected at an early stage because it frequently produces vaginal bleeding between menstrual periods or after menopause. If endometrial cancer is discovered early, removing the uterus surgically often eliminates all of the cancer.

Warning signs. Endometrial cancer may cause vaginal bleeding after menopause; prolonged menstrual periods or bleeding between periods; abnormal, nonbloody vaginal discharge; pelvic pain; pain during intercourse; and unintended weight loss.

Risk factors. Endometrial cancer is associated with:

- Never having been pregnant
- Irregular ovulation patterns, such as those that may occur with polycystic ovary syndrome, obesity and diabetes
- Late onset of menopause or prolonged estrogen therapy or tamoxifen use after menopause
- Use of hormone therapy for breast cancer
- Hereditary nonpolyposis colorectal cancer (HNPCC)

See back cover for online resource

Checkups and screening. Most endometrial cancer is detected early due to postmenopausal bleeding. A pelvic exam is done to feel for lumps or changes in the uterus, and a biopsy is typically done. Other diagnostic tests, such as a transvaginal ultrasound, may be done. If you're a woman with a personal or family history of HNPCC, ask your doctor what cancer screening tests you should undergo.

Skin cancer
Skin cancer most often develops on skin exposed to the sun. But this common form of cancer can also occur on areas of your skin not ordinarily exposed to sunlight. With early detection, you can receive successful treatment for most skin cancers, even the most aggressive forms. See page 129 for more information, including prevention tips.

Hodgkin's lymphoma
Hodgkin's lymphoma, formerly known as Hodgkin's disease, is a cancer of the lymphatic system, which is a part of your immune system. Advances in treatment have helped make this disease highly treatable, with the potential for full recovery.

Warning signs. Hodgkin's lymphoma may cause painless swelling of lymph nodes in the neck, armpits or groin; fatigue, fever or chills; night sweats; weight loss and loss of appetite; and itching.

Risk factors. Hodgkin's lymphoma is associated with:
- Family history of lymphoma
- Past infection with the Epstein-Barr virus
- Weakened immune system

Checkups and screening. A number of tests and procedures can help in diagnosis, such as a biopsy, a computerized tomography (CT) scan or X-rays, among others.

Non-Hodgkin's lymphoma
Non-Hodgkin's lymphoma is more than five times as common as Hodgkin's lymphoma. There are more than 20 types of non-Hodgkin's lymphoma. Although the incidence has increased, so has the survival rate.

Warning signs. Non-Hodgkin's lymphoma may cause painless, swollen lymph nodes; fever; night sweats; fatigue; weight loss; abdominal pain or swelling; and chest pain, coughing or trouble breathing.

Risk factors. Non-Hodgkin's lymphoma is associated with:
- Weakened immune system, such as in people who have received organ transplants or people with HIV
- Various infections, such as with *Helicobacter pylori*
- Exposure to certain chemicals, such as those used to kill insects or weeds
- Older age (age 60 and older), although the disease can occur at any age

Checkups and screening. A number of tests and procedures can help in diagnosis, such as a biopsy, a computerized tomography (CT) scan or X-rays, among others.

Other cancers
For information on cancer of the testicle, see page 140. For ovarian cancer and cervical cancer, see page 151. Information on thyroid cancer is on page 160.

FOR MORE INFORMATION
- National Cancer Institute, 800-422-6237, *www.cancer.gov*
- American Cancer Society, 800-227-2345, *www.cancer.org*
- CureSearch (children's cancer research), 800-458-6223, *https://curesearch.org*

Specific Conditions

Diabetes

Diabetes (diabetes mellitus) is a disease that affects the way your body uses blood glucose, often called blood sugar. Glucose is your body's main source of energy.

The body breaks down food and converts it into glucose. Insulin (made by the pancreas) helps move glucose from the bloodstream into cells, where it's burned for energy. But if you have diabetes, your body produces little or no insulin. Or, the insulin doesn't work very well, so you end up with too much glucose in your blood.

The most common forms of diabetes are type 1 and type 2. But there are other forms, such as gestational diabetes, which occurs during pregnancy.

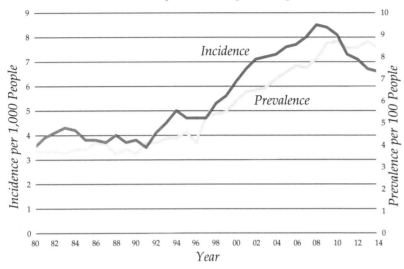

Trends in the incidence and prevalence of diabetes diagnosed in adults. Based on Centers for Disease Control and Prevention. National Center for Chronic Disease Prevention, 2016.

Type 1 and type 2: The difference

Type 1 diabetes is an autoimmune disease. Your own immune system attacks your pancreas, destroying cells, so little if any insulin is made. Without insulin to help move glucose into your cells, glucose stays in your bloodstream. Daily insulin shots are needed. The disease most often develops when you're a child or a teen, although adults can develop type 1 diabetes.

Type 2 diabetes is by far the most common form of the disease. Your pancreas may make some insulin, but your cells become resistant to insulin, so too much glucose stays in your bloodstream. Being overweight makes it harder for your body to use insulin. Type 2 diabetes usually develops in adults, but as more children and teens become overweight, the incidence of type 2 diabetes is increasing at younger ages.

Complications

Both types of diabetes can cause long-term complications, including heart and blood vessel disease (such as a heart attack and stroke), nerve damage, kidney disease and eye damage. Keeping your blood sugar close to normal — by healthy eating, physical activity and, if needed, medications — greatly reduces your risk of complications.

What's prediabetes?

Prediabetes means that your blood sugar is higher than normal but not high enough to be type 2 diabetes. The long-term damage associated with diabetes — especially to your heart and blood vessels — may already be starting if you have prediabetes.

But you can prevent or delay type 2 diabetes by making healthy lifestyle changes. In a major study on diabetes prevention, those in the lifestyle-treatment group (who ate a healthy diet, engaged in moderately intense physical activity and lost a small percentage of weight) cut their risk of diabetes in half.

See back cover for online resource ⓘ

Diabetes warning signs

Often, prediabetes has no signs or symptoms, so it's important to know your blood sugar level. Watch for these classic signs and symptoms of diabetes:

- Excessive thirst
- Frequent urination

  Other signs and symptoms may include:
- Constant hunger
- Unexplained weight loss
- Weight gain (more common in type 2)
- Flu-like symptoms, including weakness and fatigue
- Blurred vision
- Slow-healing cuts or bruises
- Tingling or loss of feeling in hands and feet
- Recurring infections of gums and skin
- Recurring vaginal or bladder infections

Are you at increased risk of type 2 diabetes?

These factors raise your risk of type 2 diabetes. The more risk factors you have, the higher your risk.

- Parent, brother or sister who has type 2 diabetes
- Overweight
- Carry excess weight around waist or upper body (apple-shaped body) rather than hips and thighs (pear-shaped body)
- Metabolic syndrome (see below)
- Not physically active — get little or no exercise
- Over age 45
- African-American, Latino, Native American, Alaska Native, Asian-American or Pacific Islander
- Gave birth to a baby who weighed more than 9 pounds
- Developed diabetes when pregnant (gestational diabetes)

Metabolic syndrome raises diabetes risk

Metabolic syndrome is a cluster of conditions that increases your risk of type 2 diabetes, heart disease and stroke. According to the American Heart Association, if you have three or more of the risk factors below, you probably have metabolic syndrome.

- **Abdominal obesity:** For women, a 35-inch waist or larger; for men, a 40-inch waist or larger
- **Triglycerides:** 150 milligrams per deciliter (mg/dL) or higher
- **High-density lipoprotein (HDL) cholesterol (the "good" cholesterol):** Women, under 50 mg/dL; men, under 40 mg/dL
- **Blood pressure:** Top number (systolic), 130 millimeters of mercury (mm Hg) or higher; bottom number (diastolic), 85 mm Hg or higher
- **Fasting blood glucose:** 100 mg/dL or higher

   If you think that you have metabolic syndrome, talk with your doctor about tests that can help determine this. Eating a heart-healthy diet, achieving a healthy weight and increasing your level of physical activity can help combat metabolic syndrome and play a role in preventing diabetes and other serious diseases. It's also important to monitor and manage your blood glucose, blood pressure and cholesterol levels.

Testing for prediabetes and diabetes

An international committee of diabetes experts recommends the A1C test (glycated hemoglobin test) for prediabetes and diabetes testing. This blood test helps determine your average blood sugar level over the past two to three months. If the A1C test isn't available or if you have a condition that can make the A1C test inaccurate, a fasting blood glucose test or an oral glucose tolerance test may be used.

A1C level*	Fasting blood glucose test	Oral glucose tolerance test	Indicates
Less than 5.7%	Under 100 mg/dL†	Under 140 mg/dL	Normal
Between 5.7% and 6.4%	100 mg/dL to 125 mg/dL	140 mg/dL to 199 mg/dL	Prediabetes
6.5% or higher	126 mg/dL or higher	200 mg/dL or higher	Diabetes

*Results indicate what percentage of your hemoglobin — a protein in red blood cells — is sugar coated (glycated).
†Milligrams of glucose per deciliter of blood

Source: American Diabetes Association, 2016.

Self-care

If you play an active role on your health care team, you can take control of your diabetes. Learn as much as you can about diabetes and self-care, including how to monitor and effectively treat your diabetes, and how to achieve a healthy lifestyle. These self-care tips can help you take charge of your diabetes.

Monitor your blood sugar

Managing your blood sugar is key to feeling your best and preventing complications. Your blood sugar goals and how often and when to test depend on your type of diabetes and treatment plan. If you take insulin, test your blood sugar at least twice a day. Your doctor may advise testing more often.

If you have type 2 diabetes and don't need insulin, test your blood sugar as often as needed to be sure it's under control. This can mean daily testing or twice a week. Discuss this with your diabetes care team.

Work closely with your team to manage your **ABCs**, as identified by the American Diabetes Association, and lower your risk of heart disease, stroke and other complications. These goals are appropriate for most people with diabetes, but ask your doctor what your goals are:

- **A = A1C.** Aim for less than 7 percent, unless your doctor advises otherwise.
- **B = Blood pressure.** Aim for less than 140/90 mm Hg.
- **C = Cholesterol.** Aim for:
  - LDL ("bad") cholesterol under 100 mg/dL (if you have heart disease or are at very high risk, your LDL goal may be under 70 mg/dL)
  - HDL ("good") cholesterol above 40 mg/dL for men or above 50 mg/dL for women
  - Triglycerides under 150 mg/dL (emerging data indicate that below 100 is ideal)

Use medications wisely

Insulin and other diabetes medications can lower your blood sugar and prevent long-term complications. But medication effectiveness depends on the timing and dose — which in large part depends on you. Learn when and how to take your diabetes medications. For example, with certain medications, timing of meals is very important. Ask about the advantages and disadvantages of your options. Also:

- Store medications properly so that they stay effective.
- Report problems to your doctor. Dosage or timing may need to be adjusted.
- Be cautious with a new medication, whether it's nonprescription or a new prescription for another condition. Ask if it can affect your blood sugar level.

If you take insulin, the type and amount that's best depends on your patterns of blood sugar levels, what you eat, how physically active you are, and whether you have other health conditions.

Your doctor may prescribe other drugs taken by injection — liraglutide (Victoza, Saxenda) or pramlintide (Symlin) — which affect how rapidly blood sugar enters the bloodstream. Follow instructions carefully and ask about potential side effects.

Choose healthier foods

A registered dietitian and diabetes educator can help you adjust your diet to meet your needs. Here are some basic tips to help you gain better control of blood sugar:

- **Stick to a schedule.** Eat three meals a day. Be consistent in the amount of food you eat and the timing of eating. If you're hungry after dinner, choose a food low in calories or carbohydrates before going to bed, such as raw vegetables.
- **Focus on fiber.** Eat a variety of fresh fruits, vegetables, legumes and whole-grain foods. These high-fiber foods help control blood sugar and are low fat and rich sources of vitamins and minerals.
- **Limit foods that are high in saturated and trans fats.** Choose lean cuts of meats and use low-fat dairy products. Use small amounts of healthy oils instead of shortening and butter.
- **Choose proteins low in saturated fat.** If you eat too much protein, your body stores the extra calories as fat. Choose fish and poultry more often than red meat.
- **Eat fewer sweets.** Candy, cookies and other sweets aren't forbidden but they're often high in fat and calories. Count them in your total carbohydrate intake.
- **Use alcohol in moderation.** An occasional alcoholic beverage is OK if your doctor says it's safe. But be mindful of how much you drink. Alcohol can affect your blood sugar and increase your calorie intake, which affects your weight.
- **Maintain a healthy weight.** Being overweight is by far the greatest risk factor for type 2 diabetes. If you're overweight, losing even a few pounds can improve your blood sugar levels.

Get more active

Regular physical activity and exercise are essential to help lower your blood sugar and improve your body's ability to use insulin or other diabetes medications. Regular exercise may even reduce the amount of diabetes medication that you need. Also, regular physical activity and exercise can help with weight loss, improve your circulation, lower your risk of heart disease and reduce your stress.

You can increase physical activity by doing simple things, such as taking the stairs instead of the elevator. Learn how to avoid blood sugar problems during exercise. Before you start a fitness program, talk with your doctor.

Specific Conditions

Handling medical emergencies

If your blood sugar goes to extremes (too high or too low), you can have serious problems. Learn the signs below and what to do if they occur. If you have a medical emergency, take action immediately.

Low blood sugar (hypoglycemia)

- **Early signs.** Sweating, shakiness, visual disturbances, nervousness, headache, weakness, hunger, dizziness, irritability, nausea, cold and clammy skin.
- **Later signs.** Slurred speech, drowsiness, drunken-like behavior, confusion.
- **Emergency signs.** Seizures, coma (which can be fatal).
- **What to do.** If blood sugar is below 70 mg/dL, eat or drink something to raise your level quickly, such as hard candy (equal to about five Life Savers), ½ cup regular (not diet) soft drink, ½ cup fruit juice, or three or four glucose tablets. If needed, repeat in 15 minutes. If there's no improvement, get medical help right away. If you use insulin, ask your doctor if you need a glucagon emergency kit.

Dangerously high blood sugar

- **Early signs.** Excessive thirst, leg cramps, dry mouth, frequent urination, dehydration.
- **Later signs.** Rapid pulse, weakness, confusion.
- **Emergency signs.** Seizures, coma.
- **What to do.** If blood sugar is over 350 mg/dL and you feel ill or stressed, call your doctor. If it's 500 mg/dL or higher, go to the emergency room if you feel ill or see your doctor immediately if you're otherwise well. If your doctor can't see you, go to the emergency room. Emergency treatment may correct the problem within hours. Without prompt treatment, this can be fatal.

High ketones (diabetic ketoacidosis)

- **Early signs.** High blood sugar, excessive thirst, dry mouth, frequent urination.
- **Later signs.** Fatigue, nausea, vomiting, abdominal pain, shallow breathing, sweet and fruity odor on your breath, blurry vision, confusion, loss of appetite, weight loss, weakness, drowsiness.
- **Emergency signs.** Seizures, coma.
- **What to do.** Ketones are the result of your body burning fat for fuel. High amounts of ketones in the body can be dangerous. Check your urine ketone level, especially if blood sugar is persistently over 250 mg/dL. If the test strip color shows a moderate or high ketone level, call your doctor right away and ask how much insulin to take. Drink plenty of water to prevent dehydration. If your ketone level is high and you can't reach your doctor, seek emergency care.

Foot care reduces the risk of injury and infection

Diabetes can damage the nerves in your feet and reduce blood flow to them. Foot care is essential:

- Check your feet every day for blisters, cuts, sores, redness or swelling.
- Wash your feet daily in lukewarm water. Dry them thoroughly and gently.
- Trim nails straight across. File rough edges.
- Don't use wart removers or trim calluses and corns yourself. See your doctor or a podiatrist.
- Wear cushioned, well-fitted shoes. Check inside shoes daily for fabric wear or rough edges.
- Wear clean, dry socks.
- Don't walk barefoot, even at home.
- Avoid tight clothing around your legs or ankles.
- Avoid exposing your feet to temperature extremes.
- Moisturize feet and ankles with lotion, but don't put lotion between your toes.

Heart disease

Your heart pumps blood to every tissue in your body through a network of blood vessels. Problems can arise in the heart muscle or valves, the electrical conduction system, the sac surrounding the heart (pericardium) or the arteries that supply blood to the heart (coronary arteries). This section focuses on the coronary arteries.

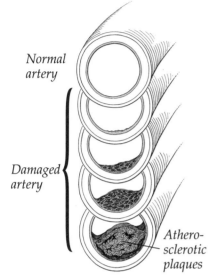

Normal artery

Damaged artery

Athero-sclerotic plaques

When you have too much cholesterol in your bloodstream, fatty deposits (plaques) can accumulate in your arteries in a process called athero-sclerosis. As these deposits build up, blood flow is reduced, putting you at risk of a heart attack or stroke. High cholesterol is one of several risk factors for heart disease.

Coronary artery disease

Your coronary arteries are major blood vessels that supply your heart with blood, oxygen and nutrients. When these arteries become damaged or diseased, usually due to a buildup of fatty deposits called plaques, it's called <u>coronary artery disease</u>.

These deposits can slowly narrow your coronary arteries, reducing blood flow to your heart and other vital organs — a condition called athero-sclerosis, which some people call "hardening of the arteries." Eventually, reduced blood flow may cause the signs and symptoms below. A complete blockage, caused either by a buildup of plaques or a ruptured plaque, can cause a <u>**heart attack**</u>. Sometimes a heart attack is the first sign that your artery is completely blocked — and in some cases there are no signs or symptoms leading up to the heart attack (see "Heart attack," page 5).

Signs and symptoms

Reduced blood flow may not cause coronary artery disease symptoms for years. But as the fatty deposits build up in your arteries, you may develop:

- **Chest pain (angina).** You may feel pressure, squeezing, burning or tight-ness in your chest, as if someone were standing on your chest. This pain, called angina, usually occurs with physical activity and is relieved within minutes of rest. If discomfort gets more frequent, severe or longer, you may have a more dangerous form of angina (unstable angina) or a heart attack. Women may have subtler symptoms, more often have symptoms at rest or with stress, or have pain in other locations (such as the upper back, jaw or arms).
- **Shortness of breath.** If your heart can't pump enough blood to meet your body's needs, you may get short of breath or tire easily doing usual daily activities. Women of any age and men over age 65 are more likely to have shortness of breath without chest discomfort.

Chronic leg pain? It could be PAD

If your leg arteries become clogged or partially blocked with fatty buildup, you likely have peripheral artery disease (PAD), often mistaken for arthritis. If you have PAD, you probably have clogged arteries in other parts of your body, increasing your risk of heart attack and stroke.

People with PAD may have no symptoms or:
- Leg cramps or pain that starts with walking and stops with rest (earlier stage)
- Leg cramps or pain even at rest (later stage)

- Leg or foot coldness
- Sores on toes, feet or legs that don't heal

A simple test, the ankle-brachial index, helps detect PAD by comparing ankle blood pressure with arm blood pressure. Even without symptoms, if you are over age 70; over 50 and have a history of diabetes or smoking; or under age 50 with diabetes and other PAD risk factors, such as obesity or high blood pressure, ask your doctor if you should be screened for PAD.

See back cover for online resource ⓘ

Risk factors

Risk factors for coronary artery disease include:

- **Age.** Simply getting older increases your risk of damaged and narrowed arteries.
- **Sex.** Men are generally at greater risk of coronary artery disease than are women. However, the risk for women increases after menopause.
- **Family history.** A family history of heart disease is associated with a higher risk of coronary artery disease, especially if a parent developed it at an early age (before age 55 for men and before age 65 in women).
- **Smoking.** Nicotine constricts your blood vessels, and carbon monoxide can damage their inner lining, making them more susceptible to atherosclerosis.
- **High blood pressure.** Uncontrolled high blood pressure can result in hardening and thickening of your arteries, reducing blood flow.
- **High cholesterol.** High levels of cholesterol in your blood can increase the risk of formation of plaques and atherosclerosis. High cholesterol can be caused by a high level of low-density lipoprotein (LDL), known as "bad" cholesterol, or a low level of high-density lipoprotein (HDL), known as "good" cholesterol.
- **Diabetes.** Diabetes is associated with an increased risk of coronary artery disease. Both conditions share similar risk factors, such as obesity and high blood pressure.
- **Obesity.** Excess weight typically worsens other risk factors.
- **Physical inactivity.** Lack of physical activity also is associated with coronary artery disease and some of its risk factors.
- **High stress.** Too much stress in your life may damage your arteries as well as worsen other risk factors for coronary artery disease.
- **Poor nutrition.** A diet that lacks essential nutrients, such as from ample fruits, vegetables and whole grains, can affect your risk.

If you have many risk factors

The more risk factors you have, the greater your risk of a heart attack. Risk factors often occur in clusters and can build on one another, such as obesity leading to diabetes and high blood pressure. When grouped together, certain risk factors put you at an ever greater risk of coronary artery disease. For example, metabolic syndrome — a cluster of conditions that includes elevated blood pressure, high triglycerides, elevated insulin levels and excess body fat around the waist — increases the risk of coronary artery disease. (See more on metabolic syndrome on page 173.)

Daily aspirin therapy: Is it right for you?

Daily aspirin therapy helps lower the risk of heart attack and stroke by reducing the tendency of your blood to clot. This helps prevent a blockage from forming in your coronary arteries. If you've had a heart attack, aspirin can help prevent future attacks. Typically the daily dose for prevention is 8l milligrams, but check with your doctor before starting.

Daily aspirin therapy is recommended if you've had a heart attack or stroke, or you're at high risk of either — for example, if you have diabetes. Even if you are not at high risk, you might benefit from aspirin therapy. Men over age 45 and women over age 55, should ask your doctors if daily aspirin therapy is appropriate.

Not for everyone

For some people, daily use of aspirin can have side effects, such as stomach bleeding. This is especially of concern if you have a history of gastrointestinal bleeding or ulcers. While daily aspirin can help prevent a clot-related stroke, it may increase your risk of a bleeding stroke (hemorrhagic stroke). Ask your doctor what's right for you.

If you have heart failure, don't take daily aspirin unless your doctor recommends it.

| **Self-care** | Several risk factors for coronary artery disease can be modified through lifestyle changes or medications. Here's what you can do to reduce your risk: |

- **Stop smoking.** If you smoke, see page 192.
- **Control your blood pressure.** See page 182.
- **Check your cholesterol.** See page 213.
- **Keep diabetes under control.** See page 172.
- **Maintain a healthy weight.** See page 206.
- **Eat healthy foods.** Ample fruits, vegetables and whole grains are key. Try to eat at least two servings (3 ounces each) a week of fish rich in heart-healthy omega-3 fatty acids, such as salmon, sardines, trout and whitefish. See page 210.
- **Increase your physical activity.** See page 215.
- **Take steps to reduce stress.** See page 221.

Medical help

In addition to the self-care steps above, your doctor may recommend:

- **Taking daily aspirin.** Don't take this without your doctor's approval. See the box on page 178.
- **Fish oil supplements.** The evidence is stronger for the heart-healthy benefits of eating fish rich in omega-3 fatty acids compared with using fish oil supplements. However, people who have heart disease may benefit from supplements and should discuss this with their doctors.
- **Prescription medications.** If you have coronary artery disease or you've had a heart attack, other medicines may lower your risk of heart disease or heart attack. Discuss medications with your doctor. Options may include cholesterol-lowering medicines, such as statins, nitroglycerin, beta blockers, angiotensin-converting enzyme (ACE) inhibitors or calcium channel blockers.
- **Procedures to restore and improve blood flow.** Options may include a procedure called angioplasty and stent placement or coronary artery bypass surgery.

Heart failure

Heart failure, also known as congestive heart failure (CHF), means your heart can't pump enough blood to meet your body's needs. You're at higher risk of heart failure if you have high blood pressure, coronary artery disease, a history of heart attack, faulty heart valves, diabetes or certain other conditions. Heart failure can be a long-term condition (chronic) or an emergency, with symptoms appearing suddenly (acute).

Signs and symptoms

Signs and symptoms may include:

- Swelling in your abdomen, legs, ankles or feet, or unexplained weight gain.
- Shortness of breath during activity or at rest. Difficulty breathing while lying flat at night.

- Rapid or irregular heartbeat.
- Feeling tired all the time and having a hard time doing daily activities.
- Persistent cough or wheezing with white or pink phlegm (mucus).

What to do

Notify your doctor if you have any of the signs and symptoms above. Treatment strategies include medications and, sometimes, surgery or implantable devices.

Lifestyle changes can help reduce symptoms and prevent the disease from worsening. These often include limiting sodium and alcohol, monitoring your fluid intake, eating healthier foods, getting physical activity, and keeping a daily weight log.

Hepatitis

Hepatitis is an inflammation of the liver. How do hepatitis A, B and C differ?

Hepatitis A

Hepatitis A is a highly contagious liver infection caused by the hepatitis A virus.

How hepatitis A is spread

You can get the hepatitis A virus by:

- Ingesting tiny amounts of contaminated feces — for example, when someone with the virus handles the food you eat without careful hand-washing after using the toilet — or by drinking contaminated water
- Eating raw shellfish from water polluted with sewage
- Being in close contact with a person who's infected
- Having sex with someone who has the virus
- Receiving a blood transfusion with blood that contains the virus (this is very rare)

Signs and symptoms

Signs and symptoms, which typically don't appear until you've had the virus for a month, may include fatigue, nausea, vomiting, abdominal pain or discomfort (especially near the liver on your right side under the lower ribs), loss of appetite, low-grade fever, dark urine, muscle pain, itching, yellow skin and eyes (jaundice).

Tests and treatment

Blood tests can detect hepatitis A. There is no treatment. Your body can clear the virus on its own. Usually the liver heals in a month or two with no lasting damage.

Prevention of hepatitis A

Children and adults in certain risk groups are advised to get the hepatitis A vaccine — see pages 226-228. See page 283 if you're traveling to a high-risk area.

Hepatitis B

Hepatitis B is a serious liver infection caused by the hepatitis B virus. For some people, hepatitis B infection becomes chronic, leading to liver failure, liver cancer or cirrhosis — a condition that causes permanent scarring of the liver.

How hepatitis B is spread

The hepatitis B virus is spread by:

- Sexual contact during unprotected sex with an infected partner
- Sharing needles and syringes contaminated with infected blood
- Accidental needle sticks with infected blood, a concern for health care workers
- Receiving hemodialysis treatments for a long period of time
- Infected mothers to children during childbirth

Signs and symptoms

Most infants and children with hepatitis B never have signs and symptoms, and this is true for some adults. Symptoms usually appear two to three months after infection and may include abdominal pain, dark urine, joint pain, loss of appetite, nausea, vomiting, weakness and fatigue, yellow skin and eyes (jaundice).

See back cover for online resource

Tests and treatment

Certain blood tests can diagnose hepatitis B infection. Your doctor can determine if you need treatment for short-term (acute) hepatitis B infection. Treatment for long-term (chronic) hepatitis B infection may include antiviral drugs or even a liver transplant if your liver has been severely damaged.

Prevention of hepatitis B

Almost anyone can receive the hepatitis B vaccine, including infants — see pages 226-228. See page 283 for vaccine advice if you're traveling to a high-risk area.

Hepatitis C

Hepatitis C is an infection caused by a virus that attacks the liver and leads to inflammation. It's generally considered the most serious type of hepatitis, but it is treatable.

How hepatitis C is spread

Examples of how you can get hepatitis C include:

- Blood transfusions and organ transplants received before 1992
- Receiving clotting factor concentrates before 1987
- Sharing needles and syringes contaminated with infected blood
- Accidental needle sticks with infected blood, a concern for health care workers
- Receiving hemodialysis treatments for a long period of time
- From body or ear piercing, tattoos, or acupuncture with unsterile equipment
- From infected mothers to children during childbirth (uncommon)
- Sexual contact during unprotected sex with an infected partner (rare)

Signs and symptoms

Hepatitis C infection usually has no signs or symptoms in its early stage. When they do occur, they're generally mild and flu-like and may include fatigue, fever, nausea, poor appetite, muscle and joint pains, and tenderness in the area of your liver.

Tests and treatment

Blood tests can diagnose hepatitis C infection. You may also need a liver biopsy to help determine disease severity. The infection is treated with antiviral medications intended to clear the virus from your body. In serious cases, a liver transplant may be warranted.

Prevention of hepatitis C

While there is no vaccine for hepatitis C, getting vaccinated against hepatitis A and B can reduce your risk of liver damage.

Stop the virus from spreading

If you're diagnosed with hepatitis A, B or C, ask your doctor for advice on how to prevent spreading the virus to others. For example, if you have hepatitis A, avoid sexual activity (condoms don't offer adequate protection), wash your hands thoroughly after using the toilet and don't prepare food for others while you're infected. Don't drink alcohol and avoid medications that may cause liver damage if you have hepatitis C.

No matter what type of hepatitis you have, prevent others from coming in contact with your blood. Cover wounds, don't share your toothbrush or razors, and advise health care workers that you have the virus. Don't donate blood, body organs, tissues or semen. Also, maintain a healthy lifestyle, including not smoking, eating healthy foods, and getting enough physical activity and rest.

High blood pressure

Most people with **high blood pressure** (hypertension) don't experience any signs or symptoms, even if blood pressure reaches dangerously high levels. That's why it's called a silent killer. Many people aren't aware that high blood pressure can have damaging effects on the arteries, heart, brain, kidneys and eyes.

What is blood pressure?

Blood pressure is the force of blood, pumped by your heart, pushing against the walls of your arteries. Your blood pressure reading has two numbers: the systolic pressure (top number) and diastolic pressure (bottom number).

Your blood pressure is highest each time your heart muscle tightens (contracts) and pumps out blood — that's your systolic blood pressure. Between beats, your heart rests, decreasing your blood pressure — that's your diastolic blood pressure. With high blood pressure, your heart has to work a lot harder than normal to pump blood throughout your body. High blood pressure becomes more common with age.

Know your numbers

Knowing your numbers and taking steps to control your blood pressure are critical to your health. If you're over 20, get your blood pressure checked at least every two years or more often if your doctor recommends it. See the chart below.

Prehypertension is the term for blood pressure that's above normal but not high enough to be defined as high blood pressure. When a cause can't be determined, high blood pressure is called **essential hypertension** or **primary hypertension.** When a cause is the result of an underlying condition, the term **secondary hypertension** is used. Causes may include medications such as oral birth control pills, kidney disorders such as kidney failure, adrenal gland tumors or certain congenital heart defects.

Your blood pressure reading

Top number (systolic)		Bottom number (diastolic)	What it means
Less than 120	and	Less than 80	Normal
120-139	or	80-89	Prehypertension
140-159	or	90-99	Stage 1 hypertension
160 or greater	or	100 or greater	Stage 2 hypertension

Note: This chart applies to adults 18 and older. Numbers are in millimeters of mercury (mm Hg). Diagnosis is based on the average of two or more readings taken at two different visits, after the initial screening. If your readings fall into two different categories, your result is the higher category.

Source: James PA, et al. 2014 Evidence-Based Guideline for the Management of High Blood Pressure in Adults: Report From the Panel Members Appointed to the Eighth Joint National Committee (JNC 8). *JAMA.* 2014;311(5):507.

See back cover for online resource ⓘ

Self-care

Lifestyle changes can help you control and prevent high blood pressure — even if you're taking blood pressure medication. Here's what you can do:

- **Eat healthy foods.** Try the Dietary Approaches to Stop Hypertension (DASH) diet, which emphasizes fruits, vegetables, whole grains and low-fat dairy foods. Get plenty of potassium, which can help prevent and control high blood pressure. (If you have kidney disease you may need to limit your potassium intake.)
- **Decrease the salt in your diet.** Salt causes the body to retain fluids and so, in many people, can cause high blood pressure. Don't add salt to food. Avoid salty foods such as cured meats, snack foods, canned foods and other processed foods, such as canned soups or frozen dinners.
- **Maintain a healthy weight.** If your body mass index (BMI) is over 25 (see page 207), lose weight, unless your BMI is due to muscle rather than fat. Losing even 5 pounds may lower your blood pressure. In some people, weight loss alone is sufficient to avoid the need to take blood pressure medications.
- **Increase physical activity.** Regular physical activity can help lower blood pressure and manage weight. Get at least 150 minutes a week of moderate aerobic activity (such as brisk walking) or 75 minutes a week of vigorous aerobic activity (such as swimming laps) spread out during the course of a week.
- **Don't smoke.** Tobacco injures blood vessel walls and speeds up the process of hardening of the arteries. If you smoke, ask your doctor to help you quit.
- **Limit alcohol.** Even if you're healthy, alcohol can raise your blood pressure. If you choose to drink alcohol, do so in moderation — no more than one drink a day for women and anyone over age 65, and a limit of two drinks a day for men.
- **Manage stress.** Reduce stress as much as possible. Practice healthy coping techniques, such as muscle relaxation and deep breathing, and get plenty of sleep.
- **Monitor blood pressure at home.** Home blood pressure monitoring can help you keep closer tabs on your blood pressure, show if medication is working, and even alert you and your doctor to potential complications.

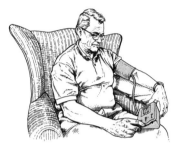

With an electronic blood pressure monitor, you simply put the cuff on your upper arm and push a button to inflate the cuff and get a reading. Home blood pressure monitoring can help track how well your treatment is working.

The use of medications

Your doctor will determine which drug or combination of drugs may work best for you. Cost, side effects, interaction between multiple drugs and how the drugs affect other illnesses may be considered. It may take time to find the most effective drug for your needs. If the first drug doesn't lower your blood pressure, a second, third or even fourth drug may be prescribed either as a substitute or as an additional drug.

Low blood pressure (hypotension)

Low blood pressure is called hypotension. It isn't uncommon to have chronic low blood pressure — when your blood pressure is below average but you don't have symptoms and it's not dangerous. But if blood pressure falls to dangerously low levels (shock), the situation can be life-threatening.

Low blood pressure can be caused by medications, pregnancy, certain heart problems, diabetes, thyroid disorders, dehydration, blood loss or other medical conditions.

One common type of low blood pressure is called postural hypotension. The key symptom is dizziness or faintness that occurs when you stand up quickly from a seated position. Typically this type of blood pressure isn't life-threatening, but it may increase the risk of falls and injury. (See "Dizziness and fainting," page 34.)

Sexually transmitted infections

Sexually transmitted infection (STI) is increasing in the United States. Most STIs are treatable, but human immunodeficiency virus (**HIV**), the cause of acquired immuno-deficiency syndrome (**AIDS**), currently has no cure. Yet when HIV is well-managed with a number of medications, some people live an almost normal life expectancy.

Although HIV can be spread through use of contaminated needles or, rarely, through blood transfusion, it usually is transmitted by sexual contact. The virus is present in semen and vaginal secretions and enters the body through small tears that can develop in the vaginal or rectal tissues during sexual activity. Transmission of the virus occurs only after intimate contact with infected blood, semen or vaginal secretions. There have been cases of HIV being passed to health care workers through needle sticks.

STIs such as **chlamydia** infections, **gonorrhea**, hepatitis B and C, **genital herpes**, **genital warts** and **syphilis** are highly contagious. Many can be spread through only one sexual contact. The microorganisms that cause STIs, including HIV, all die within hours once they're outside the body. However, none of these infections is spread through casual contact such as shaking hands or sitting on a toilet seat.

The only sure way of preventing STIs and HIV infection is through sexual abstinence or a relationship exclusively between two uninfected people. If you have several sexual partners or an infected partner, you're at higher risk of contracting an STI.

The use of condoms

Correct and consistent use of a latex or polyurethane condom and avoidance of certain sexual practices can decrease the risk of contracting HIV and other STIs, although condoms don't completely eliminate the risk. You won't be protected by the condom if either partner has a sore on the labia or scrotum. The condom doesn't cover this area, so there's a risk of exposure to the sore. Condoms sometimes are made of animal membrane, and the pores in such natural skin condoms may allow the HIV to pass through. The use of latex condoms is recommended.

To be effective, a condom must be undamaged, applied before genital contact and remain intact until removed on completion of sexual activity. Extra lubrication (even with lubricated condoms) can help prevent the condom from breaking. Use only water-based lubricants. Oil-based lubricants can cause a condom to break down.

A condom for females can help reduce the risk of getting an STI. Other types of birth control used by females — for example, the pill — don't protect against STIs.

Risky behaviors

HIV is commonly transmitted sexually by penile-anal intercourse. The receptive (passive) partner is at much higher risk of getting HIV than is the active partner, although gonorrhea and syphilis can be acquired from the passive partner's rectum. The likelihood of HIV transmission also depends on the stage of the infection.

Heterosexual vaginal intercourse, particularly with multiple partners, carries a risk of contracting HIV. The virus is believed to be transmitted easier to the woman from the man than vice versa. Oral-genital sex is also a possible means of transmitting HIV, gonorrhea, herpes, syphilis and other STIs.

Sharing needles to self-inject drugs also increases your risk of getting HIV, as well as the hepatitis B and C viruses. The hepatitis B and C viruses are also transmitted by sexual activity and exposure to infected blood.

See back cover for online resource

Sexually transmitted infections

If you think you have a sexually transmitted infection (STI), see a doctor immediately. If an STI is diagnosed, share the information with your sexual partner(s). Don't have sexual contact until the infection is completely gone. Some STIs don't cause signs or symptoms, and you may not know you're infected. (Also see lice and scabies, page 126, and HPV, page 151.)

Signs and symptoms	About the disease	How serious is it?	Medical treatment

AIDS

Signs and symptoms	About the disease	How serious is it?	Medical treatment
• Soaking night sweats • Recurring fever • Chronic diarrhea • Persistent white spots or unusual lesions on your tongue or in your mouth • Persistent, unexplained fatigue • Weight loss • Skin rashes or bumps	AIDS is caused by HIV. Unfortunately, an HIV test isn't accurate immediately after infection because it takes time for your body to develop antibodies. It usually takes 12 weeks for an HIV test to become positive.	HIV weakens the immune system to the point that diseases that your body would normally fight off (opportunistic diseases) begin to affect you. There's no cure for HIV/AIDS, although significant advances in treatment have been made.	There's no vaccine, but use of the drug emtricitabine-tenofovir (Truvada) can reduce the risk of sexually transmitted HIV infection in those at high risk. Treatment includes a combination of medications to reduce the amount of virus in your blood to low or even undetectable levels (antiretroviral medications) and medications to help prevent or treat opportunistic infections.

Chlamydia infection

Signs and symptoms	About the disease	How serious is it?	Medical treatment
• Painful urination • Vaginal discharge • Painful sexual intercourse in women • Bleeding between periods and after sex • Discharge from penis • Testicular pain • Lower abdominal pain	Chlamydia infection is caused by bacteria. The infection can cause scarring of fallopian tubes in women and prostatitis or epididymitis in men.	Touching your eye with infectious secretions can cause an eye infection. Mothers can pass the infection to newborns during delivery, causing pneumonia or an eye infection.	Antibiotics are prescribed. The infection should disappear within 1 to 2 weeks. All sexual partners must be treated, even though they may not have symptoms, to prevent reinfection.

Genital herpes

Signs and symptoms	About the disease	How serious is it?	Medical treatment
• Pain or itching in the genital area • Water blisters or open sores • Genital sores present but invisible inside the vagina (women) or urethra (men) • Recurrent outbreaks	Genital herpes is caused by the herpes simplex virus, usually type 2. Symptoms begin 2 to 12 days after exposure. Itching or burning is followed by clustered blisters and sores. The virus remains dormant and periodically reactivates, causing symptoms.	There's no cure or vaccine. The disease is very contagious whenever sores are present, and the virus can still be spread even when there are no visible lesions. Newborns can become infected as they pass through the birth canal of mothers with open sores.	The prescription oral antiviral drugs acyclovir (Zovirax), famciclovir and valacyclovir (Valtrex) help speed healing. If recurrences are frequent, an oral antiviral medication can be taken daily to suppress the virus.

Continued on p. 186

Specific Conditions

Continued from p. 185

Signs and symptoms	About the disease	How serious is it?	Medical treatment

Genital warts

• Small, flesh-colored or gray swellings in the genital area • Several warts close together that take on a cauliflower-like shape • Itching or discomfort in the genital area • Bleeding with intercourse	Genital warts are caused by the human papillomavirus (HPV). They affect men and women. People with impaired immune systems and pregnant women are more susceptible.	Genital warts are sexually transmitted. Men and women with a history of genital warts have a higher risk of anal cancer. Women have a higher risk of cervical cancer.	Warts are removed by medication, freezing (cryosurgery), surgical excision, laser or electrical current. These procedures may require local or general anesthesia.

Gonorrhea

• Thick, pus-like discharge from urethra • Burning, frequent urination • Slight increase in vaginal discharge and inflammation in women • Anal discharge or irritation • Occasionally fever and abdominal pain	Gonorrhea is caused by bacteria. In men, symptoms first appear 2 days to 2 weeks after exposure. In women, symptoms may not appear for 1 to 3 weeks.	This is a highly contagious, acute infection that may become chronic. In men, it may lead to epididymitis. In women, it can spread to the fallopian tubes and cause pelvic inflammatory disease. It may result in scarring of the fallopian tubes and infertility. It rarely causes joint or throat infection.	Many antibiotics are safe and effective for treating gonorrhea. Although treatable, gonorrhea is becoming resistant to some antibiotics. It may be cured only with the antibiotic ceftriaxone — given as an injection — in combination with either azithromycin or doxycycline, which are taken orally.

Hepatitis B

• Skin and eyes are yellowish • Urine is tea colored • Flu-like illness • Fatigue and achiness • Fever • Joint pain • Loss of appetite	Hepatitis B is caused by a virus. Some carriers never have symptoms but are capable of passing the virus to others.	Pregnant women may pass the virus to the developing fetus. Hepatitis B rarely causes liver failure and death.	Call your doctor immediately after exposure: An injection of hepatitis B immune globulin within 24 hours may help protect you. Ask your doctor if antiviral drugs are needed. Hepatitis B is preventable by vaccination.

Syphilis

• Painless sores on the genitals, rectum, tongue or lips • Enlarged lymph nodes in the groin • Rash, especially on palms and soles • Fever • Headache • Soreness and aching in bones or joints	Syphilis is caused by a bacteria. Primary stage: Painless sores appear in the genital area, rectum, tongue or lips 10 days to 6 weeks after exposure. Second stage, 1 week to 6 months later: Red rash may appear. Third stage, often after yearslong latent period: heart disease, mental deterioration.	Syphilis can be completely cured if the diagnosis is made early and the infection is treated. Left untreated, the disease can lead to death. In pregnant women, it can be transmitted to the fetus, causing deformities and death.	Syphilis is usually treated with penicillin. A single injection of penicillin can stop the disease from progressing if you've been infected for less than a year. Some people don't respond to the usual doses of penicillin. They must get periodic blood tests to make sure the infection has been destroyed.

Based on *MayoClinic.org.*

Mental Health

- **Addictive behavior**
- **Anxiety disorders**
- **Depression**
- **Domestic violence**
- **Memory loss**

This section examines a range of issues that affect the mental health of millions of Americans and their families. Get helpful information on how to deal with addictive behavior, anxiety and panic disorders, depression, domestic abuse, and memory loss.

Addictive behavior

You can become addicted to many substances and practices. The main traits of addictive behavior include a compelling need to use the addictive substance or engage in the activity, impaired control as a result of the use or activity, and continued use or activity despite adverse consequences. This section includes discussions of alcohol, drugs, tobacco and compulsive gambling.

■ Alcohol use disorder

Alcohol use disorder causes major social, economic and public health problems. Over 15 million adult Americans have alcohol use disorder to some degree. Each year, about 88,000 people die of alcohol-related causes. Alcohol misuse costs billions of dollars each year in lost productivity and health expenses.

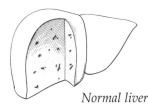

Normal liver

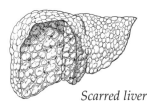

Scarred liver

Excessive alcohol intake can damage body tissues, particularly the liver. Excess use can cause scarring (cirrhosis).

How alcohol works in the body

When a person drinks alcohol, it depresses the central nervous system by acting as a sedative. In some people, the initial reaction may be stimulation, but the more they drink, the more they become sedated. Initially, alcohol affects areas of thought, emotion and judgment. In sufficient amounts, alcohol impairs speech and muscle coordination. Taken in large enough quantities, alcohol is a lethal poison — it can cause a life-threatening coma by severely depressing the vital centers of your brain.

Excessive use of alcohol can produce several harmful effects on the brain and nervous system. It can also severely damage the liver, pancreas and cardiovascular system. Alcohol use in pregnant women may permanently injure the fetus.

Being drunk (intoxicated)

The intoxicating effects of alcohol relate to its concentration in the blood. For example, if you're not a regular drinker and your blood alcohol concentration is more than 0.10 percent, you may be quite intoxicated and have difficulty speaking, thinking and moving around. As your blood alcohol level increases, mild confusion may give way to stupor and, ultimately, a coma. Regular drinkers develop a tolerance for alcohol, but they still experience impairment.

Your body size, body fat percentage, rate of drinking and alcohol tolerance affect how you respond to alcohol. Women generally have a higher blood alcohol concentration per drink than men do because of more body fat, which absorbs alcohol faster.

Most states define legal intoxication as a blood alcohol level of 0.08 percent or higher, but under some circumstances limits may be lower. Some states require drivers under 21 to have a blood alcohol level of zero. Even at levels much lower than the legal limit, you may lose coordination and reaction time.

What is binge drinking?

Binge drinking is a pattern of drinking alcohol that brings the blood alcohol level to 0.08 percent or above. This pattern of drinking usually means five or more drinks on a single occasion for men or four or more drinks for women, generally within about two hours. Binge drinking is associated with the same major health risks noted earlier. And it's the main cause of alcohol poisoning, which has become a serious, even deadly, problem on some college campuses.

Warning signs

Alcohol use disorder can be mild, moderate or severe, based on the number of symptoms you experience. Signs and symptoms may include:

- Being unable to limit the amount of alcohol you drink
- Wanting to cut down on your drinking or making unsuccessful attempts to do so
- Spending a lot of time drinking, getting alcohol or recovering from alcohol use
- Feeling a strong craving or urge to drink alcohol
- Failing to fulfill obligations at work, school or home due to repeated alcohol use
- Continuing to drink alcohol even though you know it's causing physical, social or interpersonal problems
- Giving up or reducing social and work activities and hobbies
- Using alcohol in situations where it's not safe, such as when driving or swimming
- Developing a tolerance to alcohol so you need more to feel its effect or you have a reduced effect from the same amount
- Experiencing withdrawal symptoms — such as nausea, sweating and shaking — when you don't drink, or drinking to avoid these symptoms

Seeking an evaluation

If you decide that alcohol use is a problem in your life, seek a professional evaluation. It will include questions about your symptoms, thoughts, feelings and behavior patterns.

The Diagnostic and Statistical Manual of Mental Disorders, Fifth Edition (DSM-5) is often used to diagnose mental health conditions and by insurance companies to reimburse for treatment. You may be asked specific questions from the DSM-5 to assess whether you have alcohol use disorder and, if so, how severe the disorder is for you.

Resistance to treatment

Most people who develop a problem with their drinking undergo professional assessment or enter treatment with reluctance or resistance, denying the problem. They often must be pressured to get help, such as required treatment following an arrest for driving while intoxicated (DWI). Health problems also may prompt treatment. If you're concerned about a friend or family member, discuss intervention with a professional.

Self-administered screening test

To screen for alcohol misuse, Mayo Clinic developed the Self-Administered Alcoholism Screening Test (SAAST). It consists of 37 questions. The SAAST tries to identify behaviors, medical symptoms and consequences of drinking in the person dependent on alcohol. Here are examples of questions:

1. Do you feel you are a normal drinker (that is, drink no more than average)?
2. Do close relatives ever worry or complain about your drinking?
3. Are you always able to stop drinking when you want to?
4. Has your drinking ever created problems between you and your spouse, parent or other near relative?
5. Do you ever drink in the morning?
6. Have you ever felt the need to cut down on your drinking?
7. Have you ever been told by a doctor to stop drinking?
8. Have you been arrested for driving while intoxicated?

What your answers mean

These responses suggest you may have a problem with alcohol use: 1. No; 2. Yes; 3. No; 4. Yes; 5. Yes; 6. Yes; 7. Yes; 8. Yes; 9. Yes.

If you answered three or more of the questions with the responses listed, seek an evaluation.

Individualized treatment

A wide range of treatments are available to help people with alcohol problems. Treatment should be tailored to the individual. Treatment may involve an evaluation, a brief intervention, an outpatient program or counseling, or a residential inpatient stay.

It's important to first determine whether you have an alcohol use disorder. If you haven't lost control over your use of alcohol, your treatment may involve reducing your drinking. If the disorder is mild, you may be able to modify your drinking. With a more severe disorder, cutting back is ineffective and inappropriate. Instead, abstinence from alcohol must be part of the treatment goal.

For people who aren't dependent on alcohol but are experiencing the adverse effects of drinking, the goal of treatment is reduction of alcohol-related problems, often by counseling or a brief intervention. A brief intervention usually involves certified specialists, who can establish a specific treatment plan. Interventions may include goal setting, behavior modification techniques, use of self-help manuals, counseling and follow-up care at a treatment center.

Residential alcohol treatment programs include abstinence, individual and group therapy, participation in Alcoholics Anonymous or other self-help groups, educational lectures, family involvement, work assignments, activity therapy and use of counselors (many of whom are recovering alcoholics), and multiprofessional staff.

Residential and outpatient treatment settings incorporate many approaches, including acupuncture, biofeedback, motivational enhancement therapy and cognitive behavioral therapy.

What to expect from residential treatment programs
On the next page is a list of what you might expect from a typical residential treatment program. Ask your insurance provider about coverage.

Coping with teenage drinking

Although it may take years for many adults to develop an alcohol problem, teenagers can become addicted in months. Alcohol use among teens generally intensifies with increasing age, although reports suggest alcohol use among teenagers is declining.

Alcohol is the fourth-leading preventable cause of death in the United States, as well as a major cause of disability. Alcohol is also often implicated in other teenage deaths, including drownings, suicides and fires.

For young people, the likelihood of addiction depends on the influence of parents, peers and other role models, the age they begin using alcohol, susceptibility to advertising, their psychological need for alcohol, and genetic factors (family alcoholism) that may predispose them to addiction. Look for these signs of a possible alcohol problem:
- Loss of interest in activities and hobbies
- Anxiety and irritability
- Difficulties with or changes in relationships with friends — joins a new crowd
- Dropping grades

To prevent teenage alcohol use:
- Set a good example regarding alcohol use
- Communicate with your children
- Discuss the legal and medical consequences of drinking

- **Detoxification and withdrawal.** Treatment may begin with a program of detoxification. This usually takes about two to seven days. Medications may be necessary to prevent delirium tremens (DTs) or withdrawal seizures.
- **Medical assessment and treatment.** Common problems linked to severe alcohol use disorders are high blood pressure, increased blood sugar, and liver and heart disease.
- **Acceptance and abstinence.** Effective treatment is impossible unless you accept that you're addicted and unable to control drinking, and you stop drinking.
- **Recovery programs.** Detoxification and medical treatment are only the first steps for most people in a residential treatment program.
- **Psychological support and psychiatric treatment.** Group and individual counseling and therapy support recovery from the psychological aspects of alcohol use disorder. Sometimes emotional symptoms of the disease may mimic psychiatric disorders. Clinical depression and anxiety may coexist with the alcohol problem, and treatment may prevent relapse.
- **Drug treatments.** An alcohol-sensitizing drug called disulfiram (Antabuse) is sometimes used. If you drink alcohol, the drug produces a severe physical reaction that includes flushing, nausea, vomiting and headaches. Disulfiram won't cure alcoholism, and it can't remove the compulsion to drink. But it can be a strong deterrent. Naltrexone (ReVia), a drug known to block the narcotic high, and acamprosate (Campral) have been found to reduce the urge to drink in recovering alcoholics. Unlike disulfiram, neither one makes you feel sick soon after drinking alcohol. There also is an injectable version of naltrexone (Vivitrol). People taking these medications are more likely to remain sober longer.
- **Continuing support.** Aftercare programs and Alcoholics Anonymous help recovering alcoholics maintain abstinence from alcohol, help manage any relapses and help with needed lifestyle changes.

FOR MORE INFORMATION

- Alcoholics Anonymous, New York headquarters, 212-870-3400 (check your phone directory or the AA website for a local group near you), *www.aa.org*
- Al-Anon/Alateen (for family and friends of people with drinking problems), 757-563-1600, *https://al-anon.org/*
- National Council on Alcoholism and Drug Dependence, 24-hour referral to local resources, 800-NCA-CALL (800-622-2255), *https://www.ncadd.org*

Treatment for hangover: Avoid alcohol altogether

Even small amounts of alcohol can cause unpleasant side effects. Some people develop a flushed feeling. Others are sensitive to certain ingredients and develop headaches or other reactions.

The classic hangover, although well-studied, isn't fully understood. It's probably due to dehydration, byproducts from the breakdown of alcohol, liver injury, overeating and disturbed sleep.

The best treatment for a hangover is prevention: Either avoid alcohol or keep your drinking to moderate levels.

If you have a hangover, it's too late to do much to improve your health and function. A lot of hangover remedies have been tried, but there isn't much evidence that they help — and they may hurt.

If you have a hangover, follow this advice:
- Rest and rehydrate. Drink bland liquids (water, soda, some fruit juices or broth). Avoid acidic, caffeinated or alcohol-containing beverages.
- Use over-the-counter pain medication with care (see page 258).

Smoking and tobacco use

When you inhale the smoke of a cigarette, you're letting loose a chemical parade that will march through some of your body's vital organs — lungs, heart, blood vessels and brain. Cigarette smoke delivers to your body over 60 known cancer-causing chemicals — tiny amounts of poisons such as arsenic and cyanide, and more than 7,000 other substances. More than 480,000 Americans die each year from **smoking** cigarettes or from secondhand smoke. Almost 1 of every 5 deaths in the U.S. is related to smoking.

Nicotine, one of the key ingredients in tobacco, is an addictive substance, and the cigarette is the most efficient delivery system. It's the nicotine that keeps you smoking. It increases the amount of a brain chemical called dopamine, which produces feelings of pleasure and satisfaction. Getting that "dopamine boost" is part of the addiction process, making you want to keep smoking to re-experience the pleasure.

Another reason people continue to smoke is because they've become accustomed to smoking in certain situations, and they find it very difficult to break these ingrained behaviors. This includes having a cigarette with the first cup of coffee in the morning, while driving, after meals, to relieve a stressful situation, and as a reward for completing a task or making it through a difficult event. Others value the social aspect of smoking, and their quit attempts fail when they socialize with active smokers.

How to stop smoking

Many smokers want to stop, but find it hard to stop because of tobacco's addictive hold. In fact, most people need more than one attempt before they successfully stop. Here are some suggestions to help you **stop smoking**:

Do your homework. Talk to ex-smokers. Find out how they stopped and what they found helpful. Find a treatment program. Group programs sponsored by the American Cancer Society and the American Lung Association are available in many communities. Your doctor, a tobacco treatment specialist, and your state's quit line at 800-QUIT-NOW (800-784-8669) or Smokefree.gov website at *https://smokefree.gov* can help.

Make small changes. Limit places where you smoke. Smoke outside. Don't smoke in the car. Buy cigarettes by the pack instead of the carton. Change to a brand that's less satisfying.

Pay attention to your smoking. As you prepare to stop smoking, pay attention to your behavior. When do you smoke? Where? With whom do you smoke? List your key triggers to smoking. Have a plan to cope with them when you stop. Practice coping with these situations without smoking.

Seek help. Participate in a formal program or individual counseling. The more help you get, the better your chance of success. Studies show that people who participate in formal programs are up to eight times more likely to stop smoking than those who try on their own.

Be motivated. The key to stopping is commitment. When Mayo Clinic studied the results of its own programs, it found that smokers who were more motivated to stop were twice as likely to be successful in stopping as those who were less motivated. List your reasons for stopping. To increase your motivation, add to the list regularly.

Set a stop date. Make it a day with low stress. But don't wait for a day with no stress. That may mean postponing forever. Tell your friends, spouse and co-workers your intention. Let them know how they can support your efforts.

■ Nicotine replacement therapy

The best-tested treatments currently available to help people stop smoking are based on delivering nicotine to the brain by means other than smoking, or with medications that modify brain chemistry to reduce withdrawal symptoms and other effects that nicotine has on the brain.

Over-the-counter medications

Nicotine patch. The patch delivers nicotine through your skin and into your bloodstream. Studies show people who properly use the patch are twice as likely to stop smoking. Place the patch on the least hairy areas of your body (your chest, upper arms or abdomen) in the morning. Rotate locations. Remove the old patch before putting on a new one. Heavy smokers may need to use more than one patch at a time — under the direction of a doctor. Length of use varies with individual needs. Usually six to eight weeks is necessary to establish the required behavior changes. But many people need to use the patch for a longer time. The main side effect is an itchy rash at the site of the patch. If it's a minor redness, use a small amount of hydrocortisone cream on the area after the patch is removed.

Nicotine gum. This gum-like resin delivers nicotine to the blood through the lining of your mouth. People who properly use the gum are twice as successful as those who try to stop smoking without it. Two strengths are available: 2 milligrams (mg) and 4 mg. Heavy smokers may need the higher dose. Put a piece of gum in your mouth and bite it gently a few times until you experience a tingling or peppery taste. Then park the gum between your cheek and gum. Repeat the process every few minutes. A piece should last about 30 minutes. Use the gum when you feel the urge to smoke or in situations when you know the urge will be present. Initially, you may use up to 10 to 12 pieces a day. Gradually decrease the number over a period of weeks. Rapid chewing and swallowing the saliva inactivates the nicotine and may cause nausea.

Nicotine lozenge. The lozenge is like a cough drop that delivers nicotine to your body through the lining of your mouth. You move it around in your mouth as it slowly dissolves. It's available without a prescription in 2-mg and 4-mg doses. Heavy smokers may need the higher dose. You can use a lozenge to control withdrawal symptoms or cravings. When starting, use a minimum of eight to nine lozenges a day but no more than 20 without consulting with your health care provider. Taper use after six to eight weeks.

Prescription medications

Nicotine nasal spray. The nicotine in the nasal spray is sprayed directly into each nostril, where the nicotine is absorbed through nasal membranes into veins, transported to the heart and then sent to the brain. It's a somewhat quicker delivery system than the gum or patch, although it's not nearly as quick as a cigarette. The usual dose is one spray in each nostril. Start with one to two doses an hour. The minimum is eight doses a day, and the maximum is 40 doses a day. For most people, use of the spray should be reduced six to eight weeks into the treatment. During the first days of use, the spray can be irritating to the nose, causing a runny nose, coughing and sneezing. These signs usually go away after five to seven days.

Nicotine inhaler. The inhaler looks like a short cigarette with a plastic mouthpiece, where a cartridge of nicotine is inserted. You puff on it, and it gives off small amounts of nicotine vapor in your mouth. The nicotine is absorbed slowly through the lining of the mouth — not through the lungs as smoke is — and into your bloodstream and then it goes to the brain, relieving withdrawal symptoms.

Bupropion. Bupropion is an antidepressant that is effective in helping people stop smoking. For treatment of depression, it's sold as Wellbutrin. For treating smokers, it's sold as Zyban. Bupropion is thought to increase the level of dopamine, a brain chemical boosted by smoking. Side effects include insomnia and dry mouth. Don't use bupropion if you have a history of seizures.

Varenicline. Varenicline (Chantix) is a drug that selectively attaches to the brain's nicotine receptors, mimicking the effect of nicotine and releasing dopamine. In studies, it's been found to be more effective than bupropion or nicotine patches. Side effects include nausea and vivid dreams. There have been reports of symptoms such as agitation, depressed mood, and suicidal thoughts and behavior, although a cause and effect has not been proved. If you develop these symptoms, stop the medication and call your doctor.

Combining medication with visits to your health care provider or tobacco treatment specialist for support and counseling increases your chances of stopping smoking. U.S. Public Health Service Commissioned Corps guidelines recommend using combination treatments — for example, the nicotine patch plus a short-acting nicotine medication (such as the gum or lozenge) or a nicotine medication and bupropion.

■ Coping with nicotine withdrawal

Problem	Solutions
Craving	● Distract yourself. ● Do relaxed-breathing exercises (see page 223). ● Realize that the craving will pass fairly quickly.
Irritability	● Take a few slow, deep breaths. ● Imagine an enjoyable outdoor scene, and take a minivacation. ● Soak in a hot bath.
Insomnia	● Take a walk several hours before going to bed. ● Unwind by reading. ● Take a warm bath. ● Eat a banana, or drink warm milk. ● Avoid beverages with caffeine after noon. ● See "Sleep disorders," page 44.
Increased appetite	● Make a personal survival kit that includes straws, cinnamon sticks, sugar-free candy, licorice, toothpicks, gum or fresh vegetables. ● Drink lots of water or low-calorie liquids.
Inability to concentrate	● Take a brisk walk — outside if possible. ● Simplify your schedule for a few days. ● Take a break.
Fatigue	● Get more exercise. ● Get an adequate amount of sleep. ● Take a nap. ● Try not to push yourself for two to four weeks.
Constipation, gas or stomach pain	● Drink plenty of fluids. ● Add fiber to your diet: fruit, raw vegetables, whole-grain cereals. ● Gradually change your diet. ● See "Constipation," page 58, and "Excessive gas and gas pains," page 60.

■ Teenage smoking: What can be done?

What's the harm in teens experimenting with cigarettes? It's a major problem because almost all adults who smoke daily began as teenagers. Cigarette smoking is rapidly addictive. Many teenagers believe that they can stop smoking anytime they choose. However, analyses have found that this isn't often the case. While there is a need for counseling to help teens quit smoking, prevention is the key.

Here are some strategies parents might try to help keep teens from smoking:

- Learn what your teen thinks about smoking.
- Help your teen explore personal feelings about peer pressure and smoking.
- Encourage your teen to stay physically active.
- Note the social repercussions of smoking.
- Set a personal example of not smoking.
- Help your teen find alternatives to smoking.

Chewing tobacco

Call it what you want — smokeless tobacco, spit tobacco, chew, snuff, pinch, plug or dip — but don't call it harmless. If you're considering making the switch from cigarettes to **chewing tobacco** because you think the smokeless version of tobacco won't hurt you, be warned — chewing tobacco can also cause serious health problems.

- **Addiction.** Chewing tobacco gets you hooked on nicotine, similar to the way cigarettes get you hooked. And once you're addicted, it becomes difficult to stop using chewing tobacco.
- **Cavities and gum disease.** Chewing tobacco and other forms of smokeless tobacco cause tooth decay. That's because chewing tobacco contains high amounts of sugar, which contributes to cavities, and coarse particles that can irritate your gums, scratch away at the enamel on your teeth and cause gum disease (gingivitis).

- **Heart and blood vessel (cardiovascular) problems.** Some evidence suggests that chew and other forms of smokeless tobacco may increase your risk of heart attack and stroke.
- **Precancerous mouth sores.** People who use smokeless tobacco are more likely to develop small white patches called leukoplakia (loo-koh-PLAY-key-uh) inside their mouths. These mouth sores are considered precancerous — meaning that the sores could one day develop into cancer.
- **Cancer.** Using smokeless tobacco increases your risk of oral cancer. Oral cancer includes cancers of the mouth, throat, cheek, gums, lips and tongue. Surgery to remove cancer from any of these areas can leave your jaw, chin, neck or face disfigured. Smokeless tobacco also is associated with cancer of the pancreas and cancer of the esophagus.

The dangers of secondhand smoke

The health threat to nonsmokers from exposure to tobacco smoke is well-documented. **Secondhand smoke** exposure is associated with lung cancer and heart disease in nonsmokers. That's why smoke-free workplace laws are essential.

People with respiratory or heart conditions and the very young and very old are especially at risk when exposed to secondhand smoke. Infants are three times more likely to die of sudden infant death syndrome if their mothers smoke during and after pregnancy.

Children under 1 year who are exposed to smoke have more hospital admissions for respiratory illness than children whose parents don't smoke. Secondhand smoke increases a child's risk of ear infections, pneumonia, bronchitis and tonsillitis.

So take steps to protect yourself and your loved ones from the dangers of secondhand smoke.

See back cover for online resource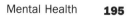

Drug use and dependency

Drug abuse, whether of prescription or illegal drugs, may be dangerous because of its long-term physical effects, its disruptive effect on family and work, and the potential risks of sudden withdrawal. Medical help is often essential to quitting.

Common drugs of abuse

Glue and other inhalants. Children and teens may sniff (huff) glue or fumes from products such as paint thinner or hair spray to get a high. This practice can damage the brain, lungs and central nervous system and cause death. Signs and symptoms of sniffing include slurred speech, dizziness, drowsiness, lack of inhibition, amnesia and sometimes hallucinations, weight loss, or loss of consciousness.

Stimulants. Stimulants, such as amphetamines and cocaine, are addictive drugs that can give a short-lived rush. But with repeated use, they can dampen the ability to feel any pleasure and cause heart and blood vessel problems, and even death. These drugs can cause users to be more talkative, energetic, anxious, hostile and paranoid. Abusing amphetamines can cause fast speech, shaky hands, hyperactivity and insomnia. Signs and symptoms of meth use include excited speech, agitation, irritability, violent behavior, paranoia and hallucinations. Cocaine can cause bizarre and violent behavior, as well as heart attacks and strokes.

Opioids. When taken as directed by a doctor, opioids can effectively manage pain. Opioids include morphine, codeine, oxycodone and related drugs. But when they're abused, these addictive drugs can be as dangerous as heroin (another opioid). Signs of abuse include sleepiness or sedation, confusion, avoidance of usual activities, and increased risky behavior, such as driving under the influence of the drug.

Marijuana and hashish. Marijuana (pot) is the dried flower of the cannabis plant. Hashish (hash) comes from the plant's resin. These drugs can cause problems with concentration, perception, learning, memory and coordination. They can also rapidly increase the heart rate and cause lung problems. Withdrawal symptoms can include irritability, sleeplessness and anxiety. Although marijuana has been legalized in some states, regular use may still result in addiction.

Hallucinogens. These drugs cause imagined experiences that seem real (hallucinations). Lysergic acid diethylamide (LSD) produces profound changes in mood and thought, with hallucinations. Panic and terrifying thoughts can occur. LSD can also cause a rapid heart rate, high blood pressure and tremors. Phencyclidine (PCP), a white granular powder, can cause anxiety, delusions, hallucinations and paranoia. In high doses, it can cause coma and death. People on PCP can be violent or suicidal.

Designer drugs and club drugs. Designer drugs are made from approved drugs, but they're chemically changed. Club drugs, including designer drugs, may be used by teens and young adults at dance clubs, bars and concerts. Examples include ecstasy (MDMA, or molly), gamma-hydroxybutyrate (GHB) and flunitrazepam (Rohypnol). These drugs are illegal and dangerous — they can cause serious medical problems and even death.

Medical help

Family and friends may need to help drug users realize that treatment is needed. Treatment may include hospitalization to get toxic drugs out of the body (detoxification), long-term outpatient programs and self-help groups to prevent a relapse.

FOR MORE INFORMATION
- National Institute on Drug Abuse, 301-443-1124, *https://www.drugabuse.gov*
- Narcotics Anonymous, 818-773-9999, *https://www.na.org*

Possible signs of drug use among teenagers

These are possible signs that your teenager is using drugs:

- **School.** Your child gradually shows an active dislike of school and looks for excuses to stay home. Contact school officials to see if your child's attendance record matches what you know about the absent days. An A or B student who suddenly starts to fail courses or gets only minimally passing grades may be using drugs.
- **Physical health.** Listlessness and apathy are possible signs of drug use.
- **Appearance.** Appearance is extremely important to teenagers. A significant warning sign can be a sudden lack of interest in clothing or looks.

- **Personal behavior.** Teenagers enjoy their privacy. However, be wary of extreme efforts to bar you from going into their bedrooms or knowing where they go with their friends.
- **Money.** Sudden requests for more money without a reasonable explanation may be a red flag.

What can you do?

Teenagers need an open line of communication with their parents. Even if your child is reluctant to share feelings, show interest in listening to your child talk about his or her experiences. Learn more about teen drug abuse, and seek professional advice if needed. (See "For more information," page 196.)

Compulsive gambling

Compulsive **gambling**, an impulse control disorder, is the uncontrollable urge to keep gambling despite the toll it takes on your life. Signs and symptoms of compulsive (pathological) gambling include:

- Gaining a thrill from taking big gambling risks
- Taking increasingly bigger gambling risks
- Being preoccupied with gambling (may become restless or irritable when trying to cut down or stop)
- Reliving past gambling experiences
- Taking time from work or family life to gamble
- Concealing gambling
- Feeling guilt or remorse after gambling
- Gambling when feeling helpless or distressed
- Borrowing money or stealing to gamble
- Failing at efforts to cut back on gambling
- Lying to hide gambling
- In severe cases, financial ruin, loss of career and family, and even suicide

Certain medications for Parkinson's disease and restless legs syndrome (RLS) have a rare side effect that may result in compulsive behavior. If you are taking medicines for Parkinson's or RLS and suddenly start gambling, talk with your doctor.

Medical help

Treatment for compulsive gambling involves three main approaches:

- **Psychotherapy.** Cognitive behavioral therapy (CBT) may be especially helpful for compulsive gamblers. CBT focuses on identifying irrational, negative beliefs and replacing them with healthy, positive ones. Group therapy also may help.
- **Medications.** Antidepressants and mood stabilizers may help emotional issues, but not necessarily the compulsive gambling. Medications called narcotic antagonists, useful in treating substance abuse, may help treat compulsive gambling.
- **Self-help groups.** Gamblers Anonymous (GA) and other groups may help as part of treatment, but GA doesn't yet have the track record of Alcoholics Anonymous. You also may find state-sponsored help groups in your phone directory or online.

Anxiety disorders

It's normal to feel anxious or worried at times. Everyone does. But millions of Americans have anxiety disorders, and many don't seek treatment. Yet treatment for anxiety disorders can be highly effective by using medication, therapy or both.

■ Generalized anxiety disorder

If you often feel anxious without reason and your worries disrupt your daily life, you may have **generalized anxiety disorder**. Generalized anxiety disorder causes excessive or unrealistic anxiety and worry — well beyond what's appropriate.

In addition to chronic worry (about almost everything), signs and symptoms vary. They may include restlessness, difficulty concentrating, fatigue, irritability, muscle tension, trouble sleeping, stomachaches, excessive sweating, shortness of breath, diarrhea and headaches. Generalized anxiety disorder can lead to or worsen depression, substance abuse, insomnia, digestive problems and headaches.

Treatment options

Treatment often includes medications (anti-anxiety medications and antidepressants) or therapy or both. Cognitive behavioral therapy can help you replace negative thoughts, beliefs and unhealthy behaviors with healthy, positive ones.

■ Social anxiety disorder

It's normal to feel nervous in some social situations, such as giving a presentation. But a **social anxiety disorder** involves an irrational anxiety or fear of situations in which you believe others are watching or judging you.

Signs and symptoms include intense fear of being around people you don't know, worrying that you'll embarrass or humiliate yourself, avoiding doing things or speaking to people out of fear of embarrassment, and having anxiety that disrupts your daily routine. Physical signs may include blushing, sweating, trembling, nausea, difficulty making eye contact, a shaky voice and stomach upset, among others.

Treatment options

Treatment is similar to that for generalized anxiety disorder. Antidepressants called selective serotonin reuptake inhibitors (SSRIs) are generally considered the safest and most effective medications for long-term symptoms of social anxiety disorder.

What is OCD?

Being a perfectionist isn't the same as having **obsessive-compulsive disorder (OCD)**. OCD is an anxiety disorder with unreasonable thoughts and fears (obsessions) that result in repetitive behaviors (compulsions).

For example, obsessions may include fear of contamination, excessive orderliness or desire for sexual images. Compulsions may include handwashing until your skin is raw, doing the same actions repeatedly (such as repeatedly checking locks) or counting in certain patterns.

If you think you have OCD, seek medical help. Medications and behavioral therapy may help control your symptoms so that they don't rule your life.

See back cover for online resource ⓘ

Phobias

A **phobia** is an overwhelming, unreasonable fear of an object or situation that poses little real danger. Some people fear open spaces (agoraphobia). Others are extremely self-conscious and can't tolerate social situations (social phobia). Some people have a specific phobia, such as fear of enclosed spaces (claustrophobia), spiders or flying.

Not all phobias need treatment, but if a phobia affects your daily life, different therapies can help you overcome your fears — often permanently. Your doctor or a mental health provider may suggest medications or behavioral therapy or both. Most adults don't get better on their own and need some type of treatment.

■ Post-traumatic stress disorder (PTSD)

Post-traumatic stress disorder (PTSD) is an anxiety disorder triggered by a traumatic event. You can develop PTSD when you experience or see an event that causes intense fear, helplessness or horror, such as sexual assault or exposure to combat.

Symptoms of PTSD typically begin within three months of the traumatic event, but, in a few cases, they may not occur until years later. Symptoms may include nightmares and flashbacks of the traumatic event, emotional numbness, intrusive memories, relationship problems, anger, guilt, shame, suicidal thoughts, and self-destructive behavior. Symptoms may come and go and get worse during times of higher stress.

Treatment options

Effective treatment often includes medication (antidepressants, anti-anxiety medications and others) and therapy. This may include supportive talk therapy and cognitive behavioral therapy. There may be professionally led support groups available.

■ Panic attacks and panic disorder

A **panic attack** is a sudden episode of intense fear for no apparent reason that triggers severe physical reactions. Panic attacks typically begin in young adulthood. An episode usually comes on suddenly and can be over in minutes or last for hours. Symptoms can include a rapid heart rate, sweating, trembling and shortness of breath. You may have chills, hot flashes, nausea, abdominal cramping, chest pain, dizziness, a tight throat or trouble swallowing. You may have a few or many symptoms.

Your chance of having panic attacks increases if a close family member has had them. Other health problems — such as an impending heart attack or hyperthyroidism — can cause symptoms similar to panic attacks. If panic attacks are frequent or if fear of them affects your activities, you may have **panic disorder**. Severe panic disorder can lead to depression and even suicidal thoughts.

Treatment options

Effective treatments include medication, therapy or both. For an attack, sedatives called benzodiazepines can help. For long-term problems, antidepressants are effective. Cognitive behavior therapy helps change thinking patterns that trigger fears and attacks.

FOR MORE INFORMATION
- National Institute of Mental Health, 866-615-6464, *https://www.nimh.nih.gov*

Depression

Almost everyone feels down from time to time — a period of several days or a week in which you seem to be in a funk. This condition usually goes away, and you resume your normal patterns. Nevertheless, the feeling is troublesome, and there are steps you can take to avoid it.

Feeling down isn't the same as having clinical depression. While minor depression is temporary and usually goes away after a short time, major depression does not.

Depression may improve eventually, but leaving it untreated typically means it will continue for many months or longer. If you're depressed, you may find little, if any, joy in life. You may have little or no energy, feel unworthy or guilty for no reason, find it difficult to concentrate, or be irritable. You might wake up after only a few hours of sleep or experience changes in appetite — eating less than usual or eating too much. You may experience a sense of hopelessness or even consider suicide (see page 202). A person with depression may have some, most or all of these symptoms. The list below shows the different signs of major and minor depression:

Signs of major depression

- Persistent lack of energy
- Lasting sadness
- Irritability and mood swings
- Recurring sense of hopelessness
- Continual negative view of the world and others
- Overeating or loss of appetite
- Feelings of unworthiness or guilt
- Inability to concentrate
- Recurrent early-morning awakening or other changes in sleep patterns
- Inability to enjoy pleasurable activities
- Feeling as though you'd be better off dead

Signs of minor depression

- Feeling down for a few days but still able to function normally in daily activities
- Occasional lack of energy, or a mild change in sleeping patterns
- Ability to enjoy some recreational activities
- Stable weight
- A quickly passing feeling of hopelessness

Self-care for minor depression

If your mood falls into the minor depression column, try these things:

- Share your feelings. Talk to a trusted friend, spouse, family member or your spiritual counselor. He or she can offer you support, guidance and perspective.
- Spend time with other people.
- Engage in activities that have interested you in the past, particularly activities that you have enjoyed.
- Do moderate physical activity on a regular basis to lift your mood.
- Get adequate rest and eat balanced meals.
- Don't undertake too much at one time. If you have large tasks to do, break them into smaller ones. Set goals you can accomplish.
- Look for small opportunities to be helpful to someone less fortunate.
- Avoid alcohol, drugs, sedatives and other mood-altering substances.

Causes of depression

Millions of Americans have depression. Occasionally, it's a side effect of a prescription drug or an illness. Imbalances of certain brain chemicals may be a factor. But often the cause is unclear.

You're at a higher risk of depression if a blood relative, such as a parent, has had it. Depression may also be preceded by a severe shock or stress in life, such as the death of a loved one or the loss of a job. Or it can arise when things are going very well. Certainly it's normal to feel sad after losses or setbacks. But if that sadness doesn't stop fairly quickly, a serious depression likely has developed.

If you've had depression once, you're at a higher risk of developing it again. Don't delay seeking medical attention if you notice that symptoms have returned. Discussing feelings with a family member or close friend may help, but it's no substitute for seeking professional help.

Seek help

Depression is a biological illness. Don't expect to snap out of it all of a sudden or be able to beat it through sheer determination. If depressive symptoms last more than a few weeks or if you're feeling hopeless or suicidal, it's time to seek help. For many people, the most effective treatment is a combination of medication and counseling.

Contact your primary care doctor or ask for a referral to a psychiatrist. A psychiatrist is trained as a medical doctor and can help you find out if a medical illness might be contributing to your symptoms.

If your symptoms are mild — but persistent — a psychologist may be helpful. Psychologists are trained in psychotherapy, which is effective in treating depression and anxiety. However, psychologists don't have medical degrees, so they don't prescribe or manage medications.

If you're being treated for depression by one clinician, let your other health care providers know so that they can collaborate and medication interactions can be avoided. In most cases, depression can be successfully treated.

Seasonal affective disorder, another form of depression, seems to be related to light exposure. The disorder is sometimes treated with increased light exposure during the day by using a light box that has a source of bright broad-spectrum light.

Helping others

If you know someone who's depressed, don't judge the person or minimize his or her feelings. Encourage and support seeking professional care. Offer reassurance that things will get better, but don't expect a person with depression to improve suddenly — it takes time.

Coping with loss: Practical suggestions

- **Express your feelings.** Write a book of memories, or even write a letter to the person who died.
- **Ask for help.** When people experience sudden loss, their friends may not know how to respond. It benefits everyone to ask for specific kinds of help.
- **Stay involved.** People who grieve may need to remind themselves about exercise, diet and rest.
- **Evaluate yourself for depression.** If the grief is extremely severe in the short run or persistent over the long run (six months or more), consider depression as a possible cause.

Treatment options

Most people who have depression improve greatly when treated with antidepressant medications. Dozens of medications are available, and some work in different ways. A doctor can select a medication that's suitable for you.

Discuss potential side effects with your doctor. If you experience side effects that concern you, call your doctor. Common side effects may include nausea, fatigue and drowsiness, dry mouth, insomnia, constipation, blurred vision, dizziness, jitteriness, weight gain, and sexual side effects. If your child is depressed, ask your child's doctor about the benefits and risks of antidepressants.

Other treatment methods include talking about your feelings with a psychiatrist, psychologist or other licensed mental health provider. There are various types of psychotherapy. Cognitive behavioral therapy — which helps you replace negative beliefs and behaviors with healthy, positive ones — can be very effective.

Treatment takes time

Remember, treatment takes time. Some signs of change may occur in as little as two weeks, but it may take eight weeks or more to get the full benefit. That can be discouraging, so it's important for friends and family to give support and encouragement during this time when medications may need adjusting. Don't quit taking your medications too soon. You may need them for at least a year or longer. Follow your doctor's advice.

Make sure that your clinician is licensed and qualified and that you feel comfortable with him or her. See "For more information," below, to find services in your area.

Warning signs of potential suicide

You're at a higher risk of **suicide** if you are an older adult, if you are widowed, divorced or single, or if you abuse alcohol or other drugs. If you or a loved one needs help, get it immediately (see the resources below).

Signs include:
- **Withdrawal.** Is unwilling to communicate and has an overwhelming urge to be alone.
- **Moodiness.** Has an emotional high one day followed by being down in the dumps, or becomes suddenly calm for no clear reason.
- **Life crisis or trauma.** Experiences a divorce, a loved one's death or an accident, or loses self-esteem after a job loss or financial setback, which leads to suicidal thinking.
- **Personality change.** Has a change in attitude, personal appearance or activities. Or an introvert suddenly becomes an extrovert.
- **Threats.** Makes threats about suicide. Take these threats seriously.
- **Gift giving.** Gives cherished belongings to friends and loved ones.
- **Depression.** Appears to be depressed and may be unable to function socially or at work.
- **Risk taking.** Starts taking risks, such as sudden involvement in high-speed driving or unsafe sex.

FOR MORE INFORMATION
- Substance Abuse and Mental Health Services Administration (SAMHSA): Behavioral health treatment services locator, 800-662-HELP (800-662-4357), *https://www.findtreatment.samhsa.gov*
- National Institute of Mental Health, 866-615-6464, *https://www.nimh.nih.gov*
- National Suicide Prevention Lifeline, 800-273-TALK (800-273-8255), 24/7 support (can refer you to the nearest crisis center), *https://suicidepreventionlifeline.org*

See back cover for online resource ⓘ

Domestic violence

Beatings, forced sex, being afraid of violence from a spouse or partner, or living in fear that your spouse or partner will harm or abuse your children: All of these situations are examples of **domestic violence**, also called domestic abuse.

Women are most often the victims of domestic violence, including being battered, raped and sometimes murdered by a husband, ex-husband or partner. But men also can be victims and need to seek help. Domestic violence can happen among people of all races, ages, income levels and religions.

Battering is the use of physical force to control and maintain power over another person. Domestic violence may also involve intimidation, psychological abuse, harassment, humiliation and threats.

Signs and symptoms of abusive behavior

You may be in an abusive relationship if you:

- Have ever been hit, kicked, shoved or threatened with violence
- Feel that you have no choice about how you spend your time, where you go or what you wear
- Have been accused by your partner of things you've never done
- Must ask your partner for permission to make everyday decisions
- Go along with your partner's decisions because you're afraid of his or her anger

Self-care

How to respond

- In an emergency, call 911 or your local emergency number.
- If you're in an abusive relationship or you worry about the potential, start by telling someone. Turn to a trusted friend, relative or licensed mental health provider for support.
- Seek support from your doctor, nurse or other health care provider.
- Call a domestic violence hotline for advice (see "For more information," below).
- Have a flight plan. Be prepared to take your children, house keys and important papers. Be alert and ready to leave at a moment's notice. Know exactly where you'll go and how you'll get there. Know the phone number of a shelter.
- Keep cash on hand in case of an emergency.
- Keep a list of phone numbers of friends who may be able to help you.

Professional help

If you call the police, request an immediate response. Some areas have a mandatory arrest law, which means the abuser will be removed from the home while the case is in court.

If you go to a shelter, expect to be safe and to receive counseling. Also ask about legal assistance (for instance, you may want a restraining order that legally requires the abuser to stay away from you or face arrest).

Contacting a national hotline, a local crisis hotline, or a counseling center or social service agency that deals with domestic violence can empower you to take action. At first, you might find it hard to talk about the abuse, but you'll likely feel some relief and receive much-needed support and advice.

FOR MORE INFORMATION

- National Domestic Violence Hotline, 800-799-7233, *www.thehotline.org*
- National Organization for Victim Assistance, 800-879-6682, *www.trynova.org*

Memory loss

Everyone forgets things. How many times have you lost track of your car keys or forgotten the name of a person you just met? This is normal.

Memory isn't just a single process. You have three types:

- **Sensory memory.** This is an initial impression that registers the impact of sight, sound, touch, taste or smell for less than a second.
- **Short-term memory.** Also called working memory, this is your temporary memory. You may look up a number in the phone book, but after you call the number you forget it. Once you've finished using the information, it vanishes.
- **Long-term memory.** This includes everything from remembering your home address and phone number to the complex procedures you use to complete tasks at work.

Possible causes of reversible memory loss include a side effect of medications, a minor head injury, depression, anxiety, stress, sleep deprivation, excessive alcohol or a vitamin B-12 deficiency. Hearing and vision problems and frequent migraines also can affect memory. Pregnant women sometimes have short-term memory problems.

Forgetfulness tends to increase with age, but there's a big difference between normal absent-mindedness and the type of memory loss associated with dementia.

Alzheimer's disease is the most common form of dementia. Symptoms include gradual loss of memory for recent events and the inability to learn new information; a growing tendency to repeat oneself, misplace objects, become confused and get lost; a slow disintegration of personality, judgment and social graces; and increasing irritability, anxiety, depression, confusion and restlessness.

Self-care to improve your memory

- **Establish a routine.** Managing your daily activities is easier when you follow a routine. Choose a set time to do household chores — clean the bathroom on Saturday, and water the plants on Sunday.
- **Exercise your 'mental muscles.'** Play word games, crossword puzzles or other activities that challenge your mental abilities.
- **Practice.** When you walk into a room, make a mental inventory of people you recognize. When you meet someone, repeat his or her name in conversation.
- **Make associations.** When driving, look for landmarks to associate with your route and name them out loud to imprint them on your memory. Example: "Turn left at the high school to get to Bob's house."
- **Write lists.** Keep track of important tasks and appointments. For example, pay your bills on a certain day each month.
- **Pay attention.** Forgetfulness may indicate nothing more than having too much on your mind. Slow down and pay full attention to the task at hand.
- **Try not to worry.** Fretting about memory loss can make it worse. Replace self-blame statements ("I'm such a scatterbrain") with positive messages ("I remember the things that are really important").

Medical help

Consult a health care provider if you're concerned about memory loss. The resources below can help if the diagnosis is Alzheimer's disease.

FOR MORE INFORMATION

- Alzheimer's Association, 800-272-3900, *www.alz.org*
- Alzheimer's & related Dementias Education & Referral Center, 800-438-4380, *www.nia.nih.gov/alzheimers*

See back cover for online resource ⓘ

Staying Healthy

- **Weight: What's healthy for you?**
- **Healthy eating**
- **Lowering your cholesterol**
- **Physical activity and fitness**
- **Keeping stress under control**
- **Screening and immunization**
- **Protecting yourself**
- **Aging and your health**

This section is filled with practical information on how you can take charge of your health by establishing and maintaining a healthy lifestyle. From eating healthier to getting the immunizations you need, there's a great deal you can do to stay healthy.

Weight: What's healthy for you?

It seems almost everywhere you turn these days, you're bombarded by diets and weight-loss schemes. Weight loss sells! However, as anyone who has tried to lose weight knows, doing so isn't easy. Success at losing weight requires the key ingredients of knowledge, commitment, healthy eating and regular physical activity.

For most overweight Americans, weight loss is a healthy goal. Losing weight often means a reduced risk of heart disease, diabetes and high blood pressure.

The risks of being overweight

Your desirable weight is the weight at which you're as healthy as possible. Your weight is only one part of the lifestyle picture that contributes to your long-term health.

Being overweight may place you at risk of:

- High blood pressure
- Heart disease
- Type 2 diabetes
- Deteriorating joints
- Abnormal blood fats
- Certain cancers
- Chronic low back pain
- Gallstones
- Respiratory problems

Losing weight can be a challenge. Of people who lose weight, especially those who lose it rapidly, a majority regain the weight within one to five years. So, what should you do? First, determine how much you're overweight, and then develop a safe and healthy weight management program.

Your body has a nearly unlimited capacity to store fat. Losing weight reduces crowding of your organs and the strain on your lower back, hips and knees.

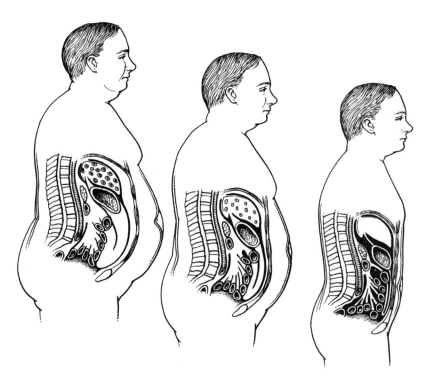

See back cover for online resource ⓘ

■ Determining your body mass index

What is a healthy weight? Do-it-yourself tools can help determine whether your weight is healthy or whether you could benefit from losing some weight.

Body mass index

The first step in determining whether your weight is healthy is to figure out your **body mass index (BMI)**. You can do that by using the chart below or the online **BMI calculator**.

A BMI under 18.5 indicates that you're underweight, 18.5 to 24.9 is considered a healthy range, 25 to 29.9 indicates overweight, and 30 or greater means you're **obese**. You're at increased risk of a weight-related disease, such as heart disease or type 2 diabetes, if your BMI is 25 or higher. But Asians with a BMI of 23 or higher may have an increased risk of health problems.

However, the BMI isn't perfect. Someone with a large amount of muscle mass may have a high BMI but not be at increased health risks.

Body mass index (BMI)

BMI	Healthy		Overweight					Obese				
	19	**24***	25	26	27	28	29	30	35	40	45	50
Height						Weight in pounds						
4'10"	91	115	119	124	129	134	138	143	167	191	215	239
4'11"	94	119	124	128	133	138	143	148	173	198	222	247
5'0"	97	123	128	133	138	143	148	153	179	204	230	255
5'1"	100	127	132	137	143	148	153	158	185	211	238	264
5'2"	104	131	136	142	147	153	158	164	191	218	246	273
5'3"	107	135	141	146	152	158	163	169	197	225	254	282
5'4"	110	140	145	151	157	163	169	174	204	232	262	291
5'5"	114	144	150	156	162	168	174	180	210	240	270	300
5'6"	118	148	155	161	167	173	179	186	216	247	278	309
5'7"	121	153	159	166	172	178	185	191	223	255	287	319
5'8"	125	158	164	171	177	184	190	197	230	262	295	328
5'9"	128	162	169	176	182	189	196	203	236	270	304	338
5'10"	132	167	174	181	188	195	202	209	243	278	313	348
5'11"	136	172	179	186	193	200	208	215	250	286	322	358
6'0"	140	177	184	191	199	206	213	221	258	294	331	368
6'1"	144	182	189	197	204	212	219	227	265	302	340	378
6'2"	148	186	194	202	210	218	225	233	272	311	350	389
6'3"	152	192	200	208	216	224	232	240	279	319	359	399
6'4"	156	197	205	213	221	230	238	246	287	328	369	410

*Asians with a BMI of 23 or higher may have an increased risk of health problems.
Based on *Circulation*, 2014; 129(suppl 2):S102; NHBLI Obesity Expert Panel, 2013

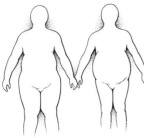

Pear shape   Apple shape

It's not only how much you weigh that's important but also where your body stores extra fat. People with an apple shape tend to have a higher risk of health problems than do people with a pear shape.

Waist size

Your waist size also is important in estimating health risks. It indicates where most of your fat is located. People who carry most of their weight around their waists are referred to as having an apple shape. Those who carry most of their weight below their waists, around their hips and thighs, are said to have a pear shape.

Generally, it's better to have a pear shape than an apple shape. Fat accumulation around your waist is associated with an increased risk of high blood pressure, diabetes, high cholesterol and triglycerides, and coronary artery disease.

A modest loss of just 3 to 5 percent of unwanted weight can have a positive effect on blood pressure, blood sugar, cholesterol and triglycerides, reducing your risk of heart and blood vessel disease and other diseases.

To determine whether you're carrying too much weight around your abdomen, measure around your waist. Find the highest point on each of your hipbones and measure across your abdomen horizontally just above those points. A measurement of more than 40 inches in men and 35 inches in women signifies increased health risks. In general, the greater your waist size is, the greater your health risks are.

■ Tips on losing weight

To lose weight, you need to modify your lifestyle. This often means making changes in your diet and physical activity level. Commit to losing weight and work to gradually change your eating and exercise habits. It's long-term changes that spell success.

Self-care

Getting started

- **Determine a good time to begin your weight-loss program.** It's best to start when you can devote some time and attention to making changes in your life. A hectic schedule, stress or depression can be barriers to a successful start.
- **Set reasonable weight-loss goals** (long- and short-term). If you want to lose 40 pounds, start with a short-term goal of losing 5 pounds.
- **Check your food intake.** It's usually reasonable to cut 500 to 1,000 calories a day from what you currently eat to lose 1 to 2 pounds a week. Starting calorie goals will vary, depending on height, activity level and whether you have medical a condition. Many women can start as low as 1,200 calories a day and many men can start as low as 1,400 calories a day. But diets of fewer than 1,200 calories a day may not meet your daily nutritional needs. (See "Healthy eating," page 210.)
- **Keep a food journal and track your diet.** People who write down everything they eat and drink are more successful at long-term weight maintenance. In addition, record factors that influence your eating behaviors, such as stress or skipping meals.

Eat healthier foods

- **Enjoy healthier foods.** See the Mayo Clinic Healthy Weight Pyramid on page 211 for healthy diet recommendations. Keep healthy foods on hand. Consider healthy snack options only if they help you from overeating at the next meal. This way you won't let hunger destroy your willpower.
- **Eat more vegetables and fruits.** They help you feel full and don't contain a lot of calories. Eat at least three fruit and four vegetable servings daily.
- **Limit high-calorie foods.** You can lower your calorie intake dramatically by eating less meat, choosing fat-free or low-fat dairy products and avoiding fried foods, rich desserts, processed foods and fatty add-ons such as butter and dressings.

- **Limit sugar and sweets.** Both are high in calories and low in other nutrients. Sweets such as candy and desserts also can be high in fat.
- **Consider what you drink.** Limit soft drinks and consume alcohol only in moderation. Low-fat milk and juices should not be consumed to excess — calories can add up quickly. Water is generally the best fluid to drink.

Change eating behaviors
- **Don't skip meals.** Eat at regular times to keep your appetite and food selections under better control.
- **Serve yourself and other family members,** rather than placing the entire dish of food on the table. This helps prevent taking second helpings.
- **Use a smaller plate.** Doing so encourages you to take smaller portions, while still appearing as though your plate is "full."
- **Focus on eating.** Don't read or watch television while you're eating.
- **Stop eating when you're full.** Contrary to what your mother may have taught you, you don't have to clean your plate.
- **Try to ride out food cravings** when they hit. They usually pass in minutes. If not, eat something healthy and low in calories.

Other suggestions
- **Track your weight.** Whether you weigh yourself frequently or occasionally, look at trends over time, not daily changes.
- **Use a daily multiple vitamin-mineral supplement** if you're limiting calories to 1,200 a day. Also, if your food selections are limited, ask your doctor or dietitian if you need a vitamin-mineral supplement.
- **Talk to your doctor about other options if needed.** For some people who are obese, medications to suppress appetite or **gastric bypass surgery** may be needed to improve health. These approaches must be carefully supervised by a doctor. But without a change in eating habits, even these more radical steps may fail.

■ Physical activity: The key to burning calories

Physical activity and exercise are important to any weight-loss program. Make changes gradually, especially if you're out of shape. If you're older than 40, you're a smoker, you've had a heart attack or you have diabetes, consult your doctor before you start an exercise program.

Self-care

- **Try to find activities that you enjoy** and can do regularly. Begin slowly and increase gradually. Your goal is to maintain moderately vigorous activity for at least 150 minutes a week.
- **You don't need maximum exertion** to get positive results. You can reach your goal through moderately vigorous, regular physical activity, such as walking.
- **Vary your exercises** to improve overall fitness and to keep it interesting.
- **Break up your activity into 10-minute increments.** Every activity counts.
- **Find an exercise partner.** It may help you stick to your schedule.
- **Little things can add up.** Park at the far end of the parking lot. Take the stairs rather than the elevator. Get off the bus a stop or two early and walk.
- **Keep a log of your activity.**
- **Stick with your exercise schedule.** Don't use lack of time as an excuse.

Healthy eating

Food provides nutrition, energy and, of course, a pleasurable experience. But getting good nutrition can be a challenge. To feel good, ward off disease and perform at a peak level, you need balanced nutrition. Many diseases, such as heart disease and diabetes, are, in part, linked to poor eating habits.

For most people, the best approach to healthy eating is to follow the principles of the Mayo Clinic Healthy Weight Pyramid, summarized below.

Self-care

- Aim for a healthy weight.
- Be physically active every day.
- Make vegetables and fruits the foundation of your diet. They're low in calories and contain many disease-fighting nutrients.
- Eat grain products, such as bread and pasta, made from whole grains.
- Consume low-fat or fat-free dairy products without added sugar.
- Eat more plant sources of protein, such as beans, lentils and peas, and less meat.
- Try to eat at least two servings (3 ounces each) a week of fish rich in heart-healthy omega-3 fatty acids, such as salmon, sardines, trout and whitefish.*
- Limit saturated fats, avoid trans fats, and choose unsaturated fats found in foods such as olive and canola oils, avocados, and nuts.
- Limit sweets to 75 calories a day or about 500 calories a week.
- If you choose to drink alcohol, do so in moderation. For healthy adults, that means up to one drink a day for women of all ages and men older than age 65, and up to two drinks a day for men age 65 and younger. Don't drink alcohol at all if you're pregnant.

*Due to mercury levels, pregnant women, nursing mothers and young children should avoid king mackerel, shark and swordfish, and limit white (albacore) tuna to 6 ounces a week.

Eat more plant foods for a healthy diet

Fruits and vegetables contain a powerhouse of nutrients that help protect your health.

Whole fresh and frozen fruits are best because they're higher in fiber and lower in calories than canned fruits, fruit juices and dried fruits are.

Most fresh fruits and vegetables contain a lot of water, which provides volume and weight but few calories. Dried fruits are less filling and relatively high in calories because their water has been removed, so the volume is much smaller.

Because different fruits provide different nutrients, variety is vital. Choices are almost unlimited: apples, bananas, blueberries, raspberries, strawberries, cherries, grapefruits, cantaloupes, honeydew melons, oranges, plums, and many more. Choose fruits at every meal and consider as a snack, if needed.

Vegetables are an excellent source of fiber and nutrients and are naturally low in fat and calories. Eat a variety for different nutrients and health benefits: salad greens, asparagus, green beans, carrots, broccoli, cauliflower, zucchini, summer squash, eggplant, mushrooms, onions, tomatoes, and many more.

Some vegetables are considered carbohydrates because they are starchy, have more calories than typical vegetables do, and function more like a carbohydrate in your body. Starchy vegetables include corn, green peas, potatoes, sweet potatoes and winter squash.

Other healthy carbohydrates include whole grains, such as brown rice, whole-wheat pasta and whole-grain breads and cereals.

Mayo Clinic Healthy Weight Pyramid

If weight is an issue for you, the Mayo Clinic Healthy Weight Pyramid can show you what foods to buy and eat when choosing foods that promote healthy weight. You'll also reduce your risk of weight-related diseases. What's more, you'll feel fuller and less hungry if you follow this approach.

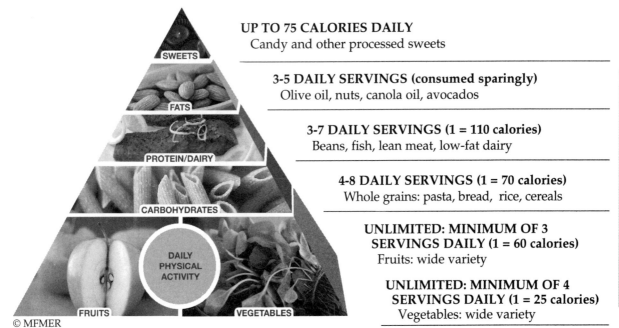

UP TO 75 CALORIES DAILY
Candy and other processed sweets

3-5 DAILY SERVINGS (consumed sparingly)
Olive oil, nuts, canola oil, avocados

3-7 DAILY SERVINGS (1 = 110 calories)
Beans, fish, lean meat, low-fat dairy

4-8 DAILY SERVINGS (1 = 70 calories)
Whole grains: pasta, bread, rice, cereals

UNLIMITED: MINIMUM OF 3 SERVINGS DAILY (1 = 60 calories)
Fruits: wide variety

UNLIMITED: MINIMUM OF 4 SERVINGS DAILY (1 = 25 calories)
Vegetables: wide variety

© MFMER

See your doctor before you begin any healthy-weight plan.

Daily serving recommendations for different calorie levels

Food group	Starting calorie goals				
	1,200	1,400	1,600	1,800	2,000
Vegetables*	4 or more	4 or more	5 or more	5 or more	5 or more
Fruits*	3 or more	4 or more	5 or more	5 or more	5 or more
Carbohydrates†	4	5	6	7	8
Protein/dairy†	3	4	5	6	7
Fats†	3	3	3	4	5

*The servings for fruits and vegetables are minimums. Potatoes are in the *carbohydrates* food group.
†The recommended servings for carbohydrates, protein/dairy, fats and sweets are maximums.

Based on *The Mayo Clinic Diet*, 2017

Healthy cooking

Healthy cooking doesn't mean you have to invest in special cookware. Simply use standard cooking methods to prepare foods in healthy ways. Change how you prepare familiar meals and try new recipes, using the tips below.

Self-care

Decrease the amount of fat, sugar and salt in your recipes. For example:
- Reduce or eliminate sugar in foods.
- Trim fat from meat before cooking and drain off fat drippings after cooking.
- De-fat soups, stews, sauces and gravies by chilling and skimming off the fat.
- Add chopped vegetables to lean ground beef, using less meat, to increase bulk.
- Minimize foods used for appearance, such as coconut and frosting, and extras such as ketchup, mayonnaise and jam.
- Use oil sparingly. When you do use it, choose olive or canola oils.
- Use herbs instead of salt.
- Use nonstick cookware or vegetable cooking sprays instead of oil or butter.
- Use these cooking methods to capture flavor and retain nutrients in food without adding too much fat: baking, braising, broiling, grilling, roasting, sautéing, steaming and stir-frying. Avoid frying foods.

Mix-and-match salads

Having a salad is a great way to include more vegetables and fruits in your diet. The next time you have a salad, don't be afraid to experiment. To prepare a nutritious and tasty salad, pick one or more ingredients from each column.

Try 1 of these greens	with 1 of these veggies	plus 1 of these proteins	plus 1 of these toppings	and 1 of these dressings
• Arugula • Baby kale • Bibb lettuce • Cabbage • Leaf lettuce • Romaine • Spinach • Spring mix	• Artichokes • Beets • Bell peppers • Broccoli • Carrots • Cauliflower • Cucumbers • Mushrooms • Onions • Radishes • Tomatoes	• Black beans • Chicken breast • Edamame • Extra-firm tofu • Chickpeas • Hard-boiled eggs • Kidney beans • Lean ground beef • Salmon • Shrimp • Turkey breast	• Croutons • Dried fruit • Fruit • Hard or sharp cheese • Nuts • Seeds	• Balsamic vinegar • Cilantro lime • Light Caesar • Light Italian • Low-fat ranch • Low-fat raspberry vinaigrette • Olive oil • Other vinegars • Salsa or taco sauce

Lowering your cholesterol

Heart and blood vessel disease (cardiovascular disease) is the leading cause of death in the United States. Many deaths occur because of narrowed or blocked arteries (atherosclerosis). Cholesterol plays a major role in this condition.

Atherosclerosis is a silent, painless process in which cholesterol-containing fatty deposits (plaques) accumulate in the walls of your arteries over many years, beginning in childhood. As plaques build up, your arteries narrow and blood flow is reduced. Decreased blood flow to your heart increases your risk of a heart attack. Reduced blood flow to your brain can cause a stroke.

Why you need cholesterol

Cholesterol is used by your body to build healthy cells, as well as some vital hormones. Your liver manufactures about two-thirds of the cholesterol in your body. You take in the rest when you eat animal products.

Cholesterol is transported throughout your body by your bloodstream. Low-density lipoprotein (LDL) cholesterol is often referred to as "bad" cholesterol. Over time, it can build up in your blood vessels and form plaques. That can cause a blockage, resulting in heart attack or stroke. In contrast, high-density lipoprotein (HDL) cholesterol is often called "good" cholesterol because it helps "clean" cholesterol from your blood vessels.

Why do you have high cholesterol?

Your genes and lifestyle influence how much cholesterol you have. Your liver may make too much LDL cholesterol or may not "clean" enough of it from your blood. Or it may not make enough HDL cholesterol. But high cholesterol is largely preventable and treatable. A high-fat diet, inactivity and smoking can increase LDL levels and reduce HDL levels.

Lifestyle changes

Lifestyle changes are essential to improve your cholesterol. To bring your "bad" cholesterol down, it's important to lose excess weight, eat healthy foods and increase physical activity. If you smoke, quit. See "Self-care" on page 214.

Drug therapy

If, despite dietary changes and physical activity, you still have too much bad cholesterol (**high blood cholesterol**) or not enough good cholesterol, your doctor may recommend drug therapy. Medications can reduce cholesterol and triglycerides, another type of blood fat.

Staying Healthy

Coronary artery angiograms taken five years apart show the kind of results that can be achieved with cholesterol-lowering medications.

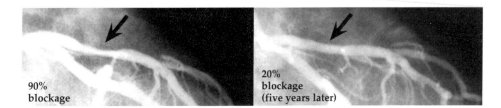

90% blockage

20% blockage (five years later)

By reducing LDL cholesterol, drugs can help prevent buildup of plaques, and reduce them or prevent them from rupturing, which can cause a blood clot that blocks an artery. Statins (Crestor, Lipitor, Zocor, others) are the most commonly prescribed drugs, but there are many others. The choice depends on your risk factors, age, health and possible side effects.

Most of these medications are well-tolerated, but there can be side effects. The statins, for example, can cause muscle pain, but this is uncommon. If you take cholesterol medication, your doctor may recommend blood tests to monitor your liver.

With weight reduction, more physical activity and a healthier diet, your doctor may be able to reduce your medication or decide that you no longer need it. But don't reduce or stop taking medication without your doctor's advice.

Know these numbers

Over the years, it's been common for doctors to utilize set targets for total cholesterol, LDL, HDL and triglycerides. However, current guidelines recommend an approach that goes beyond cholesterol levels alone and considers your overall heart risk. Be aware of these five key numbers and whether they change over time:

Category	Ideal numbers
Total cholesterol	Get your cholesterol checked and talk to your doctor about your numbers and how they impact your overall health
High-density lipoprotein (HDL) cholesterol	
Blood pressure	Less than 120/80 mm Hg*
Fasting blood sugar	Less than 100 mg/dL†
Body mass index	Less than 25

*Millimeters of mercury
†Milligrams per deciliter of blood
Based on American Heart Association, 2016

Self-care

- **Lose excess weight.** Losing even 5 to 10 pounds may help lower cholesterol.
- **Eat a diet rich in fiber and other cholesterol-lowering foods.**
  - ▸ Choose unsaturated fats, such as monounsaturated fat, found in olive, canola and peanut oils, as well as walnuts and almonds (but watch the calories).
  - ▸ Avoid trans fats, which may be listed in the ingredients as hydrogenated or partially hydrogenated vegetable oil.
  - ▸ Limit dietary cholesterol. Instead of high-fat meats, egg yolks and whole milk products, choose fish or poultry, lean meat, egg whites and fat-free milk.
  - ▸ Choose whole-grain versions of foods, such as whole-grain breads, whole-wheat pasta, whole-wheat flour, wild rice, oatmeal and oat bran.
  - ▸ Stock up on fruits and vegetables. They're rich in dietary fiber. Aim for four or more servings of vegetables and three or more servings of fruits a day.
  - ▸ Eat heart-healthy fish. See "Self-care" on page 210 for examples.
  - ▸ Consider foods fortified with plant sterols or stanols, such as certain margarine-like spreads and orange juice, but watch the calories.
  - ▸ Target foods with soluble fiber, such as psyllium seed.
- **If you smoke, stop** — to improve cholesterol and reduce risk of heart disease.
- **Increase your physical activity.** See the next section.

Physical activity and fitness

Regular physical activity — at least 150 minutes a week — can reduce your risk of many serious health problems, including heart disease, high blood pressure, stroke, diabetes, certain cancers and osteoporosis. The benefits of physical activity include:

- **Heart.** Physical activity increases your heart's ability to pump blood and decreases your resting heart rate. Your heart can pump more blood with less effort.
- **Cholesterol and triglycerides.** Physical activity improves blood-fat levels, raising your HDL ("good") cholesterol and helping lower your LDL ("bad") cholesterol.
- **Blood pressure.** Physical activity can lower blood pressure and is especially helpful if you have mild high blood pressure (hypertension). Regular physical activity can also help prevent as well as reduce high blood pressure.
- **Diabetes.** If you have diabetes, physical activity can lower your blood sugar. It can also help prevent type 2 diabetes.
- **Bones.** Women who perform weight-bearing physical activity have a better chance of avoiding osteoporosis.
- **Weight.** Physical activity lowers body fat stores.
- **General.** Regular physical activity can also relieve stress, improve your overall sense of well-being, help you sleep better and improve concentration.

■ Aerobic vs. anaerobic activity

Aerobic activity ("to be active using oxygen") occurs when you continuously move large muscle groups such as your leg muscles. This type of activity helps improve the function of the heart, lungs and muscle cells. It should not be so intense, however, that it causes pain. If you're in a good aerobic range, you should be breaking a sweat and breathing faster but still be able to exercise comfortably for 30 to 60 minutes. Aerobic activity improves your overall endurance. Walking, biking, jogging and swimming are familiar aerobic activities.

Anaerobic activity ("to be active without using oxygen") occurs when the demands made on a muscle are so great that it uses up all available oxygen and starts to burn stored energy without oxygen. This can cause pain and soreness. You can't carry on anaerobic activities very long, such as lifting heavy weights or sprinting. Anaerobic exercise builds strength and speed, but it can also help improve endurance. When starting a strength training program, work with light weights or set the machines at light resistance to avoid injuries. Supplement your anaerobic activities with aerobic activities.

What it means to be fit

You're fit if you can:
- Carry out daily tasks without fatigue and have enough energy to enjoy leisure pursuits
- Walk a mile or climb a few flights of stairs without becoming winded or feeling heaviness or fatigue in your legs
- Carry on a conversation during light to moderate exercise such as brisk walking

If you sit most of the day, you're probably not fit. Signs of deconditioning include:
- Feeling tired most of the time
- Being unable to keep up with others your age
- Avoiding physical activity because you know you'll quickly tire
- Becoming short of breath or fatigued when walking a short distance

■ Starting a fitness program

Consult your health care provider before you begin a **fitness program** if you smoke, are overweight, are older than 40 years and have never exercised, or have a chronic condition such as heart disease or a family history of heart disease, diabetes, high blood pressure, lung disease or kidney disease. The risks of physical activity stem from doing too much, too vigorously, with too little previous activity.

If you are medically able to begin a program, here are some helpful hints:

- **Begin gradually.** If you're not used to being physically active, work up to your goal. If you have trouble talking during a workout, you're pushing too hard.
- **Select the activities that work for you.** It should be activities that you enjoy.
- **Do them regularly but moderately** and never exercise to the point of nausea, dizziness or extreme shortness of breath. Your goals should be:
  - ▸ *Frequency.* Try to exercise or be physically active at least three days a week.
  - ▸ *Intensity.* See "Intensity" on page 217 to learn about simple tools you can use.
  - ▸ *Time.* Try to accumulate at least 150 minutes of moderately intense activity each week. Alternatively, spending a little as 10 minutes three times a week with intervals of harder intensity can make a difference on lowering your disease risk.
- **Always warm up and cool down.** Warm up to help loosen muscles. Cool down after to help increase flexibility and joint range of motion.

Calories burned in 1 hour

The number of calories burned varies widely depending on the type of activity, intensity level and individual, so these are estimates. If you weigh less than 160 pounds, your calories burned would be less than shown. If you weigh more than 240 pounds, calories burned would be more.

Activity (1-hour duration)	Weight of person and calories burned		
	160 pounds	200 pounds	240 pounds
Aerobics, low-impact	365	455	545
Bicycling, < 10 mph, leisure	292	364	436
Golfing, carrying clubs	314	391	469
Hiking	438	546	654
Jogging, 5 mph	606	755	905
Skiing, cross-country	496	619	741
Skiing, downhill	314	391	469
Stair treadmill	657	819	981
Swimming, laps, light/moderate	511	637	763
Tennis, singles	584	728	872
Walking, 2 mph	204	255	305
Walking, 3.5 mph	314	391	469

Based on Ainsworth BE, et al. 2011 Compendium of Physical Activities: A second update of codes and MET values. *Medicine & Science in Sports & Exercise.* 2011;43:1575.

Walk your way to fitness

Less than half of American adults are physically active on a regular basis. Yet a brisk walk, 30 to 60 minutes each day, can help you attain the fitness level associated with a longer, healthier life. Physical activity doesn't have to be intense. Even walking slowly can lower your risk of heart disease. Faster, farther or more frequent walking offers greater health benefits.

First things first

The best walking program takes advantage of your fitness goals while being safe, convenient and fun. Here are tips to get the most out of walking:

- **Set realistic goals.** What do you want to gain from regular physical activity? Are you 45 and concerned about warding off a heart attack? Are you 75 and wanting to enjoy recreational activities and prolong independence? Do you want to lose weight? Lower blood pressure? Relieve stress? Maybe you just want to feel better. Walking can help achieve these goals. Decide what's most important and be specific about how to reach your goal. Don't say, "I'm going to walk more." Say, "I'm going to walk from 7 to 7:30 on Tuesday, Thursday and Saturday mornings."
- **Buy good shoes.** You don't need to spend a lot of money on shoes designed specifically for walking. You do need to wear shoes that provide protection and stability.
- **Dress right.** Dress in loosefitting, comfortable clothes. Choose materials appropriate for the weather — a windbreaker for cool and windy days, layers of clothing in cold weather. Wear bright colors trimmed with reflective fabric or tape. Avoid rubberized material — it doesn't allow perspiration to escape. Protect yourself from the sun with sunscreen (at least 30 SPF), sunglasses and a hat.
- **Drink water.** When you're physically active or exercise, you need extra water to maintain your normal body temperature and cool working muscles. To help replenish the fluids you lose during exercise, drink water before and after activity. If you take a brisk walk for more than 45 minutes, drink water every 15 to 20 minutes, especially in hot weather.
- **See your doctor.** If you're age 40 or older or have a chronic health problem, review your physical activity and exercise goals with your doctor before starting.

Planning your program

If you put out a little more physical effort than usual, your body responds by improving its capacity for physical activity. By gradually increasing the amount of activity, you can improve your fitness level in eight to 12 weeks. To condition your heart and lungs safely, include intensity, frequency and duration in your fitness plans.

- **Intensity.** Remember, physical activity doesn't have to be strenuous to be healthy. But what is a desirable range of exercise intensity for you? Here are two simple tools to help you find out:
  - *Talk test.* While you walk, you should be able to carry on a conversation with a companion. If you can't, you're probably pushing too hard. Slow your pace.
  - *Target heart rate.* If you'd rather get specific, use your heart rate to estimate intensity. Many people aim for a target heart rate of 50 to 80 percent of their maximum heart rate. If you're not fit or you're just starting an activity program, you may need to aim for 40 to 50 percent of maximum heart rate. As your fitness improves, increase the intensity of your workouts.

If you're aiming for a target heart rate of 50 to 80 percent:

1. Subtracting your age from 220 = your maximum heart rate.
2. Your maximum heart rate multiplied by 0.5 = your lower limit.
3. Your maximum heart rate multiplied by 0.8 = your upper limit.

- **Frequency.** Try to walk at least three times a week. For conditioning and health benefits, your goal is eventually to walk three to four hours a week.
- **Duration.** Gradually work your way up to walking at least 150 minutes a week. If you've never exercised regularly or you haven't been physically active for a long time, start at a level that's comfortable for you, even if it's just five minutes. Track how many steps or miles you walk and how long it takes. A pedometer is a great tracking tool.

Check your pulse to get your heart rate

To get your heart rate, you can check your pulse in two ways. To check your pulse over your carotid artery, place your index and third fingers on your neck, at the side of your windpipe.

To check your pulse at your wrist, follow these steps:

1. Place two fingers between the bone and the tendon over your radial artery, which is located on the thumb side of your wrist.
2. When you feel your pulse, look at your watch and count the number of beats in 10 seconds.
3. Multiply this number by 6 to get your heart rate per minute.

A good physical activity program includes three phases:

- **Warmup.** Before each walk, spend about five minutes preparing your body for walking. For the first three to five minutes, walk at a slower pace to gradually increase your heart rate, body temperature and blood flow to the exercising muscles. Stretching also develops and maintains muscle flexibility and joint range of motion. Use the stretching and flexibility exercises on the next page.
- **Conditioning.** Walking develops your aerobic capacity by increasing your heart rate, depth of breathing and muscle endurance. You'll also burn calories. Calories burned depend on how fast and how long you walk and how much you weigh (see "Calories burned in 1 hour," page 216).
- **Cool-down.** At the end of your walk, slow your pace for three to five minutes to gradually reduce your heart rate and blood pressure. Then, repeat the same stretching exercises you used for warmup to help improve your range of motion.

A well-rounded exercise program

To get the most health benefits, have a well-rounded routine. Include these elements in your exercise plan:

- **Aerobic exercise** for a healthy heart and lungs
- **Stretching** to improve your flexibility and help prevent injury
- **Strength training** to build strong bones and muscles
- **Core exercises** to strengthen core muscles (abdominals, back and buttocks), which helps protect your back and gives you more stability

---

Stretching exercises for walkers
Stepping out safely

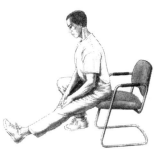

Hamstring stretch
Position yourself as shown above. Slowly straighten your left knee until you feel a stretch. Hold for 30 to 45 seconds. Don't stretch to the point of experiencing pain. You may apply gentle downward pressure with your hands. Repeat with your right leg.

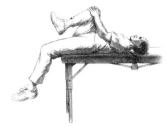

Hip stretch
Lie on a sturdy table or bed. Hold both your knees to your chest. Release your left leg and slowly straighten, allowing it to hang off the table or bed. Hold for 30 to 45 seconds. Feel the stretch in your left hip. Repeat with your other leg.

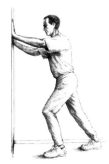

Calf stretches
1. Lean against a wall as shown. While maintaining a straight right knee, bend your left knee as if moving it toward the wall. Hold for 30 to 45 seconds. Feel the stretch in your right calf. Repeat with your other leg.

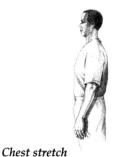

Chest stretch
1. Position yourself in a neutral posture as shown above.

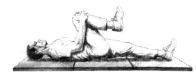

Back stretches
1. Position yourself as shown above. Slowly pull your right knee up toward your chest. Keep your left leg relaxed. Hold for 30 to 45 seconds. Feel the stretch in your low back and hip. Repeat with your left leg.

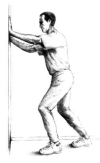

2. Position yourself similar to the previous exercise, but with your right knee bent instead of straight. Bend your left knee as if to move it toward the wall. Hold for 30 to 45 seconds. Feel the stretch in the deep calf muscle. Repeat with your other leg.

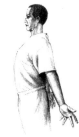

2. Move your arms backward while rotating your palms forward. Squeeze shoulder blades together, breathe deeply, and lift your chest upward. Hold for 30 to 45 seconds. Return to starting position.

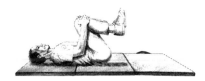

2. Position yourself as shown above. Pull both knees up toward your chest. Hold for 30 to 45 seconds. This variation usually provides a more intense low back stretch.

Congratulations! You've committed to a regular walking program. You're confident of the benefits you'll gain. But beware of the "terrible toos" — doing too much, too hard and with too little preparation

Foot or heel pain is common. Problems such as these can derail your walking program and sap your motivation. Here's how to walk without wearing yourself out:

- **Progress gradually.** If you haven't been active in the past two months, start slowly. In the first two to three weeks, do low-intensity walking. Gradually increase intensity only after you're walking comfortably for your desired length of time.
- **Listen to your body.** Expect to feel some mild muscle soreness after adding time to your schedule. However, gasping for breath and feeling sore joints are signals to slow down. Muscle stiffness lasting several days means you went too far. *See your doctor immediately* if you notice any symptoms suggesting heart or lung disease, such as chest pain, chest pressure, unusual fatigue lasting several hours, heart irregularity, dizziness or unusual shortness of breath.
- **Replace worn-out shoes.** Shoes begin to lose their cushioning ability after 300 to 500 miles of use and should be replaced. In addition, invest in a new pair when soles start to separate from uppers. Check for loss of stability by lining up your shoes side by side. Then look to see if either shoe tilts to the right or left.
- **Choose your course carefully.** Check out the route you plan to walk. Avoid paths with cracked sidewalks, potholes, low-hanging limbs or uneven turf. Don't walk at night along a road. When possible, walk with a companion and carry identification.
- **Don't overdo it.** If physical activity begins to feel like an obligation, take a day off each week. Use the time to do some other recreational activity that you enjoy.

Consider interval training

High-intensity interval training (HIIT) is an efficient way to achieve many of the same benefits of continuous moderate exercise. HIIT involves exercising as hard as you can for about 30 seconds, then resting with low-level activity for about three to four minutes, then repeating this cycle three or four times.

An entire session may not take more than 20 minutes, with only around two minutes of intense activity. However, this type of exercise, has been shown to be very effective in producing beneficial change for the cardiovascular system. It also helps improve metabolic factors and aids in weight loss.

HIIT has shown to be well-tolerated in people with heart disease and obesity, and many people find this type of exercise enjoyable and easy to fit into their days. If you have joint pain or arthritis, make sure the exercise you perform your intervals in is low-impact, such as with a stationary bicycle or elliptical trainer, or in the water.

Just move more

Physical activity isn't just exercise, it's any movement you make that burns calories — from gardening to walking up stairs. To include more physical activity in your day:

- Take a brisk walk around your neighborhood before or after work.
- Do housework at a pace fast enough to get your heart pumping.
- Involve the family. Play catch or ride your bikes.

- Take daily walks with your dog.
- Walk or bike to work, if feasible. If you ride the bus, get off a few blocks early and walk.
- Take the stairs instead of the elevator.
- Start a lunchtime walking group with co-workers.

Schedule physical activity as an appointment. Don't change your plans unless you absolutely have to. Regular physical activity is critical to your health.

Keeping stress under control

Stress is something that most people know well and experience often. It's that feeling of pressure, often resulting from having too much to do and too little time to do it. In today's busy world, stress is unavoidable.

Stress may be caused by positive events — a job promotion, vacation or marriage — as well as negative events — the loss of a job, a divorce or the death of a loved one. Stress is your response to an event — not the event itself.

When you experience stress, especially severe stress, a physical response occurs to meet the perceived energy demands of the situation. Your heart beats faster, your breathing quickens, and your blood pressure rises. In addition, your blood sugar rises, and blood flow to your brain and large muscles increases. After the threat passes, your body slowly relaxes again.

Stress may be short term (acute) or long term (chronic). Chronic stress is often related to situations that aren't easily solved, such as relationship problems, loneliness, financial worries or long workdays. You may be able to handle an occasional stressful event, but when stress occurs regularly, the effects multiply and compound over time.

Stress produces a variety of physical, psychological and behavioral symptoms. And it can lead to illness — aggravating an existing health problem or possibly triggering a new one, if you're already at risk of that condition.

That's why **stress management** is so important. Stress management gives you the tools to reset your alarm system. Without stress management, your body is always on red alert. Over time, that level of stress leads to serious health problems. Don't wait until then to combat stress. Start learning stress management techniques now.

The following sections explain the health effects associated with stress, showing how critical it is to learn how to manage your stress.

Stress suppresses immune system

The hormone cortisol produced during the stress response may suppress your immune system, increasing your susceptibility to upper respiratory viral infections such as a cold or the flu (influenza) and other infections.

Stress can also worsen the symptoms of autoimmune diseases, such as triggering a flare-up of lupus.

Stress increases risk of heart and blood vessel disease

High levels of cortisol due to stress can raise your heart rate and blood lipid (cholesterol and triglyceride) levels. These increased levelsare risk factors for both heart attacks and strokes.

If you experience a distressing event, your blood pressure may dramatically increase due to the temporary increase in cortisol and adrenaline. But once the stressor disappears, your blood pressure returns to normal. However, even temporary spikes in blood pressure — if they occur often enough — can damage your blood vessels, heart and kidneys.

Stress worsens other illnesses

Other relationships between illness and stress aren't as clear-cut. However, stress may worsen your symptoms if you have any of the following conditions:

- **Asthma.** A stressful situation may make your airways overreactive, precipitating an asthma attack.
- **Gastrointestinal problems.** Stress may trigger or worsen symptoms associated with some gastrointestinal conditions, such as irritable bowel syndrome or non-ulcer dyspepsia.
- **Chronic pain.** Stress can heighten your body's pain response, making chronic pain associated with conditions such as arthritis, fibromyalgia or a back injury more difficult to manage.
- **Mental health disorders.** Stress may trigger depression in people who are prone to the disorder. It may also worsen symptoms of other mental health disorders, such as anxiety and insomnia.

Signs and symptoms of stress

Your first indications that your body and brain are feeling pressured may be associated symptoms of stress — headache, insomnia, upset stomach and digestive changes. An old nervous habit such as nail biting may reappear. Another common symptom is irritability with people close to you. Occasionally, these changes are so gradual that you or those around you don't recognize them until your health or relationships change.

Some signs and symptoms of stress

Physical	Psychological	Behavioral
Headaches	Anxiety	Overeating or loss of appetite
Grinding teeth	Irritability	Impatience
Tight, dry throat	Feeling of impending danger or doom	Argumentativeness
Clenched jaws	Depression	Procrastination
Chest pain	Slowed thinking or racing thoughts	Increased use of alcohol or drugs
Shortness of breath	Obsessive thinking	Increased smoking
Pounding heart	Feeling helpless	Withdrawal or isolation
High blood pressure	Feeling hopeless	Avoidance and neglect of
Muscle aches	Feeling worthless	responsibilities
Indigestion	Feeling a lack of direction	Poor job performance
Constipation or diarrhea	Feeling insecure	Burnout
Increased perspiration	Sadness	Poor personal hygiene
Cold, sweaty hands	Defensiveness	Change in religious practices
Fatigue	Anger	Change in family or close relationships
Insomnia	Hypersensitivity	
Frequent illness	Apathy	

Relaxation techniques to manage stress

Relaxed breathing

With practice, you can breathe in a deep and relaxing way. At first, practice lying on your back while wearing clothing that's loose around your waist and abdomen. Once you've learned this position, practice while sitting and then while standing.

- Lie on your back on a bed or padded surface.
- Place your feet slightly apart. Rest one hand comfortably on your abdomen and the other hand on your chest.
- Inhale through your nose while pushing your abdomen out. Then slowly exhale through your nose while pushing your abdomen in.
- Concentrate on your breathing for a few minutes and become aware of the hand on your abdomen rising and falling with each breath. Make each breath a smooth, wavelike motion.
- Gently exhale most of the air in your lungs.
- Inhale while slowly counting to four, about one second per count.
- As you breathe in, imagine the warmed air flowing to all parts of your body.
- Pause one second after inhaling.
- Slowly exhale to a count of four. While you're exhaling, your abdomen will slowly fall.
- As air flows out, imagine that tension also is flowing out.
- Pause one second after exhaling.
- If it's difficult to inhale and exhale to a count of four, shorten the count slightly and later work up to four. If you feel lightheaded, slow your breathing or breathe less deeply.

- Repeat the slow inhaling, pausing, slow exhaling and pausing five to 10 times. Inhale slowly: 1, 2, 3, 4. Pause. Exhale slowly: 1, 2, 3, 4. Pause. Inhale: 1, 2, 3, 4. Pause. Exhale: 1, 2, 3, 4. Pause.

If it's difficult to make your breathing regular, take a slightly deeper breath, hold it for a second or two, and then let it out slowly through pursed lips for about 10 seconds. Repeat this once or twice and return to the other procedure.

Progressive muscle relaxation

- Sit or lie in a comfortable position, and close your eyes. Allow your jaw to drop and your eyelids to be relaxed but not tightly closed.
- Mentally scan your body, starting with your toes and working slowly to your head. Focus on each part individually: Imagine tension melting away.
- Tighten the muscles in one area of your body and hold them for a count of five, relax, and move on to the next area.

Imagery

- Allow thoughts to flow through your mind, but don't focus on any of them. Suggest to yourself that you are relaxed and calm, that your hands are warm (or cool if you are hot) and heavy, and that your heart is beating calmly.
- Breathe slowly, regularly and deeply.
- Once you're relaxed, imagine you're in a favorite place or in a spot of great beauty.
- After five or 10 minutes, rouse yourself from the state gradually.

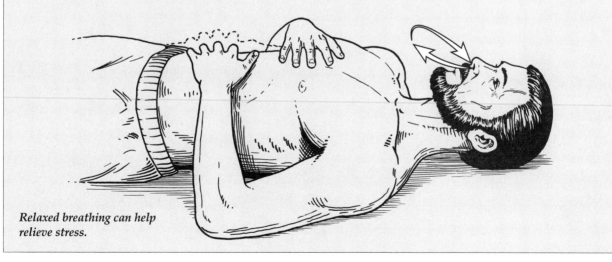

Relaxed breathing can help relieve stress.

Self-care

- **Learn to relax.** Techniques such as guided imagery, meditation, muscle relaxation and relaxed breathing can help you relax (see page 223). Your goal is to lower your heart rate and blood pressure while reducing muscle tension.
- **Discuss your concerns with a trusted friend.** Talking helps to relieve strains and put things in perspective, and it may lead to a healthy plan of action.
- **Plan your work in a step-by-step manner.** Accomplish small tasks.
- **Deal with your anger.** Anger needs to be expressed, but carefully. Count to 10, compose yourself, and respond to the anger in a more effective manner.
- **Get away.** A change of pace can help develop a new outlook.
- **Be realistic.** Set realistic goals. Prioritize. Concentrate on what's important. Unrealistically high goals invite failure.
- **Avoid self-medication.** At times people seek to use medication or alcohol for a feeling of relief. Such substances only mask the problem.
- **Get plenty of sleep.** A healthy body promotes good mental health. Sleep helps people tackle problems in a refreshed state.
- **Keep physically active.** Exercise is good for your body, and it helps burn off the excess energy that stress can produce. Even short periods (10 to 20 minutes) of physical activity can help reduce tension and improve your mood.
- **Eat well.** Junk food increases your stress level. Enjoy healthy meals and snacks.
- **Limit caffeine.** Too much coffee, tea or soda will increase your stress level.
- **Make time for activities you enjoy.** These may include going to the movies, joining a book club, going golfing with friends or getting together for a game of cards.
- **Nurture your inner spirituality.** This can be done through nature, art, music, meditation, prayer or attending religious services.
- **Develop a support network.** Family members, friends and co-workers whom you can turn to for emotional and practical support can be very important when coping with stress.
- **Seek help.** Contact your doctor or a mental health professional if stress is building or you're not functioning well.

Screening and immunizations

■ Adult screening tests and procedures

Screening recommendations apply to those in good health and without symptoms of illness. Symptoms, previous diagnosis or family history may change recommendations.

Recommended age-specific tests for women

Test	Ages 18-39	Ages 40-50	Older than age 50
Blood cholesterol test	Baseline at age 20, then every 4-6 years	Every 4-6 years	Every 4-6 years
Blood pressure measurement	Every 3-5 years	Annually	Annually
Breast cancer screening (mammogram)	Ask your doctor	Baseline at age 40, then ask your doctor	Every 1-2 years
Cervical cancer screening (Pap test), may be combined with HPV test	Every 3 years to age 29, then every 3-5 years	Every 3-5 years	Every 3-5 years until age 65
Colorectal cancer screening	Ask your doctor	Ask your doctor	Usually every 5-10 years until age 75
Dental checkup	Annually	Annually	Annually
Diabetes screening	Ask your doctor	Baseline by age 45, then every 3 years	Every 3 years
Eye exam	Ask your doctor	Baseline at age 40, then every 2-4 years	Every 2-4 years to age 54, then annually
HIV screening	At least once between ages 15-65		

Other tests women should consider

Test	Ages 18-39	Ages 40-50	Older than age 50
Bone density test	Ask your doctor	Ask your doctor	Baseline at age 65
Clinical breast exam	Ask your doctor	Ask your doctor	Ask your doctor
Full-body skin exam	Ask your doctor	Ask your doctor	Ask your doctor
Hearing test	Ask your doctor	Ask your doctor	Baseline by age 60
Hepatitis B and C screening	Ask your doctor	Ask your doctor	Ask your doctor
STI screening	Ask your doctor	Ask your doctor	Ask your doctor
Thyroid-stimulating hormone test	Ask your doctor	Ask your doctor	Ask your doctor
Tuberculosis screening	Ask your doctor	Ask your doctor	Ask your doctor
Lung cancer screening	At least one between ages 55-80 in current or recent smokers		

Recommended age-specific tests for men

Test	Ages 18-39	Ages 40-50	Older than age 50
Blood cholesterol test	Baseline by age 20, then every 4-6 years	Every 4-6 years	Every 4-6 years
Blood pressure measurement	Every 3-5 years	Annually	Annually
Colorectal cancer screening	Ask your doctor	Ask your doctor	Usually every 5-10 years until age 75
Dental checkup	Annually	Annually	Annually
Diabetes screening	Ask your doctor	Baseline by age 45, then every 3 years	Every 3 years
Eye exam	Ask your doctor	Baseline at age 40, then every 2-4 years	Every 2-4 years to age 54, then annually
HIV screening	At least once between ages 15-65		(continued on next page)

Other tests men should consider

Test	Ages 18-39	Ages 40-50	Older than age 50
Bone density test	Ask your doctor	Ask your doctor	Baseline at age 70
Full-body skin exam	Ask your doctor	Ask your doctor	Ask your doctor
Hearing test	Ask your doctor	Ask your doctor	Baseline by age 60
Hepatitis B and C screening	Ask your doctor	Ask your doctor	Ask your doctor
Prostate cancer screening	Ask your doctor	Ask your doctor	Ask your doctor
Syphilis screening	Ask your doctor	Ask your doctor	Ask your doctor
Thyroid-stimulating hormone test	Ask your doctor	Ask your doctor	Ask your doctor
Tuberculosis screening	Ask your doctor	Ask your doctor	Ask your doctor
Lung cancer screening	At least once between ages 55-80 in current or recent smokers		
Ultrasound of abdominal aorta	Once between ages 65-75 in men who have ever smoked		

■ Adult immunizations

Review the chart below and the details on page 227. Talk with your doctor about any **vaccines** that you may need. For international travel vaccines, see pages 282-283.

Recommended adult immunization schedule

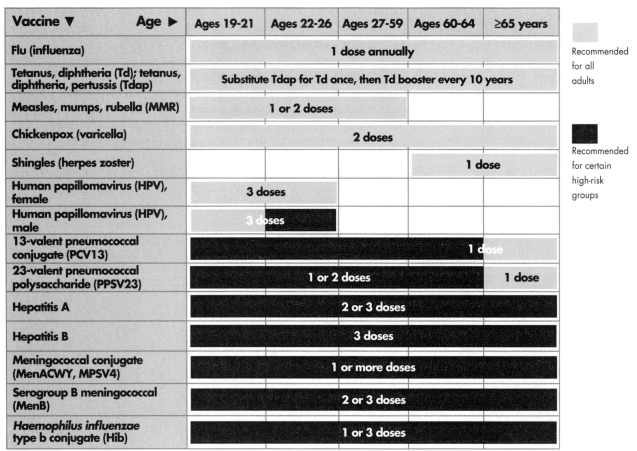

Vaccine ▼ Age ▶	Ages 19-21	Ages 22-26	Ages 27-59	Ages 60-64	≥65 years
Flu (influenza)	1 dose annually				
Tetanus, diphtheria (Td); tetanus, diphtheria, pertussis (Tdap)	Substitute Tdap for Td once, then Td booster every 10 years				
Measles, mumps, rubella (MMR)	1 or 2 doses				
Chickenpox (varicella)	2 doses				
Shingles (herpes zoster)				1 dose	
Human papillomavirus (HPV), female	3 doses				
Human papillomavirus (HPV), male	3 doses				
13-valent pneumococcal conjugate (PCV13)					1 dose
23-valent pneumococcal polysaccharide (PPSV23)	1 or 2 doses				1 dose
Hepatitis A	2 or 3 doses				
Hepatitis B	3 doses				
Meningococcal conjugate (MenACWY, MPSV4)	1 or more doses				
Serogroup B meningococcal (MenB)	2 or 3 doses				
Haemophilus influenzae type b conjugate (Hib)	1 or 3 doses				

Recommended for all adults

Recommended for certain high-risk groups

Source: Advisory Committee on Immunization Practices, Centers for Disease Control and Prevention, 2017

See back cover for online resource ⓘ

Vaccines for adults

Vaccine	Recommendation
Tetanus, diphtheria (Td); tetanus, diphtheria, pertussis (Tdap)	Needed every 10 years and after a deep or dirty wound if the most recent booster was over five years ago. Boosters needed as soon as possible after injury. A tetanus, diphtheria and whooping cough (pertussis) vaccine is also recommended; almost all teens and adults ages 19 to 64 should get one adult lifetime dose of Tdap instead of Td.
Human papillomavirus (HPV)	Protects against cervical cancer and genital warts. Two injections in six months for girls and boys ages 11 to 12 (could start as early as age 9), and three doses for females and males ages 13 to 26 who haven't been vaccinated. Most effective if given before becoming sexually active.
Chickenpox (varicella) (2-shot series)	Susceptible adults — health care workers without immunity or adults without known disease.
Shingles (herpes zoster)	Age 60 or older, whether or not you've had shingles before. Single injection of live vaccine. Doesn't guarantee you won't get shingles, but if you do, vaccine will likely reduce length, severity and risk of postherpetic neuralgia, a painful complication of shingles. Not recommended if you have certain medical conditions or weakened immunity.
Measles, mumps, rubella (MMR)	Two shots for adults born after 1956 without proof of previous vaccination or immunity. Not to be given during pregnancy or to women planning pregnancy within four weeks.
Flu (influenza)	Every year for anyone who wants to avoid the flu. Especially important for adults 50 and older and others at high risk — health care workers, people living in long-term care facilities, those with chronic illnesses or weakened immunity, or those living with people at high risk. Children 6 months old to 18 years old also receive the vaccine. Adults of any age need the vaccine if they live with young children because children are at high risk of the flu.
13-valent pneumococcal conjugate vaccine (PCV) and 23-valent pneumococcal polysaccharide vaccine (PPSV23)	Protects against severe infections due to *Streptococcus pneumoniae.* PCV13 is recommended for all adults age 65 and older and also for adults age 19 and older with conditions that weaken the immune system. PPSV23 is recommended for all adults age 65 and older, and for adults ages 19 to 64 who smoke or who have asthma.
Hepatitis A (two-shot series)	Travelers and people in high-risk groups (people with chronic liver disease, men with male sex partners, intravenous drug users, people who've had contact with someone who has hepatitis A). Now routinely given to infants. Those children don't need the vaccine as adults.
Hepatitis B (three-shot series)	Health care workers, high-risk groups (people with more than one sex partner or a sex partner who's a carrier, or men with male sex partners), and others who might be exposed to infected blood or body fluids. Now routinely given to infants (see page 228). Those children don't need the vaccine as adults.
Meningococcal conjugate and serogroup B meningococcal	Children ages 11 to 12, with a booster dose at 16. Teens and young adults (ages 16 through 23) may also receive a serogroup B meningococcal vaccine. For people who haven't been vaccinated, consider for certain foreign travelers (see page 283), for young college students living in dorms, or for people who don't have a spleen (or their spleen isn't functioning)

Well-child immunization schedule

The next page lists the **vaccine schedule for children**. Vaccines for infants include the rotavirus vaccine, which protects them against severe diarrhea. Health insurance usually covers most of the cost. A federal program called Vaccines for Children Program provides free vaccines to children who don't have health insurance coverage and to certain other groups of children. Ask your doctor about this program.

 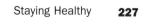

Recommended immunization schedule for children ages 0-6 years

Vaccine ▼ / Age ▶	Birth	1 month	2 months	4 months	6 months	12 months	15 months	18 months	19-23 months	2-3 years	4-6 years
Hepatitis B (HepB)	1st dose	2nd dose			3rd dose						
Rotavirus (RV1 or RV5)			1st dose	2nd dose	3rd dose*						
Diphtheria, tetanus, pertussis (DTaP)			1st dose	2nd dose	3rd dose		4th dose				5th dose
Haemophilus influenzae type b conjugate (Hib)			1st dose	2nd dose	3rd dose†	3rd or 4th dose					■
Pneumococcal conjugate (PCV13)			1st dose	2nd dose	3rd dose	4th dose					■
Inactivated poliovirus (IPV)			1st dose	2nd dose	3rd dose						4th dose
Flu (influenza)					Influenza (yearly, 1 or 2 doses)						
Measles, mumps, rubella (MMR)					■	1st dose					2nd dose
Chickenpox (varicella)						1st dose					2nd dose
Hepatitis A (HepA)						2 doses				■	
Meningococcal conjugate (Hib-MenCY, MenACWY)			■	■	■	■	■	■	■	■	
Pneumoccal polysaccharide (PPSV23)										■	

*Third dose for RV5 series only
†Hib may be given as a two- or three-dose primary series (followed by booster) depending on the vaccine used.

Legend:
- Range of recommended ages (light gray)
- Certain high-risk groups (black)

Recommended immunization schedule for children ages 7-18 years

Vaccine ▼ / Age ▶	7-8 years	9-10 years	11-12 years	13-15 years	16 years	17-18 years
Tetanus, diphtheria, pertussis (Tdap)			1 dose			
Human papillomavirus (HPV)		■	2 doses			
Meningococcal conjugate (Hib-MenCY, MenACWY)	■		1st dose		2nd dose	
Pneumococcal conjugate (PCV13)	■	■	■	■	■	■
Flu (influenza)			1 dose annually			
Hepatitis A (HepA)	■	■	■	■	■	■
Serogroup B meningococcal (MenB)		■	■	■		
Pneumococcal polysaccharide (PPSV23)	■	■	■	■	■	■

Legend:
- Range of recommended ages (light gray)
- Certain high-risk groups (black)
- May be recommended for non-high-risk group (medium gray)

Source: Advisory Committee on Immunization Practices, Centers for Disease Control and Prevention, 2017

Note: For more information on the HPV vaccine to protect against cervical cancer, see page 151. For more details on childhood, adolescent and adult immunizations, visit the website of the Centers for Disease Control and Prevention (CDC) at *www.cdc.gov* and type "immunization schedules" in the search box.

Protecting yourself

Over 130,000 deaths in the United States each year result from unintentional injuries (accidents). Accidents are the most common cause of death of people ages 1 to 44. In the following pages, you'll find a variety of safety tips that may help you prepare for potentially dangerous circumstances. For workplace safety, see page 241.

■ Emergency preparedness

Many people face emergencies at one time or another, from a car breakdown to a kitchen fire. Major emergencies from a natural disaster, toxic spill, flu epidemic or act of terrorism are rare but affect more people at once. A major emergency potentially involves death or injury, lack of food and water, and the loss of public utilities, transportation and services. Your survival may depend on how prepared you are.

Need for action

An emergency requires quick decisions: Should you stay where you are? Or is your best choice to evacuate? How will you connect with family and friends? Your decisions will depend on common sense and your knowledge of the immediate danger. Steps you may take to be better prepared include:

- **Being informed.** Determine the likely disaster scenarios that could take place in your area, for example, floods, wildfires, infectious diseases or hazardous spills. Learn how you'll be notified of emergencies. There may be special sirens, radio or television broadcasts, or emergency workers going door to door. Consider buying a weather alert radio, which can provide early warning for emergencies.
- **Staying in touch.** Choose a common emergency contact phone number — the home of a friend or relative, for example — that all family members can use to stay in touch during emergencies. Note that when there are major disruptions, it's often easier to contact someone far away than nearby.
- **Deciding whether to shelter in place or evacuate.** Government officials will give you guidance on whether to evacuate or stay in place. If you stay in place, you will need to rely on your emergency supplies.
- **Planning for evacuation.** If you must evacuate, determine locations where you and your family can meet, both within and outside the community. Know how to turn off the home utilities — water, electricity and gas. Plan to take pets with you, if possible. Always keep your vehicles' gas tanks at least half full.
- **Staying calm.** Major emergencies are generally unexpected, unfamiliar and uncontrollable. Stress from these events causes panic and confusion. Your ability to make sound decisions may depend on:
  - ‣ Practicing your emergency plan
  - ‣ Knowing your community's resources
  - ‣ Including your children in preparations and practice

Disaster supplies kit

Emergency preparations include gathering supplies that are ready to use in the event of a disaster. Keep in mind that water, food and clean air are your highest priorities. You may customize the kit to fit your needs and preferences, and to handle the most likely disasters.

There should be enough supplies for everyone for at least three days. Store the kit in a dry, cool place, preferably out of the sun. Pack items in easy-to-carry, easily accessible containers for use in your home or if you need to evacuate.

Basic items include:

- **Water.** Plan on 1 gallon a person per day, for drinking and for sanitation. Store water tightly sealed in clean plastic containers.
- **Food.** Select foods that require no refrigeration or preparation, that have a long shelf life, and that require little or no water.
- **Hygiene and sanitation items.** Pack dust masks, moist towelettes, alcohol-based hand sanitizer, toothpaste and toothbrushes, toilet paper, heavy-duty garbage bags and ties.
- **Tools.** Include a manual can opener, eating utensils, a flashlight, a battery-powered radio, extra batteries, matches (in a waterproof container), plastic sheeting and duct tape, a knife, a wrench or pliers, scissors and a whistle.
- **First-aid kit.** Pack adhesive bandages, cleansing agent (soap or towelette), antibiotic ointment, a thermometer, a tweezers, burn ointment, eyewash solution, sterile dressing, tape, elastic wrap, and aspirin or other pain reliever.
- **Family items.** Don't forget cash and coins, a supply of regularly used medications, bank numbers, important documents, medical prescriptions, driver's licenses and passports, and extra sets of keys.

Additional items include: cooking and eating accessories, blankets or sleeping bags, a change of clothing and footwear, bathing supplies, items for infants (if necessary), a compass, a tent, a camp shovel, a fire extinguisher, paper towels, disinfectant or household chlorine bleach, pet supplies, special needs items, inhalers, contact lenses, extra eyeglasses, hearing aid batteries, and feminine supplies.

Preparing for a flu epidemic

Whether it's the seasonal flu or a pandemic flu, take these steps to protect yourself and others:

- Get your seasonal flu shot, and ask your doctor if you're a candidate for a pandemic flu shot if there is a vaccine available.
- Practice good respiratory and hand hygiene to limit transmission of the disease. Keep your hands out of your eyes, nose and mouth. Cover your cough. See page 234 for good hand-washing techniques.
- Stay home if you're sick. Don't expose others if you're ill. Take care of yourself so that you can care for others, if needed. Eat healthy foods, and get plenty of rest. If symptoms are serious, call, rather than visit, your doctor for advice.

- Be prepared at home. Have a supply of nonperishable, easy-to-prepare food on hand. If you or a loved one is ill, you may not be able to get to a store. Also have enough of your prescription and nonprescription drugs on hand.
- Plan for possible school and child care closures.
- Have a plan for alternate transportation if you use buses or other public transportation.

If you have other serious medical illnesses, you may need to be on an influenza antiviral medication, either as a preventive or for treatment of symptoms. If you suspect influenza, seek early testing (within 48 hours) as you may be eligible for an antiviral medication.

FOR MORE INFORMATION
- Department of Homeland Security, 202-282-8000, *www.dhs.gov*
- CDC: Emergency preparedness and response, 800-232-4636, *https://emergency.cdc.gov*
- CDC: Influenza (flu), 800-232-4636, *www.cdc.gov/flu*

Reduce your risk on the road

Thousands of people die on roads and highways every year. To reduce your risk:

- **Always wear a seat belt,** even when you're traveling a short distance.
- **Place children in car seats and secure the seats properly.**
- **Drive defensively.** Be aware of other traffic at all times.
- **Consider the weather,** and adjust your speed according to weather conditions.
- **Don't drive while impaired** — after drinking alcohol or if deprived of sleep.
- **Avoid distractions.** Don't let the radio or a roadside attraction distract you. Don't talk or text on your cellphone at all while driving.
- **Keep your car properly serviced** to reduce the risk of breakdowns.
- **Carry an emergency kit.** A kit may include a cellphone, flashlight, first-aid supplies, jumper cables, flares, a candle and matches, and supplies for extreme weather.

Keep your children safe in the car

- Strap infants and toddlers into rear-facing car safety seats (infant seats or convertible seats) until they are at least 2 years of age or they reach the highest weight or height requirements allowed by the car seat manufacturer.
- Toddlers and preschoolers who have outgrown the rear-facing weight or height limit for their convertible seats should use forward-facing seats with harnesses for as long as possible, up to the highest weight or height allowed by the car seat manufacturer.

- Younger school-age children whose weights and heights exceed the forward-facing limit for their car seats should use belt-positioning booster seats until the vehicle seat belts fit properly, typically when they have reached 4 feet 9 inches in height and are 8 to 12 years of age.
- When children are old enough and large enough for vehicle seat belts to fit them correctly, they should always use lap and shoulder seat belts for the best protection. All children younger than 13 years of age should ride in the back seat.

Reduce your risk at home

Use this safety checklist to make your home a safer place.

- ❑ Household emergency preparedness plan and kit (See pages 229-230.)
- ❑ Fire escape plan reviewed with all occupants
- ❑ Smoke detectors installed on each floor and working
- ❑ Carbon monoxide detectors installed on each floor and working
- ❑ Fire hazards removed: flammable items away from open flame or heat source
- ❑ Poisonous or dangerous substances locked up or out of the reach of children
- ❑ Poison control, other emergency numbers and home address posted near phone
- ❑ Dangerous objects away from children: tools, firearms, and electrical or hot objects
- ❑ Electrical equipment away from water; cords and equipment in good condition
- ❑ Walkways and stairs well-lighted, free of slippery surfaces, and foreign objects
- ❑ Night lights and visual aids in place for use at night
- ❑ Handrails and nonslip surfaces in bathrooms, in showers and on stairs
- ❑ Allergen sources removed: gutters cleaned, drains clear, damp areas cleaned of mold and mildew, a dehumidifier installed; and dusty spots, carpets and rugs vacuumed
- ❑ Emergency shut-off valves for water and gas and master switch for electricity location and function known and accessible
- ❑ Protective gear accessible — safety goggles, hearing protection, gloves and masks

Preventing falls

Trips and <u>falls</u> pose a danger to everyone, but especially to young children and older adults. Falls are a common cause of injury among older adults — sometimes resulting in death. Balance problems, poor vision, illness, medications and other factors can cause falls. Develop a plan that reduces risk and prevents injury.

Self-care

Here are some tips to prevent falls:

- **Have your vision and hearing checked regularly.** If vision and hearing are impaired, you lose important cues that help you maintain balance.
- **Exercise regularly.** Exercise improves your strength, muscle tone and coordination. This not only helps prevent falls but also reduces the severity of injury if you do fall.
- **Be wary of drugs.** Ask your doctor about the drugs you take. Some drugs may affect balance and coordination.
- **Avoid alcohol.** Even a little alcohol can cause falls, especially if your balance and reflexes are already impaired.
- **Get up slowly.** A momentary decrease in blood pressure, due to drugs or aging, can cause dizziness if you stand up too quickly.
- **Maintain balance and footing.** If you feel unsteady, use a cane or walker. Wear sturdy, low-heeled shoes with wide, nonslip soles.
- **Eliminate loose rugs or mats.**
- **Install adequate lighting,** especially night lighting.
- **Block steps** for infants and toddlers, and install handrails for older people.

Lead exposure

Approximately 535,000 children in the United States ages 1 to 5 years have levels of lead in their bloodstream that are worth noting, according to the Centers for Disease Control and Prevention. <u>Lead poisoning</u> can affect nearly every system in the body. Children are more sensitive to lead poisoning than adults are. Blood testing is important for children at ages 1 and 2. Some local health departments serving high-risk areas recommend testing for lead poisoning at age 6 months if you think that your home has high lead levels, and after that as recommended by your doctor.

Here are some potential sources of lead poisoning:

- **Soil.** Lead particles that settle on the soil from paint or gasoline used years ago can stay there for many years. High concentrations of lead in soil can be found around old homes and in some urban settings.
- **Household dust.** This can contain lead from paint chips or soil brought in from outside.
- **Water.** Lead pipes, brass plumbing fixtures and copper pipes soldered with lead can release lead particles into tap water. If you have such plumbing, let cold water run 30 to 60 seconds before drinking it. Hot water absorbs more lead than does cold water. The Environmental Protection Agency (EPA) warns against making baby formula with hot tap water from old plumbing systems.
- **Lead paint.** Although now outlawed, lead paint is still on walls and woodwork in many older homes — often those built before 1978. When sanding or stripping in an older home, wear a mask and keep children away from dust and chips.

See back cover for online resource ⓘ

Carbon monoxide poisoning

Carbon monoxide is a poisonous gas produced by incomplete burning of fuel. It has no color, taste or odor. Carbon monoxide builds up in red blood cells, preventing oxygen from being carried and starving your body of oxygen.

Each year, hundreds of Americans die of unintentional **carbon monoxide poisoning**. A few simple measures can help prevent poisoning:

- **Know the signs and symptoms.** They include headache, fever, red-appearing skin, dizziness, weakness, fatigue, nausea, vomiting, shortness of breath, chest pain and trouble thinking. Symptoms of carbon monoxide poisoning often come on slowly and may be mistaken for a cold or the flu. Clues include similar symptoms being experienced by everyone in the same building or improvement of symptoms when you leave the building for a day or more and then a return of the symptoms when you come back to the building.
- **Be aware of possible sources.** The most common sources are gas and oil furnaces, wood stoves, gas appliances, pool heaters, and engine exhaust fumes. Cracked heat exchangers on furnaces, blocked chimneys, flues or appliance vents can allow carbon monoxide to reach living areas. An inadequate supply of fresh air to a furnace also can allow carbon monoxide to build up in living spaces. Tight home construction also may increase your risk because less fresh air gets in.
- **Get a detector.** It sounds a warning when carbon monoxide builds up. Look for UL 2034 on the package, an indication the detector meets industry standards.
- **Know when to take action.** If the alarm sounds, ventilate the area by opening doors and windows. If anyone is experiencing poisoning symptoms, evacuate immediately and call for emergency medical assistance from a nearby phone. If no one is experiencing symptoms, continue to ventilate, turn off all fuel-burning appliances, and have a qualified technician inspect your home.

Indoor air pollution

The EPA rates indoor air pollution among the top environmental health risks. Others are outdoor air pollution, toxic chemicals in the workplace and contaminated drinking water. The most dangerous pollutants found in indoor air include:

- **Tobacco smoke.** Smoking causes lung cancer. Even if you don't smoke but live with someone who does, you have a 20 to 30 percent higher risk of lung cancer than someone who lives in a smoke-free home. Air-filtering devices help, but they remove mainly solid particles in smoke, not the gases.
- **Radon.** This naturally occurring gas is made by the radioactive decay of uranium in rocks and soil. You can easily overlook radon because you can't see, taste or smell it. Yet, radon can seep into your home and other buildings through basement cracks, sewer openings, and joints between walls and floors. After chronic exposure at high levels, radon may lead to lung cancer. To check your home's radon level, contact your local health department, to ask if they may have a testing program, or buy a radon detector. If your radon level is high, call the National Radon Helpline at 800-55RADON (800-557-2366).
- **Household chemicals.** When using chemical compounds indoors such as glues, paints, cleaners, solvents and drain openers, be sure to ventilate the area.
- **Asbestos.** Asbestos is a natural mineral product that resists heat and corrosion.

It was used extensively in the past in products such as insulation, fire-retardant materials, cement and some vinyl floor tiles. **Asbestosis** is a breathing disorder caused by inhaling asbestos fibers. Prolonged accumulation of these fibers in your lungs can cause scarring of lung tissue and shortness of breath. Asbestosis symptoms can range from mild to severe, and usually don't appear until years after exposure. Severe cases can lead to lung cancer or other serious health problems. Most people with asbestosis got it on the job (in mining, milling, manufacturing, or installation or removal of asbestos) before the government began regulating asbestos use in the mid-1970s. Asbestos removal is best done by a professional.

Hand-washing

Americans spend billions of dollars annually to fight infections. With today's high-tech approach to health care, it's easy to forget the simplest way to avoid infection — wash your hands.

Why is it important?

Most cases of the common cold, flu (influenza), diarrhea, vomiting and hepatitis are caused by inadequate **hand-washing**. Germs accumulate on your hands as you perform daily activities. By not washing your hands, you can acquire or pass on a host of ailments.

Infections claim more lives than any other diseases except for heart disease and cancer. Pneumonia and flu are leading causes of death in the United States.

What is proper hand-washing?

Follow these steps:

- Place your hands under running water. Water temperature isn't essential. Water that's warm enough (about 110 F) to cut through grease is best. Water that's hot enough to kill germs can harm your hands.
- Apply soap or detergent to your hands.
- Rub vigorously for at least 10 seconds.
- Clean around your cuticles, under fingernails and in the creases of your hands.
- Rinse all soap from your hands to remove as many microorganisms as possible.

If you don't have time to wash with soap and water, use a waterless hand cleaner. Alcohol-based hand rubs significantly reduce the number of microorganisms on your skin and are fast-acting. Place a quarter size amount of the hand sanitizer liquid in your hand and spread over your hands for 15 seconds. Rub the solution into your skin.

When should you wash?

It's impossible to keep your hands germ-free, but there are times when it's critical to wash your hands. Always wash:

- Before you handle or eat food
- After you use the toilet
- After changing a diaper
- After playing with a pet or handling pet equipment, such as brushes, aquariums or litter boxes
- After handling garbage
- After handling money
- After blowing your nose, sneezing or coughing into your hand
- After handling uncooked food (especially raw meats)
- Before entering a hospital room and after leaving it

Aging and your health

How age can affect your health

If you're older than age 40, you've undoubtedly confronted some realities of **aging**. You've probably peeked into a mirror at a face that has developed a few more wrinkles. You may have noticed that aches and pains linger a little longer after you exercise or spend time doing yardwork. Until adults reach the fourth or fifth decade of life, aging rarely means much to them — even though it's a lifelong process that begins at birth.

Most adults experience common physical changes as they get older. Here are a few common examples:

- Your systolic blood pressure — the top number — increases as artery walls thicken and become less flexible.
- Your body redistributes fat, and your muscle mass declines.
- Your ability to hear high-frequency sounds decreases, starting around age 20, and low-frequency sounds become more difficult to hear during your 60s.
- Your maximum breathing capacity declines.
- Your brain sustains loss and damage of nerve cells.
- Your bladder loses capacity, leading to more-frequent urination and, sometimes, leakage.
- Your kidneys become less efficient in removing waste from your bloodstream.
- Your risk of falls increases.

How long can you expect to live?

This chart shows how many more years, on average, a person can expect to live, based on current age, sex and race. Of course, these are just general estimates. If you smoke or drive without a seat belt, you lower your odds. If you have a healthy lifestyle, you might increase your odds.

Average number of years remaining

Current age	White male	White female	Black male	Black female	Hispanic male	Hispanic female
50	29.9	33.4	27.1	31.5	32.0	35.6
55	25.7	29.0	23.1	27.3	27.6	31.0
60	21.7	24.7	19.5	23.3	23.5	26.5
65	18.0	20.5	16.3	19.6	19.6	22.2
70	14.4	16.6	13.3	16.0	15.8	18.1
75	11.2	12.9	10.5	12.7	12.4	14.3
80	8.3	9.7	8.1	9.7	9.3	10.8
85	5.9	6.9	6.0	7.3	6.7	7.8

Based on *National Vital Statistics Reports*, 2016;65:3

Maintaining your health as you age

Successful aging involves many factors that are within your control. Begin with strategies to maintain your overall health.

Adopt a positive attitude. Remember that your attitudes color the quality of your life. You're old only when you think you are. True, your body will age. Yet your mind, for the most part, will stay as young as you feel. In all of life, stay focused on what's important and shrug off what isn't. A sense of humor and an ability to adapt to change are golden assets. Also see "Keeping stress under control," page 221.

Eat well. Numerous studies indicate that a healthy diet, when combined with regular physical and mental activity, can help you live longer and better. As you age, however, you may need to make certain adjustments in your approach to eating. In addition to the guidelines for "Healthy eating," starting on page 210, keep these suggestions in mind:

- To allow for the fact that your metabolism slows down, consider limiting serving sizes and calories to maintain a healthy weight.
- To help prevent heart and blood vessel disease, reduce the amount of saturated fat, cholesterol and sodium that you consume. Also limit the amount of sugar that's added to foods and beverages.
- If you drink alcohol, do so in moderation — in general, for healthy adults, up to one drink a day for women of all ages and for men older than age 65, and up to two drinks a day for men age 65 and younger.
- Remember that as you get older, your thirst mechanism declines. Make it a habit to drink plenty of fluids (nonalcoholic) every day.

Avoid tobacco. Smoking has been linked to gum disease, high blood pressure, heart disease, stroke, lung cancer and a variety of other cancers. If you smoke or chew tobacco, make a plan to quit. For ideas, see page 192.

Keep physically active. Regular exercise can help reduce your risk of coronary artery disease, high blood pressure, stroke, diabetes, depression, falls and some cancers. Fitness also reduces the lifestyle-limiting effects of osteoporosis and arthritis.

It's never too late to become more active. But before you begin an exercise program that's more vigorous than walking, get a medical evaluation from your health care provider.

Stay mentally sharp. Your brain is like a muscle. To keep it strong, use it. Participate in community activities such as tutoring, serving on boards or volunteering.

Stay socially connected. Having strong ties with family and friends is always important. With age, those connections become even more crucial. Studies indicate that if you have few social ties, your risk of premature death is greater than that of people who cultivate many caring relationships.

Seek out spirituality. Research supports the wisdom of believing in something larger than yourself as a way to cope with whatever life hands you. People who attend religious services are more likely to enjoy better health, live longer and recover from illness sooner.

Everyone defines spirituality differently. For some people, it's organized religion. For others, spirituality is expressed through meditation, music or art — any source of meaning and purpose that allows you to withstand suffering and experience serenity in daily life.

Your Health and the Workplace

- Health, safety and injury prevention
- Stress relievers
- Coping with technology

This section focuses on ways to improve your well-being in the work environment. You'll find practical information on a variety of basic health and safety issues. There also are tips on managing stress, as well as strategies to deal with computer-related pains and strains.

Health, safety and injury prevention

■ Protect your back

Your back moves in several directions and you use it in weight-bearing activities. Back pain, especially low back pain, is one of the most common problems reported, both in the workplace and at home. The good news is that with as little as five to 10 minutes of exercises a day — along with following some simple guidelines when lifting — you can prevent many back problems.

Self-care

Take care of your back by following these tips:
- **Maintain a healthy weight.** A healthy weight minimizes stress on your back.
- **Exercise regularly.** Do strengthening and stretching exercises that target your back muscles. These exercises are called core strengthening because they work both your abdominal and back muscles. Strong and flexible muscles will help keep your back in shape, improve posture and combat low back pain. Core exercises may include floor exercises, Pilates or fitness balls. The benefits of core exercises depend on proper technique, so get help from a trained professional if needed. See page 55 for examples of back-strengthening exercises.
- **Lift properly.** For help in using proper lifting technique, see page 54.
- **Adopt healthy work habits.** Look at the setup of your office or work area. Think about how you could modify repetitive job tasks to reduce physical demands. Try to maintain healthy, safe postures. If you work at a computer, make sure that your monitor and chair are positioned properly. For more tips on reducing the risk of back injury and pain, see "Preventing back injuries in the workplace," page 53.
- **Avoid more back pain.** If you have back pain, there are several steps you can take to feel better without going to the doctor or chiropractor. See "Self-care," pages 51-52. Also see "Medical help," page 52, to find out when you should see a doctor.

■ Hand and wrist care

Carpal tunnel syndrome

The <u>carpal tunnel</u> is a narrow passageway in your wrist. This tunnel protects a main nerve to your hand and the tendons that bend your fingers. When the tissues in the carpal tunnel become swollen or inflamed, they put pressure on the nerve, which affects your thumb and index, middle and ring fingers. This pressure produces the numbness, pain and, eventually, hand weakness that characterize <u>carpal tunnel syndrome</u>.

If the condition is left untreated, nerve and muscle damage can result. Fortunately, for most people who develop carpal tunnel syndrome, proper treatment usually can relieve the pain and numbness and restore normal use of their wrists and hands. For more details, including symptoms and self-care, see page 96.

See back cover for online resource (i)

Coping with arthritis at work

Here are tips for dealing with arthritis at work:

- Allow time to warm up and loosen joints before starting work.
- Arrange your workspace so that you have to do minimal reaching, lifting or carrying.
- Try to organize your work activities to minimize significant repetitive motion. Alternate tasks requiring more physical effort with lighter tasks.
- Consider using special tools, modified equipment and assistive devices to make your job easier. For example, ergonomic chairs, electric staplers, enlarged pen grips and floor mats (if you'll be standing for a long time) may be helpful.
- Communicate special needs to your employer. Sometimes this is best done through the department of employee health or the department of occupational health, if available, or with the help of your doctor. Minor changes in your work environment or a different routine may be just what you need.
  See pages 161-164 for more tips on managing arthritis.

Exercises for office workers

Sitting at work for eight hours a day can cause fatigue, stress, back pain and even blood clots. These stretches will help — and could improve — your job performance.

Three five-minute stretch breaks a day can perk you up, relax your muscles and improve your flexibility. You can do the following exercises without leaving your desk. Hold each stretch for 10 to 20 seconds. Repeat each exercise once or twice on both sides.

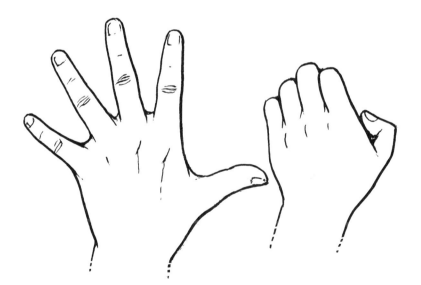

1. Stretch your fingers out as far as you can. Hold for 10 seconds. Relax. Now bend your fingers at the knuckles and squeeze.

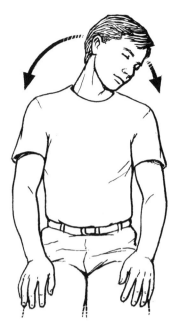

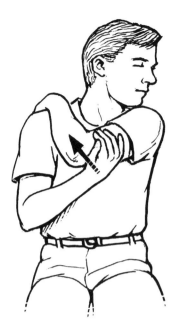

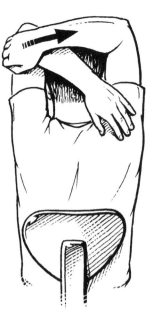

2. *Slowly tilt your head to the left until you feel a stretch on the side of your neck. Repeat to the right and forward.*

3. *Hold your left arm just above the elbow with your right hand. Gently pull your elbow across your chest toward the right shoulder while turning your head to look over the left shoulder. Repeat with your other arm.*

4. *Raise your left elbow above your head and put your left palm on the back of your neck. Now grasp your left elbow with your right hand. Gently pull your elbow behind your head and toward your right shoulder until you feel a nice stretch in your shoulder or upper arms. Repeat with your other arm.*

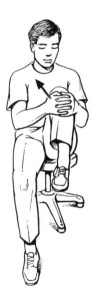

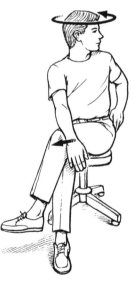

5. *Hold your left leg just below the knee. Gently pull your bent leg toward your chest. Hold it as shown and pull it toward your right shoulder. Repeat with your right leg.*

6. *Cross your left leg over your right leg. Cross your right elbow over your left thigh. Gently press your leg with your elbow to twist your hip and lower and middle parts of your back. Look over your left shoulder to complete the stretch. Repeat on the other side.*

Safety in the workplace

Protect yourself and others by following these safety rules and guidelines:

- **Protective eyewear.** If your job carries a risk of eye injury, your employer is required by law to provide you with protective glasses, and you are required to wear them. If they interfere with your efficiency, try another design.
- **Protection from noise.** In conditions of excessively loud noise, your employer should regularly measure noise levels or provide protective devices. Specially designed earmuffs are available. Some types close out the outside world; others are fitted with earphones and a microphone that enable you to communicate with other workers. Commercially available earplugs made of foam, plastic or rubber or custom-molded plugs also effectively decrease your exposure to excessive noise. Don't use cotton balls. They can get stuck deep in your ear canal.
- **Fumes, smoke, dust and gas hazards.** Many respiratory symptoms can result from exposure to toxic fumes, gases, particles and smoke in the workplace. The exposure may be long term with low levels of chemicals, or it may be accidental, in which high levels of industrial toxic chemicals are inhaled for a short time. Wear proper clothing, air-filtration masks, eye gear and other appropriate protection. Be sure ventilation is adequate. If you use a respirator at work, it should be fitted to you before first use and retested at least once a year.

If you are pregnant or are trying to become pregnant, avoid any exposure to hazardous chemicals. Review your exposure risk with your company safety officer and your obstetrician.

If you suspect that you're being exposed to dangerous smoke, fumes, dust or chemicals in your workplace, talk with your doctor. Many permanent respiratory ailments develop slowly as a result of industrial exposure over a period of years. Small exposures that may seem harmless can result in chronic disease. If you think that you or your co-workers are at unnecessary risk, talk with your company safety officer. Additional information can be obtained from the Occupational Safety and Health Administration (OSHA) or from your union, if you have one.

Medication and alcohol use. Don't consume alcohol before or during working hours. Do not operate machinery when you are taking medications that might make you drowsy. If you're taking medications, ask your doctor or pharmacist how these substances might affect your job.

Emergency preparedness. Make sure you understand the steps you need to take in case of an emergency at your place of employment. Many companies have plans that outline what to do in various types of emergencies. If your company doesn't have such a plan, talk to a supervisor about preparing one.

Sleeping tips for shift workers

Changing your normal rhythm of waking and sleeping, as a result of switching shifts, requires a period of adjustment. If your job requires constant changing of shifts, your body will have more difficulty adjusting and readjusting as you get older.

Here are some suggestions to try:

- If you can work it out with your manager, try to work the same shift for at least three weeks at a time, rather than rotate to a different shift every week.

- If you work rotating shifts, on the last few days of your current shift, adjust your bedtime and wake-up time by one to two hours as the new shift nears.
- Change the sequence, if possible. A more normal sleep pattern results when the shift sequence is day-evening-night rather than day-night-evening.
- Tolerance to shift rotation varies among people. If you experience major difficulty with falling asleep, ask your doctor about a short-acting sleeping pill. If you have trouble making the adjustment, consider changing your job. Getting enough sleep is challenging, but it needs to be your main goal.

For more information, see page 44.

Drugs, alcohol and work

Street drugs and alcohol can affect your health and safety in the workplace, as well as the safety of your co-workers. The problem is extensive.

Consider the following:
- An estimated 70 percent of adult illegal drug users are employed.
- Substance abusers are more likely to be involved in a workplace accident and file a workers' compensation claim than other employees.
- Workers with alcohol problems are 2.7 times more likely than are workers without alcohol problems to have injury-related absences.

If you have a problem with substances, get help. Many employers have support programs for their employees that are nondisciplinary. If you know of a co-worker with a problem, encourage him or her to get help. If you believe that conditions in the workplace are unsafe because of an impaired worker, it's important to report the issue.

Self-assessment

Do you have a problem with alcohol or drugs? Ask yourself these questions:
- Have I used an illegal drug in the past six months?
- Have I misused a prescription drug because of its effect (to sleep or calm myself, or for pleasure)?
- Have I done something unsafe or taken risks while under the influence of alcohol or drugs, such as driving a car, operating heavy equipment or making decisions that affect the safety of others?
- Have relatives, friends, my doctor or others expressed concern about my drug or alcohol use?
- Has my drug or alcohol use negatively affected my relationships, my health or my ability to work?

If you answered yes to any of these questions, you're showing signs of substance abuse and should take action.

Self-care

- If you or a family member is dependent on alcohol, see "Alcohol use disorders," page 188.
- If you or a family member has problems with drug addiction, refer to "Drug use and dependency," page 196.
- Many large corporations offer confidential employee assistance programs to help workers deal with drug and alcohol abuse. Ask about their availability through your personnel or human resources department.
- If your company doesn't offer an alcohol or drug rehabilitation program, contact your health care provider or a mental health professional for a confidential referral.

Stress relievers

Burned out? Get a tuneup

If you dread going to work or feel burned out or stressed, you're facing a situation that could affect your professional and personal relationships and even your livelihood. Overwhelming frustration or indifference toward your job, persistent irritability, anger, sarcasm, and being quick to argue are indicators of a condition that you need to deal with. Consider these strategies:

- **Take care of yourself.** Eat regular, balanced meals, including breakfast. Get enough sleep and physical activity.
- **Develop friendships at work and outside the office.** Sharing unsettling feelings with people you trust is the first step toward resolving them. Limit activities with "negative" friends who reinforce negative feelings.
- **Take time off.** Take a vacation or a long weekend. Plan private time each week when you don't answer calls, texts or pages. During the workday, take short breaks.
- **Set limits.** When necessary, learn to say no in a friendly but firm manner.
- **Choose battles wisely.** Don't rush to argue every time someone disagrees with you. Keep a cool head, and save your argument for things that really matter. Better yet, try not to argue at all.
- **Take advantage of on-the-job training.** Workshops and courses can spur your interest and improve your satisfaction and productivity.
- **Keep your eye on opportunities within your company.** Check internal postings that will challenge your mind and that might better match your skills and interests.
- **Have an outlet.** Read, do a hobby, exercise or get involved in some other activity that gets your mind off work and is relaxing.
- **Seek help.** If none of these steps relieves your feelings of stress or burnout, talk with an employee assistance counselor, if available, or other health care provider.

Co-worker conflict: 6 steps to make peace

It's best to deal with differences directly, that is, talk with the person with whom you have a conflict. But the mood of that discussion is crucial. Here are some tips:

- **Discuss the matter privately.** Choose neutral territory at a specific time that each person agrees on. Approach the other person in a nonthreatening manner, such as "I'd like to talk something over with you. I'm feeling ..." Or "I'd like to check something out with you when you have a chance to talk."
- **Don't blame the other person.** Use "I" statements. It will make the other person feel less defensive or angry.
- **Listen closely to the other person.** Understanding the other person's point of view may help you feel less stressed or angry.
- **Consider whether this is a personality-driven problem or a system problem.** For example, maybe the person wasn't adequately trained and needs more training.
- **Focus on ways to resolve the problem.** Don't get sidetracked in an argument.
- **Seek help.** Talk with an employee assistance counselor, who can help develop ground rules for such discussions and promote respectful communication.

5 tips for managing time

Here are some tips to ensure you're managing your time as wisely as possible:
- Create realistic deadlines for yourself, and set regular progress reviews.
- Throw away all but the important papers on your desk. Prepare a master list of tasks. Pitch files older than six months.
- Throughout the day, scan your master list and work on tasks in priority order.
- Use a planner. Store addresses and telephone numbers there. Copy master list items onto the page for the day on which you expect to do them. Evaluate and prioritize daily.
- For especially important or difficult projects, reserve an interruption-free block of time behind closed doors.

Get to know your boss: Build a healthy relationship

If you and your boss mix like oil and water, don't despair. To revive your relationship, work on getting to know him or her better. Here's how:
- **Show respect.** Try to understand the business from your boss's perspective.
- **Think about what the boss really needs.** Is it more important to him or her that you stay on schedule while producing fair-to-good results, or is sacrificing a deadline OK if it means making a project perfect? Learn your boss's preferences and use the information to make life easier for both of you.
- **Know what your boss expects.** If the person you report to isn't clear about expectations, be direct in asking what they are.
- **Determine your boss's personal style.** Formal or informal? Big picture or details? Without becoming a clone, try to adapt your behavior. If your styles differ, consider whether you can discuss this to see if there is room for compromise.
- **Be positive.** When things go wrong, communicate with questions, and if possible, solutions, instead of complaints.
- **Don't be afraid of your boss.** Your performance contributes to his or her success.
- **Welcome feedback.** Ask your boss for advice to help you grow in areas that need development.

Halt hostility: Talk it out

To head off hostility, the most important thing to do is to talk with someone to release tension and possibly gain a new perspective.

When a conflict is already brewing:
- Talk about solutions as well as problems. Work with others to resolve the issues.
- Try to put off your anger until you've heard all the facts.
- If you feel an outburst coming on, take a break. Count to 10, breathe deeply, go for a walk — whatever it takes to cool off and avoid doing something you might regret later.
- Use active listening skills and calmly repeat back what you've heard. ("Let me make sure I understand you. ...")
- When an angry confrontation seems inevitable, seek a neutral third party to help talk it through.

Coping with technology

■ Computer screens and eyestrain

There you sit, peering at your computer screen. If you're one of a growing number of people for whom using a computer is key to their work, you may be peering for the multiple hours today. And like many computer users, you may be experiencing eye-strain as a result.

Symptoms may include:
- Sore, tired, burning, itchy or dry eyes
- Blurred or double vision
- Distance vision blurred after prolonged staring at the monitor
- Headache or sore neck
- Difficulty shifting focus between monitor and source documents
- Difficulty focusing on the screen image
- Color fringes or afterimages when you look away from the monitor
- Increased sensitivity to light

Try to ease the strain

Eyestrain associated with computer monitors isn't thought to have serious or long-term consequences, but it is disruptive and unpleasant. Although you probably can't change every factor that may cause eyestrain, here are some things you can try to ease the strain:

- **Take eye breaks.** Look away from the screen and into the distance or at an object several feet away for 10 seconds every 10 minutes.
- **Change the pace.** Try to move around at least once every two hours, giving both your eyes and your body a needed rest. Arrange noncomputer work as breaks from the screen. Consider standing while doing such work.
- **Blink often.** Dry eyes can result from prolonged computer use, especially for contact lens wearers. Some people blink only once a minute when doing computer work (once every five seconds is normal). Less blinking means less lubrication from tears, resulting in dry, itchy or burning eyes. So blink more often. If that doesn't help, consider using an eyedrop form of artificial tears available over-the-counter.
- **Close them periodically.** If possible, lean back and close your eyes for a few moments once in a while. You may not want to do this at your desk and risk being accused of sleeping on the job.

Everything in its place

Monitor. Position your monitor 18 to 30 inches from your eyes. Many people find that putting the screen at arm's length works well. If you have to get too close to read small type, consider using larger font sizes.

The top of the screen should be at eye level or below so that you look down slightly at your work. Place the monitor too high and you'll have to tilt your head back to look up at it, a recipe for a sore neck, and for dry eyes because you may not close your eyes completely when you blink.

Dust on the screen cuts down contrast and may contribute to glare and reflection problems. Keep it clean.

Keyboard. Put your keyboard directly in front of the monitor. If you place it at an angle or to the side, your eyes will be forced to focus separately, a tiring activity.

Source documents. Put reading and reference material on a copy stand beside the monitor and at the same level, angle and distance away. That way, your eyes aren't constantly readjusting as they go back and forth.

Surrounding light and glare. To check glare, sit at your computer with the monitor off. You'll be able to see the reflected light and images you don't normally see — including yourself. Note any intense glare. The worst problems likely will be from sources above or behind you, including fluorescent lighting and sunlight.

If possible, place your monitor so that the brightest light sources are off to the side, parallel with your line of sight to the monitor. Consider turning off some or all overhead lights. If you can't do that, tilting the monitor downward a little may reduce glare. Closing blinds or shades also may help. A hood or glare-reducing screen is an option, but be sure you aren't sacrificing the intensity of whites on your screen. Adjustable task lighting that doesn't shine into your eyes as you look at the screen can reduce eyestrain. Overall, the surrounding light should be darker than the whitest white on your screen.

Glasses. The proper correction can help. If you wear glasses or contacts, make sure the correction is right for computer work. Most lenses are fitted for reading print and may not be optimal for computer work. For example, many bifocal wearers are constantly craning their necks to look through the bottom half of the lenses, bringing on a backache or neck ache. Glasses or contact lenses designed to focus correctly for computer work may be worth the investment.

When to seek help

See an eye care professional if you have:

- Prolonged eye discomfort
- A noticeable change in vision
- Double vision

Don't let technology rule your life

Technology can make your life easier. But it can also make it harder if you're a multitasker whose multiple devices constantly compete for your attention. Being tied to your cellphone, tablet, laptop, numerous social networking tools, TV and other types of technology can hurt your concentration and increase stress.

Determine your priorities, and don't overload yourself with gadgets. And periodically take a break from screens.

The Healthy Consumer

- You and your health care provider
- Home medical testing kits
- Your family medical tree
- Medications and you
- Dietary supplements
- Integrative medicine
- The healthy traveler

In this section, you'll learn how to be a savvy health care consumer. You'll find out how to best communicate and work with your doctor, the value of your family's medical history, and the effectiveness of home medical testing kits. The proper use of medications is covered, along with easy-to-read descriptions of cold remedies and over-the-counter pain medications.

What to include in your family's medicine cabinet and first-aid kit also is covered, as well as the potential health risks associated with travel.

You and your health care provider

Medical care is becoming increasingly complex. And finding the right health care provider for you and your family can be a challenge. You may be in good health and not need a doctor immediately. But when you do, it's good to have someone who knows you and who can quickly and efficiently coordinate your care. In this section, you'll find tips on selecting the health care team that's right for you.

■ Start with primary care

You'll likely begin by looking for a doctor who is a generalist — a primary care doctor who often leads a team that includes medical assistants, physician assistants, nurses and nurse practitioners. A primary care doctor and his or her team can do the following:

- Be the point of first contact for urgent and acute care.
- Provide preventive care, such as blood pressure monitoring, cancer screening and vaccinations.
- Provide telephone and email consultation when advice is needed but an office visit isn't required.
- Provide continuity of care. This is especially important if you or someone in your family has a chronic condition.

  Here are examples of primary care specialties:
- **Family medicine specialist.** Provides care to people of all ages and may also provide obstetric care
- **Internal medicine specialist.** Provides care focused on the general needs of adults, including older adults
- **Geriatrician.** Provides care focused on the general needs of older adults
- **Pediatrician.** Provides care for children and adolescents
- **Gynecologist.** A provider of specialty care, but many gynecologists provide primary care for adult females

■ How to find a doctor

Once you have an idea about what kind of primary care provider you want, identify several candidates. Talk with friends and co-workers about their experiences with doctors in your community. In addition, consider whether you want one primary care doctor for all family members or more-focused care from a pediatrician or gynecologist.

If you're on a managed care insurance plan, you'll probably be limited to the doctors on the insurance plan's list. If so, make sure you have the current list.

Verify credentials

Before you visit a doctor, make a phone call or visit a website to confirm the doctor's credentials. If your doctor is board certified in a specialty, such as family practice, internal medicine or geriatrics, you can confirm this by checking with the American Board of Medical Specialties. You can call this organization at 312-436-

2600 or visit the website *www.abms.org*. The American Medical Association also has a website that identifies specialists. It's called AMA DoctorFinder, *https://apps.ama-assn.org/doctorfinder/home.jsp*

To determine if any disciplinary action has been taken or may be pending against a doctor, call your state medical licensing board. For the number, look under state government listings in your phone book or call directory assistance. Keep in mind, however, that even the best doctors occasionally have legal problems. So don't let this be the only factor in your decision.

Visit the doctor's office

Once you've selected two or three doctors, set up get-acquainted visits. Tell the receptionist you're looking for a doctor and you'd like to speak with someone who could answer a few questions about the doctor and office procedures.

A good place to start is to find out if the doctor is accepting new patients. Next, ask if the doctor accepts your medical insurance plan.

Here are some additional questions you might ask:

- What's the doctor's training and special field of practice?
- What are your office hours?
- How many days a week does the doctor see patients?
- Are evening or weekend appointments possible?
- If I call the office with a medical question, can I speak with the doctor?
- How does the doctor arrange to answer medical questions after hours?
- How far in advance do people have to make an appointment? (If the doctor seems overloaded, you might want to look elsewhere.)
- How long do people generally have to wait in the office?
- How willing is the doctor to refer people to a specialist?
- How long will you be able to visit with the doctor? (Some HMOs restrict total time to less than 30 minutes.)

Trust your instincts

If you don't feel compatible with the doctor, try the next one on your list. You're more likely to follow the advice of a doctor with whom you feel comfortable. Doctors know this, so don't worry about offending them. Concentrate on your needs.

Specialists you may need

How do you know when you need a specialist or other health care provider, such as a physical therapist, a physician assistant or a nurse practitioner? Generally, your primary care doctor will refer you to a specialist when you have a problem that warrants it. If you're concerned that you have medical problems not being adequately cared for by your primary care doctor, you might want to seek a specialist whose training and experience match the problem.

If you visit a specialist, ask that the records of your diagnosis and treatment be sent to your primary care doctor, who needs to keep track of your overall health care. Ask for a copy of the records for yourself. Also, next time you visit your primary care doctor, be sure to give a report of what the specialist did for you.

Specialists

Here's a list of specialists you might need along with the systems, diseases, conditions or therapies that they can help you with:

Allergist, immunologist. Treats allergies and diseases of the immune system

Anesthesiologist. Administers and monitors anesthetics

Audiologist. Tests hearing and treats hearing disorders

Cardiologist. Treats disorders of the heart, blood vessels and circulation

Dermatologist. Treats skin diseases

Emergency medicine specialist. Evaluates and treats trauma, emergencies

Endocrinologist. Treats problems with the glands, including diabetes

Family physician. Treats all family members and conditions

Gastroenterologist. Treats digestive diseases

Geneticist. Specializes in inherited diseases

Gynecologist. Specializes in care of women

Hematologist. Treats diseases of the blood

Infectious diseases specialist. Treats infectious diseases, immunization

Internist. Involved in diagnosis and nonsurgical treatment of disease in adults

Neonatologist. Treats newborn babies

Nephrologist. Treats kidney problems

Neurologist. Specializes in nervous system disorders (brain, spinal cord, nerves)

Obstetrician. Specializes in pregnancy and delivery

Oncologist. Specializes in cancer

Ophthalmologist. Treats eye disorders

Orthopedist. Treats bone disorders and injuries with surgery

Otorhinolaryngologist. Treats ear, nose and throat disorders

Pathologist. Studies bodily fluids and tissues

Pediatrician. Provides preventive care to children and teens; treats diseases

Physiatrist. Treats disorders of the nervous and musculoskeletal systems

Preventive medicine specialist. Focuses on preventing disease and injury

Psychiatrist. Treats mental health conditions

Psychologist. Specializes in psychological assessment and counseling therapy

Pulmonologist. Treats respiratory disorders and also sleep disorders

Radiologist. Uses imaging techniques to diagnose and treat disease

Rheumatologist. Treats problems of the joints, muscles and connective tissue

Surgeon. Treats various conditions with surgery; many subspecialties

Urologist. Specializes in disorders of the urinary and urogenital tracts

Other health care providers

Nurse. If you're in the hospital, you'll probably see nurses more frequently than doctors because nurses provide most of the care. The nurses observe symptoms and listen to you describe them, help carry out the treatment plan and evaluate the results.

The initials *R.N.* after a nurse's name mean registered nurse. To be an R.N., a person must complete a bachelor's or an associate's degree in nursing or a similar program, and then pass a licensing examination. Some registered nurses have postgraduate degrees.

The initials *L.P.N.* mean licensed practical nurse. The L.P.N. course of study is shorter, and the L.P.N. generally works under the supervision of an R.N.

Some nurses specialize. They might focus on pediatrics or cardiology. Some not only specialize but also become a nurse practitioner (N.P.). A nurse practitioner usually has at least a master's degree and performs many of the same basic tasks as a doctor — examining and treating people as well as writing prescriptions.

Occupational therapist. If you're injured or disabled, an occupational therapist helps you regain your ability to carry out everyday tasks, such as the activities required to make a living. The word *occupational* is misleading because the therapy isn't aimed solely at helping you get back to work, but also at regaining the ability to do daily tasks wherever you are, at home or on the job: eating, dressing, bathing, homemaking and recreational skills. This therapist may recommend physical changes to your home or workplace — such as rearranging furniture or adding ramps and railings — to make it easier for you to get around and carry out your daily tasks.

Pharmacist. Your pharmacist is an excellent source of information about your medicine, whether it's prescription or nonprescription drugs. Since the pharmacist keeps a record of all prescriptions you buy at his or her pharmacy, it's helpful to use the same pharmacy for all your prescription drugs. This provides a double-check, to make sure you don't take a medication that reacts with something else you're taking. The pharmacist can also help you select nonprescription drugs that are best for you.

Physical therapist. Similar to an occupational therapist, a physical therapist also helps injured and disabled people regain lost physical functions, using techniques such as exercise, massage and ultrasound. The focus here is to maximize physical ability and compensate for physical functions that have been impaired or lost.

Physician assistant. Like a nurse practitioner, a physician assistant (P.A.) often works with a doctor by diagnosing and treating people with some of the more common health care problems. Most P.A.s have at least a bachelor's degree. They generally work under the supervision of a doctor, performing work assigned by the doctor. Working as part of the health care team, they take medical histories, treat minor injuries that may require stitches or casting, order and interpret lab tests and X-rays, and make diagnoses. In most states they can also write prescriptions.

In some clinics, most of the routine care is given by P.A.s. You may not see the doctor unless you have a major problem.

Selecting a surgeon

Your primary doctor can help you find a good surgeon should you ever need surgery. If you need a joint replacement, for example, you'll probably be referred to an orthopedic surgeon, who specializes in surgery involving joints, muscles and bones. When choosing a surgeon, try to select one who has performed many surgeries of the same type that you'll be having.

Given the potential risks and costs of many surgeries, it often makes good sense to get a second opinion. Either you or your primary doctor can make the decision to get that second opinion. So don't feel you need to be secretive about visiting a second surgeon. Keep your primary doctor informed.

Questions to ask before surgery

Whether your regular doctor or a surgeon recommends surgery, ask several questions:

Are there alternatives to surgery? Sometimes surgery is the only way to correct the problem. But one option might be watchful waiting, to see if the problem gets better or worse.

What is done during the surgery? Ask for a clear description of the surgery. Ask if there's a brochure with more details and pictures. Or consider asking the doctor to draw a picture to help explain exactly what the surgery involves.

How will surgery help? A hip replacement, for example, may mean you'll be able to walk comfortably again. To what extent will the surgery help, and how long will the benefits last? You'll want realistic expectations.

What are the risks? All surgeries carry some risk. Weigh the benefits against the risks. Ask also about the side effects of the surgery, such as the degree of pain you might expect and how long that pain might last.

What kind of experience have you had with this surgery? How many times has the doctor performed this surgery, and what percentage of the patients had successful results? To reduce your risks, you want a doctor who is thoroughly trained in the surgery and who has plenty of experience doing it.

Where will the surgery be done? Many surgeries today are done on an outpatient basis. You may go to a hospital or a clinic for the surgery and return home the same day.

Will I be put to sleep for the surgery? Your surgery may require only local anesthesia, which means that just part of your body is numbed for a short time. If you need general anesthesia, you're put to sleep.

How long will recovery take? You'll want to know when most people are able to resume their normal activities, such as doing chores around the house and returning to work. You may think there would be no harm in lifting a sack of groceries after a week or two. But there might be. Follow your doctor's advice as carefully as possible.

What will it cost me? Health insurance coverage varies. You may not have to pay anything. You might have a deductible to meet. Or you may have to pay a percentage of the cost. The doctor's office can usually give you information about this, but also check with your insurance company.

Find out if you're responsible for a flat copay — a set amount for the surgery — or if you have to pay a percentage of the bill. There's may be a big, and expensive, difference.

Home medical testing kits

Your pharmacy or drugstore has kits that can be used to perform medical tests at home, without the involvement of a physician or other health care provider.

Like most tests in a laboratory, home tests use urine, blood or stool. Some of them are relatively inexpensive and can be performed more than once.

Examples of kits

- **Pregnancy tests** to determine whether you're pregnant
- **Ovulation prediction tests** to help determine the best time for intercourse that may lead to conception
- **Blood sugar tests** to monitor how well your diabetes is controlled
- **Cholesterol tests** to determine your total cholesterol level
- **Urine tests**, such as for excess protein or diabetes-related toxic acids known as ketones
- **Tests to detect blood** in the stool, which may indicate a problem in the intestinal tract, such as a tumor in the colon
- **Human immunodeficiency virus (HIV) tests** to check for antibodies to HIV, the virus that causes AIDS

Disadvantages of home tests

- **There's the risk of simply doing the test wrong** and, therefore, getting a misleading result. You must follow the instructions exactly, or the test won't work properly. Professionals in a medical laboratory are less likely to make a mistake because they have more experience and better equipment.
- **Medical tests don't always work correctly.** This is true for tests done at home and for tests performed in a medical laboratory. A certain percentage of test results suggest that something is present when it's not (false-positive). For example, a false-positive test result would indicate that you're pregnant when you aren't.
- **False-negative results** can occur. A certain percentage of test results indicate that something isn't present when it is, which is called a false-negative. For example, a false-negative test result would indicate that your blood sugar concentration is normal when it is not. A doctor is in a better position to judge false-negative and false-positive test results on the basis of other medical evidence, training and experience.
- **You may interpret the result incorrectly.** Changes in the appearance of the test result, such as the color, may be confusing. And often you need to see your doctor or have the test repeated by a medical laboratory no matter what the result.
- **Indecision** is a factor. After performing the test, it's often difficult to decide what to do next. For example, if you're certain there is blood in your stool but the test indicates otherwise, should you still see your doctor? (In this example, yes, do not delay care.)

Caution

When used appropriately, many home test kits can be accurate, but use them carefully. They're not a substitute for appropriate medical care, especially when you think you may be at risk of a serious medical condition. Follow up on worrisome, unexpected test results with your health care provider.

Your family medical tree

Family gatherings are an ideal time to catch up on family news. They're also an opportunity to learn more about your family health history.

A small percentage of people with colon cancer have an inherited form. Children of alcoholics are much more likely to become addicted to alcohol or other drugs than children whose parents aren't alcoholics. A family history of high blood pressure, diabetes, some cancers and certain psychiatric disorders significantly increases all family members' odds of developing the condition.

If blood relatives have had a particular disease or condition, are you destined to get it? Usually not. But it may mean that you're at an increased risk.

Many major diseases have a hereditary component. Medical trees reveal patterns of inherited illness. With the information that a medical tree provides, your doctor may prescribe tests to determine if you have a particular condition, discuss the pros and cons of genetic testing (if it applies to your situation), or use the tree as a basis for recommending lifestyle changes to reduce your risk.

When you know that you're at increased risk of a disease, you may be able to take steps to prevent it — or at least detect it early, when the odds for a cure may be in your favor.

Creating a family medical tree

- **Learn who's who.** Research your parents, siblings and children. Then add information about grandparents, aunts, uncles, cousins, nieces and nephews. The more relatives you include, the better.
- **Dig for details.** Interview relatives by phone or email, or mail them questionnaires.
- **Look into the past.** Information about any condition — from allergies to difficulty walking — could prove helpful. Pay special attention to serious but potentially preventable conditions, such as cancer, high blood pressure, heart disease, diabetes, depression and alcoholism. Note the age of the relative when the condition was diagnosed. What kind of lifestyle did the person lead — for example, their tobacco use, activity level and diet?
- **Put it all together.** Organize your chart so that you can view the health histories of several relatives at once. Assign each medical condition a letter, and then write this letter next to the person's name or figure. Include the person's age at death.
- **Talk it over.** Ask your doctor to review your medical tree. The information it provides may suggest the need for additional or earlier screening tests.

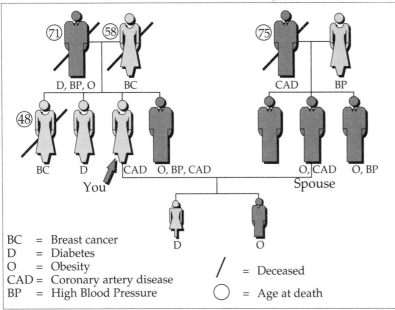

BC = Breast cancer
D = Diabetes
O = Obesity
CAD = Coronary artery disease
BP = High Blood Pressure

/ = Deceased
○ = Age at death

A family tree showing how you can chart a family medical history

Medications and you

Follow these important rules when taking medications:

- **Advise your health care provider about any over-the-counter products** you're taking, including laxatives or antacids; pain relievers; cough, cold or allergy medicines; weight-loss or weight-gain products; mineral and vitamin supplements; or herbal preparations. Nonprescription products can be potent, and some can cause serious reactions when mixed with prescription drugs.
- **Be informed.** Know what medications you take and why you're taking them.
- **Read labels and provided information carefully.** Ask your health care provider and pharmacist about potential side effects, about any dietary restrictions you should follow, whether you should avoid alcohol while taking the drug or about other concerns you have. If you get a prescription refilled and it appears different from what you had been taking, ask your pharmacist why.
- **Follow instructions.** Anyone who uses more than the recommended dosage is in danger of an overdose. The "more is better" theory doesn't apply to drugs.
- **Don't stop taking a prescribed drug** just because your symptoms seem to lessen. Take your medication for the entire length of time prescribed, even if symptoms have disappeared, unless instructed otherwise by your physician.
- **Keep a list** of what you take if you're taking several medications on a daily basis. Carry it in your purse or wallet. In addition, list allergies and drug intolerances.
- **Inform your health care provider of side effects.** Be alert to headaches, dizziness, blurred vision, ringing in your ears, shortness of breath, hives and other unexpected effects.
- **Inform your health care provider if you're pregnant, trying to become pregnant or are breast-feeding.** Some medications can be harmful to a fetus or may be excreted in breast milk, which could harm your baby.
- **Have prescriptions filled at one pharmacy.** Using one pharmacy can help you avoid problems with drug interactions. Your pharmacist can help monitor the mix of medications, even if they're prescribed by different doctors. Let your pharmacist know if you have any chronic conditions, to make sure your medications won't worsen your condition or become toxic in your body.
- **Properly store medications.** Most require a dry, secure place at room temperature and out of direct sunlight. Some drugs need refrigeration. A bathroom cabinet is a poor place to store medications because of temperature and moisture variations.
- **Discard outdated drugs.** Medicine deteriorates over time and can sometimes become toxic. Never take leftover medicine.
- **Be concerned for children.** Keep prescription and nonprescription drugs safely away from the reach of children. Buy child-resistant packages, especially if you have young children, grandchildren or very young guests.
- **Keep medicines in their original containers.** Prescription containers are designed to protect medications from light and provide vital information. If the label gets separated from a medicine container and there's any doubt as to its contents, discard the medicine immediately.
- **Don't lend or share prescription drugs.** What helps you might harm others.
- **Don't mix medications and alcohol.** The two can produce a harmful interaction.
- **Don't let cost discourage you.** If the cost of a drug is more than you can pay, ask your doctor or pharmacist if there's a less expensive alternative medication.

Healthy Consumer

Ordering medications on the internet

Ordering prescription drugs online can save you time and sometimes money. Many online pharmacies provide information about drug interactions. Some even email alerts when a drug is recalled or a generic equivalent becomes available.

But you must be careful. Questionable online pharmacies may ship expired drugs or those that haven't been stored properly. Others don't require a prescription or check for drug interactions. Some sites skirt the edge of legality and may even sell counterfeit products.

To safeguard your health and finances, here are some things to remember:

- **Consult your doctor.** Your doctor can determine if a particular drug is safe for you or if another treatment would be better. Make sure your doctor knows all the medications you're taking, including over-the-counter and prescription drugs.
- **Use a licensed pharmacy.** The National Association of Boards of Pharmacy can tell you whether a particular online pharmacy is licensed and in good standing. Some sites carry a seal of approval from Verified Internet Pharmacy Practice Sites (VIPPS). To gain this approval, sites must maintain state licenses and allow inspections by the National Association of Boards of Pharmacy.
- **Insist on access to a registered pharmacist.** Reputable sites offer toll-free access to registered pharmacists for help answering your medication questions. Some online pharmacies have traditional physical locations as well. If you have questions about a medication after you begin taking it or you're concerned about drug reactions, it may be especially valuable to speak with a pharmacist in person.
- **Read the privacy and security policies.** Before placing an order, be confident that your credit card number, personal health information and other personally identifiable information will be protected.
- **Compare prices.** You may find great deals online. But there aren't any guarantees. Your local drugstore might beat the online price.
- **Be cautious of sites based in foreign countries.** Legitimate international sites exist. But there are risks. The product label or instructions may be in a language you don't understand. The medication may not be held to rigorous safety standards. A medication sold in the United States may be a different product with the same name in another country. Some foreign sites sell drugs that are illegal in the U.S.
- **Avoid sites that bypass prescriptions.** Only your doctor can safely prescribe medication for you and safely monitor side effects.
- **Avoid sites that give risky prescriptions.** Avoid sites that allow you to consult with a doctor online who never met you, doesn't know your case or what other medications you're taking, but still writes you a prescription to be mailed to you.
- **Get an address and phone number.** Steer clear of sites that don't provide a street address and phone number or list only foreign information. An email address isn't enough.
- **Be wary of false claims.** Don't buy medication from sites that advertise "miracle cures" or that use impressive terminology to disguise a lack of good science.
- **Look for misspelled drug names.** Drug names that aren't spelled correctly are often a sign that a site isn't legitimate.
- **Report problems.** If your order doesn't arrive, you find unauthorized charges on your credit card or you have another problem with an online pharmacy, report it to the Food and Drug Administration. Speaking up can help promote a safer marketplace for everyone.

Pain relievers: Matching the pill to the pain

All nonprescription oral pain relievers contain one of these ingredients — salicylates (including aspirin), acetaminophen, ibuprofen or naproxen sodium. For pain relief, the differences among products are generally more subtle than significant.

Pain relievers are called analgesics (from the Greek words *an*, meaning "without," and *algos*, meaning "pain"). Over-the-counter (OTC) oral analgesics often relieve mild to moderate pain associated with headaches, colds, toothaches, muscle aches, backaches, arthritis and menstrual cramps. They also reduce fever. Common OTC analgesics (see page 258 for more details) include:

- **NSAIDs.** Ibuprofen and naproxen sodium reduce inflammation and are called nonsteroidal anti-inflammatory drugs (NSAIDs). They're most helpful for pain associated with conditions such as arthritis and tendinitis. Common side effects include stomach upsets, ulcers and bleeding.
- **Aspirin.** Although traditionally considered a type of NSAID, aspirin works differently from other NSAIDs. In addition to pain and inflammation relief, it can be used preventively to reduce stroke and heart attack risk.
- **Acetaminophen.** Acetaminophen doesn't relieve inflammation. Because it's relatively free of side effects at recommended doses, it may be an alternative for long-term use or when taking NSAIDs presents a risk.

All regular-strength doses of OTC pain relievers provide comparable relief for everyday pain such as headaches or sore muscles. For menstrual pain, ibuprofen and naproxen sodium may offer better relief.

Separating help from hype

OTC pain medications come in a great variety of forms. Sometimes a less expensive generic form is all you need. If you have questions, ask a pharmacist or your doctor.

Here's a guide for sorting through different forms of drug delivery:

- **Buffered.** A buffered analgesic contains an antacid to reduce acidity. It's controversial whether these products actually protect your stomach.
- **Enteric-coated.** A special coating allows pills to pass through your stomach and dissolve in the small intestine. This helps reduce stomach irritation. Consider an enteric-coated product if you need daily relief for chronic pain. Because the coating delays absorption, it's not the best choice for quick relief (such as for a headache).
- **Timed-release.** Also called extended-release and sustained-release, these products dissolve slowly. They prolong relief by maintaining a constant level of analgesic in your blood. Use them if you need lasting, not immediate, relief.
- **Extra-strength.** A single dose of these preparations contains more pain-relieving medicine than regular-strength products do — typically 500 milligrams (mg) of aspirin or acetaminophen vs. 325 mg. They're more convenient when it takes more than one regular-strength dose to improve your symptoms, but you should take them less often.
- **Combination formulas.** Some products are paired with caffeine or an antihistamine to boost their effect. Studies show that the addition of caffeine to aspirin or acetaminophen does improve pain relief.
- **Tablet, caplet, gelcap, gum or liquid.** If you have trouble swallowing a round tablet or oval caplet, a smooth gelcap might work better. Other options include taking aspirin in liquid or chewable form, as an effervescing pain reliever plus antacid (Alka-Seltzer), or chewing aspirin as a gum (Aspergum).
- **Generic.** Consider generic pain relievers, which typically cost less than brand-name drugs. Discuss medication effectiveness with your doctor and pharmacist.

Self-care

- **Know your special risks.** In general, don't take NSAIDs if you also take a blood thinner or if you have kidney disease, ulcers, a bleeding disorder or an allergy to aspirin. If you have high blood pressure, talk to your doctor before using NSAIDs on a regular basis because daily use could elevate blood pressure.
- **Avoid drug interactions.** If you take other OTC or prescription medications, talk with your doctor or pharmacist about which pain reliever is best.
- **Don't exceed the recommended dose,** unless your doctor advises it.
- **Avoid alcohol.** Mixing alcohol with aspirin, ibuprofen or naproxen sodium increases the chance of stomach upset and bleeding. In combination with higher than recommended doses of acetaminophen, alcohol increases the risk of serious damage to your liver.
- **Take NSAIDs with milk and food** to help minimize stomach upset.
- **Don't take longer than necessary.** Periodically re-evaluate your need for pain relievers.
- **Always read and follow label instructions.**

Over-the-counter oral pain relievers

	Aspirin	Acetaminophen	Ibuprofen	Naproxen sodium
Sampling of brand names	Bayer, Bufferin, Ecotrin	Tylenol	Advil, Motrin IB	Aleve
Reduces pain and fever	Yes	Yes	Yes	Yes
Reduces inflammation	Yes	No	Yes	Yes
Side effects	Stomach pain, heartburn, gastrointestinal (GI) bleeding	Rare when taken as directed for short periods (days to weeks)	Stomach pain, heartburn, GI bleeding, dizziness	Stomach pain, heartburn, GI bleeding, dizziness
Special cautions	Don't take if you have asthma, a bleeding disorder, gout, ulcers or allergy to aspirin.	Overdoses can be toxic to the liver. Alcohol enhances toxic effects of high doses.	Don't take if you have liver, heart or kidney disease, a bleeding disorder, or stomach problems.	Don't take if you have liver, heart, or kidney disease, a bleeding disorder, or stomach problems.
Children's use	Can cause Reye's syndrome* in children with chickenpox, the flu or other viral illness.	Available for children. Dosages based on age and weight. Consult your doctor.	Available for children. Dosages based on age and weight. Consult your doctor.	Don't give to children younger than 12 except on advice of a doctor.

*Reye's syndrome is a potentially fatal swelling of brain tissues.

Note: This list is not comprehensive and is not an endorsement. We rely on data available from the manufacturers.

Cold remedies: What they can and can't do

There's no cure for the common cold. Yet drugs used to treat the effects of the common cold — runny nose, fever, congestion and cough — are the largest segment of the over-the-counter market for America's pharmaceutical industry. Some of these medications are also formulated as allergy medicines to treat itchy eyes and sneezing.

Most people don't need any medication for a cold. However, if your cold is particularly bothersome, certain medications may help. Regarding a cough, guidelines developed by the American College of Chest Physicians state that nonprescription cough expectorants and suppressants often don't help relieve symptoms. If your cough is persistent, severe or accompanied by a fever, see your health care provider.

Over-the-counter cold remedies

	Antihistamines	Decongestants	Cough-cold combinations
Sampling of brand names	Benadryl Claritin Zyrtec	Afrin Neo-Synephrine Sudafed Sudafed PE	Actifed Children's Dimetapp Sudafed Cold & Cough
Symptoms relieved	Sneezing, runny nose, itchy eyes, congestion due to allergies	Congestion, stuffiness	Depends on ingredients: sneezing, runny nose, congestion, stuffiness, cough, general discomfort
Side effects and cautions	Drowsiness, dry mouth, may dry secretions, making mucus harder to clear. Alcohol may enhance drowsiness.	Insomnia, jitters, palpitations, may raise blood pressure. Don't use nasal decongestants more than three days.	May contain three or more ingredients. Side effects depend on ingredients.
Time of maximal benefit	Early in a cold when sneezing and watery, runny nose are common.	When nose is stuffed up.	When a variety of symptoms are prominent. For limited symptoms, consider using individual products.

Note: There are many different formulations of cold remedies. This list is not comprehensive and is not an endorsement. We rely on data available from the manufacturers.

Healthy Consumer

Here's some helpful advice on the use of cold medicines:

- **Always read the labels** to determine the active ingredients and side effects.
- **A single-symptom medication may be better** than a combination medication.
- **Most combination cold medications contain some form of analgesic,** such as aspirin, ibuprofen or acetaminophen (see page 258). Therefore, you don't need to take a separate analgesic.
- **Don't mix** various cold medications or take with other medications without consulting your health care provider or pharmacist.
- **Avoid alcohol** when taking cold medications.
- **Consult your physician** before giving any cold medicine to a child.
- **Decongestants should not be used in infants or young children.**
- **If you have high blood pressure, glaucoma or an enlarged prostate,** avoid cough and cold medications, unless directed by your health care provider. Some ingredients can make these conditions worse.

■ Home medical supplies

When an emergency or medical problem occurs in the home, you often don't have time to search for supplies. Keep your medical supplies in a place that's easily accessible to adults but out of the reach of children. Remember to replace items after their use to make sure the kit is always complete.

Here's what you need to be prepared for accidents and common illnesses. Check your supplies yearly for outdated items that may need replacing. Check expiration dates on medications twice yearly. Also make sure to include a first-aid manual.

- **For cuts.** Bandages of various sizes, gauze, paper or cloth tape, an antiseptic solution to clean wounds, and an antibacterial ointment to prevent infection.
- **For burns.** Cold packs, gauze, burn spray and an antiseptic cream.
- **For aches, pain and fever.** Thermometer, aspirin (for adults only) or a nonsteroidal anti-inflammatory drug, and acetaminophen for children or adults.
- **For eye injuries.** Sterile eyewash (such as a saline solution), an eyewash cup, eye patches and eye goggles.
- **For sprains, strains and fractures.** Cold packs, elastic wraps for wrapping injuries, finger splints and a triangular bandage for making an arm sling.
- **For insect bites and stings.** Cold packs to reduce pain and swelling. Hydrocortisone cream (0.5 or 1 percent), calamine lotion or baking soda (combine with water to form a paste) to apply to site until symptoms subside. Antihistamines (Benadryl, Zyrtec, others). If a family member is allergic to insect stings, include a kit containing an EpiPen — a syringe containing epinephrine (adrenaline). Your doctor can prescribe one. Check the expiration date regularly.
- **For ingestion of poisons.** Keep the Poison Help line — 800-222-1222 — on a sticker on your landline telephone and programmed into your cellphone.
- **For general care.** Sharp scissors, tweezers, cotton balls and cotton-tipped swabs, plastic bags, safety pins, tissues, soap, cleansing pads or instant hand sanitizer, latex or synthetic gloves for use if blood or body fluids are present, anti-diarrheal medication, and a medicine cup or spoon.

Dietary supplements

To stay healthy and help prevent disease, it's important to eat a balanced diet — one rich in fruits, vegetables and whole grains and low in saturated fat. But what about <u>dietary supplements</u> — pills, capsules and other products — that claim to fight off illness or improve disease symptoms? In some instances, supplements may be beneficial. In other cases, there's no clear proof that they are of any benefit.

Here's an overview of some of the more popular dietary supplements.

Antioxidants

Vitamins C and E and carotenoids, including beta carotene, are antioxidants. Antioxidants may help counter oxidation, a process that damages cells and can accelerate aging and lead to heart and blood vessel disease and cancer. It's better to get antioxidants from food rather than from supplements. Supplements touted to fight diseases of aging include:

- **Vitamin C.** Studies have shown that people whose diets are high in vitamin C, found mainly in citrus fruits, have lower rates of cancer and heart disease. But neither vitamin C nor vitamin E supplements reduce the risk of heart and blood vessel disease (see below).
- **Vitamin E.** One major report shows that neither vitamin E nor vitamin C supplements help decrease the risk of heart and blood vessel disease. Another study shows that taking megadoses of vitamin E may do more harm than good. Researchers reviewed 19 studies and found that people who took more than 400 international units (IU) of vitamin E daily died at a higher rate than those who didn't take the supplements. The cause isn't clear. Until more is known, don't take more than 400 IU of vitamin E daily. The best approach is to get the vitamin from dietary sources (nuts, vegetable oils, whole grains).
- **Carotenoids.** Several studies have found that supplements of beta carotene — which is converted into vitamin A in your body — offer no protection against heart and blood vessel disease. Two studies found an increased risk of lung cancer among smokers who took beta carotene supplements. Instead of taking supplements, you'll get more benefits by eating orange vegetables. You'll find other carotenoids in deep yellow, dark green, and red vegetables and fruits.

Other vitamins

- **Folic acid and B complex vitamins.** Studies show that raising homocysteine levels by giving supplements of vitamin B-12 and folic acid doesn't result in lower rates of heart and blood vessel disease. Instead of supplements, eat a healthy diet that includes at least five servings of fruits and vegetables daily. However, if you're of childbearing age and can become pregnant, ask your doctor about taking a multivitamin with folic acid to help prevent birth defects.
- **Vitamin D.** Vitamin D helps absorb calcium for stronger bones — this helps slow or prevent osteoporosis. Your body makes vitamin D from sunlight, but skin cancer is a risk. You can get vitamin D from food such as fatty fish (for example, herring, salmon and sardines), as well as vitamin D-fortified milk and other foods fortified with vitamin D. Because of sunscreen use (important in preventing skin cancer) and declining milk consumption, many people don't get enough vitamin D. Many experts feel that current vitamin D recommendations are too low. Ask your doctor how much vitamin D you need and whether you should take supplements.

Fish oil

The American Heart Association recommends eating fish (particularly fatty fish such as mackerel, lake trout, herring, sardines, albacore tuna and salmon) at least twice weekly. Young children and women still capable of having children should avoid fish with a high mercury content, such as shark, swordfish, king mackerel or tilefish. Fish oil supplements may be appropriate for people with heart and blood vessel disease. Ask your doctor how much to take. Make sure the supplements are high quality and free of contaminants.

Herbs

People take **herbal supplements** for a host of reasons. Here's a look at some of the most popular ones, what they claim to do and what research says about them.

- **Black cohosh.** While some studies suggest that black cohosh may help relieve hot flashes, headaches and other menopausal symptoms, other studies do not. Research is ongoing. For the most part, studies haven't found it to cause serious side effects. However, it's best not to take black cohosh for longer than six months.
- **Echinacea.** Derived from the purple coneflower, echinacea is typically used to prevent colds and flu. Despite all of the claims, the latest research suggests echinacea isn't an effective method for prevention or treatment of upper respiratory infections. While some studies have found modest benefits, echinacea hasn't been found to deliver significant decreases in the length or severity of colds. Some experts recommend limiting the use of echinacea to no more than eight weeks.
- **Ephedra (ma-huang).** Don't take this potent herb. Once found in a number of "natural" weight-loss and energy-boosting products, ephedra may increase your risk of a heart attack, seizure, stroke and sudden death. It's been taken off the market by the Food and Drug Administration (FDA).
- **Feverfew.** See "What the research shows," page 271.
- **Garlic.** While early research found small reductions in total blood cholesterol and in low-density lipoprotein (LDL), or "bad" cholesterol, from garlic use, more-recent studies have found garlic to be less effective. Some studies suggest that consuming garlic as a regular part of your diet may lower the risk of certain cancers, including stomach and colon cancers. Research also suggests that garlic may slow hardening of the arteries and reduce blood pressure in people with hypertension. However, bleeding has been associated with long-term garlic use, so caution is warranted for people taking anti-clotting medication.
- **Ginger.** Studies show that ginger may help ease nausea from pregnancy when used for short periods. However, results on the effectiveness of ginger in preventing or relieving nausea from chemotherapy and anesthesia have been inconsistent. Ginger is generally considered safe when taken in small amounts and for a short time. High doses can cause abdominal discomfort. Also, ginger may increase bleeding risk.
- **Ginkgo.** Studies have produced some encouraging results for the use of ginkgo as a treatment for certain circulation disorders and what are sometimes called cerebral insufficiencies — symptoms such as absent-mindedness and confusion — that may be associated with Alzheimer's disease. However, studies have found that ginkgo isn't an overall "brain booster," as once thought, and its effectiveness hasn't been proved. Don't take it during pregnancy or if you're taking anti-clotting medication such as warfarin (Coumadin, Jantoven).

- **Ginseng.** Studies report that ginseng may modestly improve mood, reaction times, and thinking, attention and learning performance in healthy middle-aged people. There is also some evidence that it may have a positive effect on cognitive performance in people with Alzheimer's disease. Some evidence suggests that ginseng may improve quality of life for those who have cancer. Don't use ginseng for more than six months or exceed the recommended dose, and avoid taking it if you're pregnant.
- **Kava.** Also called kava kava, this herb looked promising as a treatment for anxiety, insomnia and other problems. However, kava is linked to serious liver problems even with short-term use at a normal dose. It's banned in several countries.
- **St. John's wort.** Some studies suggest that St. John's wort may work as well as some antidepressant drugs for mild to moderate depression, and with fewer side effects. See "What the research shows," page 271.
- **Saw palmetto.** Some research indicates that saw palmetto may improve urine flow and bladder emptying in men with noncancerous enlargement of the prostate gland. See "What the research shows," page 271.

Hormones

Hormones are chemicals made by your body to regulate the activities of vital organs. Because hormone levels decline with age, some scientists speculate that hormones may play a role in the aging process. Proponents of hormone products tout that these products can set back your body's clock.

- **DHEA.** Dehydroepiandrosterone (DHEA) is converted by your body into estrogen and testosterone. Proponents of DHEA supplements claim the products slow aging, increase muscle and bone strength, burn fat, and improve cognition. There's no proof that the supplement does any of these. DHEA was banned in 1985 by the FDA, but it reappeared as an unregulated dietary supplement in 1994.
- **Melatonin.** This hormone helps improve your ability to fall asleep and sleep quality, and it may help overcome jet lag. But claims that it can slow or reverse aging, fight cancer and enhance sexuality are far from proved. Little is known of the long-term effects of melatonin. In general, treat it as you would any form of sleeping pill, and use it under your doctor's supervision.

Others

- **Coenzyme Q10.** Coenzyme Q10 (CoQ10) is an antioxidant normally produced by the body. CoQ10 has many dietary sources, including meat, fish and whole grains. Claims that the supplements can slow aging and stop cancer spread are not proved. However, CoQ10 may be beneficial for treating conditions such as congestive heart failure, high blood pressure and Parkinson's disease. It may also help prevent a condition that can arise from use of statin cholesterol medications (statin-induced myopathy).
- **Glucosamine and chondroitin.** Glucosamine is a natural compound in your body that helps make cartilage strong and rigid. Chondroitin is part of a large protein molecule that gives cartilage elasticity. Evidence conflicts, but some studies show that people with osteoarthritis pain experience less discomfort and improved joint function. Early research suggests that glucosamine may reduce rheumatoid arthritis-related pain when compared with a placebo. If you have an allergy to shellfish, you shouldn't take glucosamine. If you take blood thinners (anticoagulants), chondroitin may affect the levels.

- **SAMe.** S-adenosyl-L-methionine (SAMe) occurs naturally in all human tissue and organs. It helps produce and regulate hormones and cell membranes. Studies indicate that SAMe may relieve osteoarthritic pain in some people as well as nonsteroidal anti-inflammatory drugs (NSAIDs) can, but with fewer side effects. However, SAMe can negatively interact with antidepressant medications and shouldn't be taken if you're taking monoamine oxidase inhibitors (MAOIs). It may also worsen Parkinson's disease.

Whole foods are your best source

Benefits of whole foods

Whole foods — fruits, vegetables, grains, lean meats and dairy products — have three main benefits you can't find in a pill:

- **Whole foods are complex.** They contain a variety of the nutrients your body needs — not just one — giving you more bang for your nutrition buck. An orange, for example, provides vitamin C but also beta carotene, potassium and other nutrients. A vitamin C supplement lacks these other nutrients.
- **Whole foods provide dietary fiber.** Fiber can be found in plant-based foods such as fruits, vegetables, whole grains and beans. It's important for digestion, making you feel full and preventing certain diseases and conditions, including heart disease, diabetes and constipation.
- **Whole foods contain other substances that may be important for good health.** Fruits and vegetables, for example, contain naturally occurring food substances called phytochemicals, which may help protect you against cancer, heart disease, osteoporosis and diabetes. If you depend on supplements rather than eating a variety of whole foods, you miss the potential health benefits of phytochemicals.

The bottom line

Concentrate on getting your nutrients from food, not supplements, as much as possible. Whole foods provide an ideal mix of nutrients, fiber and other food substances. It's likely that all these work in combination to keep you healthy.

Should you take supplements?

The Academy of Nutrition and Dietetics and other major medical organizations all agree that the best way to get the vitamins and minerals you need is through a nutritionally balanced diet. But sometimes a supplement may be appropriate.

Talk with your physician about taking supplements. Sometimes too much of a vitamin, mineral or certain type of supplement can be harmful. A supplement may be appropriate if:

- **You're a female beyond menopause.** It can be difficult to get the recommended amounts of calcium and vitamin D without supplementation. Both calcium and vitamin D supplements have been shown to protect against osteoporosis. Vitamin D helps you absorb calcium. Even if you're a younger woman or you're a male, you may benefit from calcium and vitamin D supplementation.
- **You don't eat well.** If you don't eat the recommended five or more servings a day

of fruits and vegetables, taking a multivitamin supplement may be reasonable. Your best course of action would be to adopt better eating habits.

- **You're on a very low-calorie diet.** If you eat less than 1,200 calories a day, you may benefit from a vitamin-mineral supplement. Remember: A very low-calorie diet limits the types and amounts of foods you eat and, in turn, the types and amounts of nutrients you get. Very low-calorie diets should be undertaken only with guidance from your doctor.
- **You smoke.** Tobacco decreases absorption of many vitamins and minerals, including vitamin B-6, vitamin C, folic acid and niacin.
- **You drink alcohol excessively.** People who have alcoholism have impaired digestion and absorption of thiamin, folic acid and vitamins A, D and B-12. Altered metabolism also affects minerals such as zinc, selenium, magnesium and phosphorus. If you drink excessively, you may also substitute alcohol for food, resulting in a diet lacking in essential nutrients. Excessive drinking is defined as more than one drink a day for women of all ages and men older than age 65, and more than two drinks a day for men age 65 and younger.
- **You're pregnant or breast-feeding.** During these times, you need more of certain nutrients, especially folic acid and iron. Folic acid helps prevent neural tube defects in your baby, such as spina bifida. Iron helps prevent fatigue by helping you make the red blood cells you need to deliver oxygen to your baby. Your doctor can recommend a supplement — usually a prenatal vitamin. It's important to start taking a supplement before becoming pregnant.
- **You eat a special diet.** If your diet has limited variety because of a medical condition or personal preference, you may benefit from a vitamin-mineral supplement. In addition, if you are a vegetarian who does not eat any meat or dairy products, you may need to supplement your diet with calcium and vitamins B-12 and D. Ask your doctor or dietitian.
- **You're age 50 or older.** As you get older, health problems can contribute to a poor diet, making it difficult for you to get the vitamins and minerals you need. You may lose some of your ability to taste and smell. If you eat alone, you may not eat enough to get all the nutrients you need from food. In addition, as you get older, your body may not be able to absorb vitamins B-6, B-12 and D like it used to, making supplementation necessary.

■ Vitamins and minerals: How much do you need?

You may be confused about how much of a specific vitamin or mineral you need. Here's how to figure out what you need:

- **Dietary Reference Intakes (DRIs)** describe the average amount of each vitamin and mineral needed each day to meet the needs of nearly all healthy people. They're determined by the Food and Nutrition Board of the Institute of Medicine, part of the National Academy of Sciences. Recommendations for DRIs for some vitamins and minerals vary according to your sex or age, or both.
- **Daily Values (DV)** are used on food and supplement labels. They're set by the Food and Drug Administration (FDA). The FDA bases DVs on a 2,000-calorie-a-day diet. Of course, the 2,000-calorie-a-day standard is just a guideline. Individual needs may vary. Many women and older adults may actually need only about 1,600 calories a day. Active women and most men may need about 2,200 calories a day. Active men may need about 2,800 calories a day. If your

calorie needs are greater or less than 2,000 a day, your DVs for various nutrients generally rise or fall accordingly.

- **Percent Daily Value (%DV)** tells you what percentage of the DV one serving of a food or supplement supplies — that is, how it measures up as a percentage of the daily recommendation. For example, if the label on your multivitamin bottle says that your multivitamin provides 30 percent of the DV for vitamin E, you still need 70 percent to meet the recommended goal. The higher the %DV, the greater its contribution to meeting nutrient goals.

■ Choosing and using supplements

Supplements aren't substitutes. They can't replace the hundreds of nutrients in whole foods that you need for a nutritionally balanced diet. If you do decide to take a vitamin or mineral supplement, here are some factors to consider:

- **Avoid supplements that provide 'megadoses.'** In general, choose a multivitamin-mineral supplement that provides about 100 percent DV of all the vitamins and minerals instead of one that supplies, for example, 500 percent DV of one vitamin and only 20 percent DV of another. Doses above 100 percent DV don't give extra protection in most cases, but they do increase your risk of toxic side effects. Most cases of nutrient toxicity stem from high-dose supplements. Certain conditions may be treated with large doses, such as high cholesterol, which is sometimes treated with large doses of niacin, but such treatment is not common. For calcium, you may need to take several tablets to reach recommended levels. If one tablet contained 100 percent of the DV, it would be too large to swallow.
- **Consider buying generic.** Generic brands are generally less expensive and equally as effective as name brands, but ask your pharmacist or doctor to be sure. Compare the list of ingredients and the %DV among products.
- **Look for a 'USP,' 'NSF' or 'CL' symbol on the label.** This ensures that the supplement meets the standards for strength, purity and disintegration established by the testing organizations U.S. Pharmacopeia (USP), NSF International and Consumer Lab.
- **Beware of gimmicks.** Synthetic vitamins are the same as so-called natural vitamins. Don't give in to the temptation of added herbs, enzymes or amino acids — they add nothing but cost.
- **Look for expiration dates.** Supplements can lose potency over time, especially in hot and humid climates. If a supplement doesn't have an expiration date, don't buy it.
- **Store all vitamin and mineral supplements out of the sight and reach of children.** Put them in a locked cabinet or other secured location. Don't leave them sitting out on the counter or rely on child-resistant packaging. Be especially careful with any supplements containing iron. Iron overdose is a leading cause of poisoning deaths among children.
- **Explore your options.** If you have difficulty swallowing, ask your doctor whether liquid or children's chewable vitamin and mineral supplements might be right for you.
- **Play it safe.** Before taking anything other than a standard multivitamin-mineral supplement of 100 percent DV or less, check with your doctor or a registered dietitian. This is especially important if you have a health problem or are taking

medication. High doses of niacin, for example, can aggravate a stomach ulcer. In addition, supplements may interfere with medications. Vitamin E, for example, isn't recommended if you're taking blood-thinning medications because it can complicate blood thinning. If you're already taking an individual vitamin or mineral supplement and haven't told your doctor, discuss it at your next checkup.

Supplements and digestive health problems: What you need to know

If you have a digestive health problem, such as a disease of your liver, gallbladder, intestine or pancreas, or you've had surgery on your digestive tract, you may not be able to digest and absorb nutrients properly. Your doctor may recommend a vitamin or mineral supplement. Some conditions that may require you to take supplements include:

- **Crohn's disease.** A chronic inflammation of the intestine. It commonly involves the lower part of the small intestine (ileum). It can also affect your colon or any other part of your digestive tract. Your ability to absorb nutrients often is limited with **Crohn's disease**, particularly if the disease affects large portions of your small intestine or if you've had portions of your small intestine removed surgically. If you have Crohn's disease, doctors often advise that you take a standard multivitamin that provides 100 percent DV. Your doctor may also advise specific replacement of certain vitamins or minerals, if there's deficiency. If you have Crohn's disease, you may not be able to absorb vitamin B-12. Left untreated, a deficiency of this vitamin can lead to anemia, nerve disease and other problems. If this occurs, you can get the vitamin B-12 you need with monthly injections.
- **Primary biliary cirrhosis.** A condition characterized by chronic inflammation and scarring of the microscopic bile ducts within the liver. This inflammation and scarring can cause bile flow to become blocked, which can interfere with absorption of fat-soluble vitamins (A, D, E and K). If you have **primary biliary cirrhosis**, your doctor may prescribe supplements for these vitamins in a special form that's easier to absorb.
- **Pancreatitis.** An inflammation of the pancreas, which can be short term (acute) or long term (chronic). In chronic **pancreatitis**, your pan-

creas gradually becomes less able to secrete the enzymes you need to properly digest dietary fats. This also affects your ability to absorb fat-soluble vitamins. If you have chronic pancreatitis, your doctor may prescribe pancreatic enzyme supplements to help improve digestion and absorption. In addition, a multivitamin or specific vitamins or mineral supplements may be recommended, if there's evidence of deficiency.

- **Gastric bypass surgery.** Weight-loss surgery that limits your ability to absorb calories. **Gastric bypass** also limits the amount of nutrients you can absorb. Your doctor may recommend that you take calcium supplements, vitamin D, vitamin B-12 shots and at least one and often two multivitamins. If you're a premenopausal woman or develop iron deficiency, you may also be advised to take additional iron.
- **Gastroparesis.** A condition in which stomach muscles don't function normally. **Gastroparesis** can interfere with digestion, cause nausea and vomiting, interfere with blood sugar levels, and cause a deficiency in vitamin B-12, iron, calcium and other nutrients. Treatment typically includes dietary changes and medications. A liquid vitamin and mineral supplement can help supply missing nutrients, but shouldn't be used as a substitute for meals.
- **Intestinal pseudo-obstruction.** A rare condition with symptoms like those caused by a bowel blockage (such as cramps, pain, vomiting, bloating), but no blockage is found. Symptoms are caused by nerve or muscle problems that affect the movement of food and fluid through the intestines. Treatment depends on the type and severity of the problem and may involve nutritional support, medications, surgery or other procedures.

Healthy Consumer

Integrative medicine

Start sneezing and before you know it, your friends are suggesting you try this or that herb or homeopathic remedy. You wonder if you should follow their advice. You've heard about **integrative medicine** — sometimes called complementary and alternative medicine (CAM) — but you don't know that much about it. Before you decide, get the facts. Make sure to talk with your doctor before you try something new — especially if you are pregnant or breast-feeding, take medications, or have chronic health problems.

What is integrative medicine?

Most of what we call integrative or complementary treatments aren't new. Many have been practiced for thousands of years. They include a broad range of healing philosophies, approaches and therapies, including meditation, massage, acupuncture, and the use of herbs and dietary supplements. Often, though not always, the practices are used in conjunction with traditional medical treatment.

The term *alternative medicine* refers to practices not typically used in conventional Western medicine. Exactly what's considered alternative medicine changes constantly as more treatments are studied and move into the mainstream. When an alternative medicine therapy is used in addition to — not instead of — conventional therapy, it's called *complementary medicine*. By definition, *integrative medicine* is the practice of using conventional medicine alongside evidence-based complementary treatments.

The promise — and peril — of new treatment options

You have many treatment options — conventional, complementary, alternative and integrative — available to you. But you also face greater risk of confusion and harm.

You can't always accept the claims of complementary or alternative medicine practitioners at face value. True, the vast majority of these practitioners are well-intentioned, and many have specialized training. Yet quack treatments have always existed, and some unscrupulous people may falsely claim to be experts in complementary or alternative medicine. Even practitioners with the best of intentions may be undertrained, uninformed or both.

Arm yourself with two strategies

If you decide to use integrative treatments, take steps to protect your health, and your wallet. When deciding on any unconventional treatment — or conventional, for that matter — consider its safety and effectiveness. Safety means its benefits outweigh its risks. Effectiveness is the likelihood the treatment will be of benefit when used appropriately.

Research various treatments. Learn about the major forms of integrative medicine. Find out what they are and what benefits they may provide.

- Natural products — including herbs, vitamins, minerals and probiotics
- Mind-body medicine — including yoga, chiropractic and osteopathic manipulation, meditation, massage therapy, acupuncture, relaxation techniques and others
- Other complementary health approaches — including ayurvedic medicine, homeopathy and naturopathy

Take responsibility for your own care. See "5 steps in considering any treatment," pages 278-279.

See back cover for online resource ⓘ

Check out claims of treatment success

Ask your doctor for information on research results to help you make an informed decision about using a particular treatment. You can also find information on your own, but it's important to understand the quality of research. If you dig into the medical literature for studies about integrative treatments, you'll see several terms that describe different types of research. For example:

- *Clinical studies* are those that involve human beings as subjects — not animals. They're usually preceded by studies that demonstrate safety and effectiveness of the treatment in animals.
- In *randomized, controlled trials*, participants are usually divided into two groups. The first group receives the treatment under investigation. The second is a control group — they receive standard treatment, no treatment or an inactive substance called a placebo. Participants are assigned to these groups on a random basis. This helps to ensure that the groups will be similar.
- In *double-blind studies*, neither the researchers nor the human subjects know who will receive the active treatment and who will receive the placebo.
- *Prospective studies* are forward-looking. Researchers establish criteria for study participants to follow and then measure or describe the results. Information from these studies is usually more reliable than that of retrospective studies. Retrospective studies involve looking at past data (for example, asking participants to recall information), which leaves more room for errors in interpretation.
- *Peer-reviewed journals* only publish articles that have been reviewed by an independent panel of medical experts.

Identify the best research

Prospective double-blind studies that have been carefully controlled, randomized and published in scientific (peer-reviewed) journals provide the best information. When these involve large numbers of people (several hundred or more) studied over several years, they gain even more credibility. Doctors also like to see studies that are replicated — repeated by different investigators with generally the same results.

To date, few integrative treatments have been researched according to rigorous standards. For the majority of unconventional treatments, the jury is still out on whether they're helpful.

Most commonly used integrative therapies

More than 1 in 3 U.S. adults report using integrative therapies.

10 most common therapies

1. Nonvitamin, nonmineral dietary supplements
2. Deep-breathing exercises
3. Yoga, tai chi or qi gong
4. Chiropractic or osteopathic manipulation
5. Meditation
6. Massage
7. Special diets
8. Homeopathy
9. Progressive relaxation
10. Guided imagery

Source: Clark TC, et al. Trends in the use of complementary health approaches among adults: United States, 2002-2012. National health statistics reports; No. 79. Hyattsville, Md: National Center for Health Statistics. 2015.

Natural products

Although popularly thought of as "natural" and less risky than prescription drugs, herbal supplements aren't subject to the same rigorous quality control as drugs. There has been careful study of some of these treatments, but it's a good idea to be cautious when considering a supplement.

Limited FDA regulation

Herbs, vitamins and minerals are all considered dietary supplements by the Food and Drug Administration (FDA). These substances aren't considered either a food or a drug, and as such, aren't subject to usual regulatory and safety guidelines.

Manufacturers don't have to seek FDA approval before putting dietary supplements on the market. In addition, companies can claim that products address a nutrient deficiency, support health or are linked to body functions — if they have supporting research and they include a disclaimer that the FDA hasn't evaluated the claim.

However, manufacturers must follow good manufacturing practices to ensure that supplements are processed consistently and meet quality standards. These regulations are intended to keep the wrong ingredients and contaminants out of supplements, as well as make sure that the right ingredients are included in appropriate amounts.

Once a dietary supplement is on the market, the FDA is responsible for monitoring its safety. If the FDA finds a product to be unsafe, it can take action against the manufacturer or distributor or both, and may issue a warning or require that the product be removed from the market.

Regulations provide assurance that herbal supplements meet certain quality standards and that the FDA can intervene to remove dangerous products from the market. The rules do not, however, guarantee that herbal supplements are safe for anyone to use.

Use herbs safely

If you're considering taking an herbal treatment, keep these points in mind:

- **Discuss with your doctor what you're taking.** Some herbs may interfere with the effectiveness of prescription or nonprescription drugs or have other harmful effects. (See "Choosing and using supplements," pages 266-267.) Make sure you don't have an underlying medical condition that calls for treatment by your doctor.
- **Follow directions.** Like over-the-counter (OTC) and prescription drugs, herbal products have active ingredients that can affect how your body functions. Don't exceed the recommended dosages. Some herbs can be harmful if taken for too long. Get advice from your doctor and other reputable resources.
- **Keep track of what you take.** Take one type of supplement at a time to try to determine its effect. Make a note of what you take, how much and how it affects you. Does it do what it claims to do? Do you experience any side effects, such as drowsiness, sleeplessness, headache or nausea?
- **Read the label for content.** Quality and strength can vary greatly by brand. Look for third-party verification of the quality of the product (for example, United States Pharmacopeia Verified, or USP Verified), which indicates the supplements meet certain standards of quality.
- **Avoid herbs if you're pregnant or breast-feeding.** Unless your doctor approves, don't take any medications — prescription, OTC or herbal — when you're pregnant or breast-feeding. They can harm your baby.

- **Be cautious about herbal products manufactured or purchased outside the United States.** In general, European herbs are well-regulated and standardized. Toxic ingredients (including lead, mercury and arsenic) and prescription drugs (such as prednisone) have been found in some herbal supplements manufactured in other countries, particularly China and India.
- **Avoid dangerous herbs.** According to the FDA, these include belladonna, broom, coltsfoot, comfrey, liferoot, lobelia and pennyroyal. Goldenseal and licorice root are other controversial herbs that can cause serious health problems.

Ephedra has been banned by the FDA (see page 262) and another popular herb, called kava, reportedly has been associated with liver damage in some people (see page 263). There may be other harmful herbs. Overdoses of any of these herbs can be fatal.

The effectiveness of many herbs still hasn't been established. Few studies have investigated the risks of taking several different herbs at the same time. Of all the unconventional treatments, herbal therapies may present the greatest potential for harm. This is especially true when people self-prescribe herbs, or products are mislabeled or contaminated.

What the research shows

If you're thinking about using **herbal supplements**, read information on clinical studies about safety and effectiveness. From the examples below, you'll see why it's important to tell your doctor if you're using herbal products so that you can work out an effective treatment plan.

- Although studies conflict, overall evidence indicates that **St. John's wort** is useful for mild to moderate depression and produces results similar to some prescription antidepressants. However, if your depression is serious, don't treat it yourself. St. John's wort also appears to cause fewer side effects than older antidepressants, and it may cause slightly fewer side effects than newer antidepressants.

  A concern is that the herb can dangerously alter the effects of a number of prescription drugs. Until more is known, don't mix St. John's wort with any medication without discussing it in advance with your doctor.

- Some studies (but not all) have shown that the herb **saw palmetto** improves urinary symptoms such as poor urine flow, inflammation and frequent nighttime urination in men with noncancerous enlargement of the prostate gland (benign prostatic hyperplasia, or BPH). Saw palmetto does not appear to interfere with the results of the prostate-specific antigen (PSA) test, a tool that helps detect prostate cancer. However, if you take saw palmetto, mention it to your doctor before the test.

- Research suggests that taking an oral **feverfew** supplement can help prevent migraines by reducing inflammation and preventing the blood vessels from constricting, both of which can lead to headaches. However, more and better quality studies are needed to confirm effectiveness and safety. Feverfew should not be taken during pregnancy.

Healthy Consumer

■ Mind-body medicine

These treatments are based on the idea that mind and body function as a unified field. With some, such as biofeedback or hypnosis, practitioners may hold that negative thoughts and feelings can produce symptoms in your body. Treatment often aims to help you detach from these thoughts and feelings, or to actively change them.

Some other types of mind-body practices involve human touch. Examples are chiropractic treatment, osteopathy, massage, therapeutic touch and acupuncture.

Biofeedback

This practice uses technology to teach you how to control certain body responses. During a biofeedback session, a trained therapist applies electrodes and other sensors to various parts of your body. The electrodes are attached to devices that monitor your responses and give you visual or auditory feedback. For example, you might see patterns on a monitor that display your levels of muscle tension, brain wave activity, heart rate, blood pressure, breathing rate or skin temperature.

With this feedback, you can learn how to produce positive changes in body functions, such as lowering your blood pressure or raising your skin temperature. These are signs of relaxation. The biofeedback therapist may use relaxation techniques to further calm you, reducing muscle tension or slowing your heart rate and breathing even more.

You can get biofeedback treatments in several settings — physical therapy clinics, medical centers and hospitals. Increasingly, biofeedback programs are available for home use using sensors and a home computer.

Hypnotherapy

Hypnotherapy produces a state of deep relaxation, but your mind stays alert. During hypnosis, you can receive suggestions designed to decrease your perception of pain or to help you stop habits such as smoking. No one knows exactly how hypnotherapy works, but experts believe it alters your brain wave patterns in much the same way as other relaxation techniques.

The success of hypnotherapy depends on the expertise of the practitioner, your understanding of the procedure and your willingness to try it. You need to be strongly motivated to change. Some people eventually develop the skills to hypnotize themselves.

Psychiatrists and psychologists occasionally practice hypnotherapy. There are also professional hypnotists, but beware, because this field is poorly regulated.

Yoga

People do yoga for many reasons. For some, yoga is a spiritual path. For others, yoga is a way to promote physical flexibility, strength and endurance. In either case, you may find that yoga helps you to relax and manage stress.

Americans generally associate the term *yoga* with one particular school of this ancient discipline — hatha yoga. In most cases, hatha yoga combines gentle breathing exercises with movement through a series of postures called asanas.

Yoga teachers commonly offer instruction in meditation. According to an ancient yoga text, the purpose of yoga is to calm the mind in preparation for meditation.

One principle of meditation is that stress comes with a racing mind. Meditators observe the flow of thoughts without judging them, a process that helps the mind to slow down naturally.

Tai chi

One sophisticated and enjoyable method to improve physical and emotional balance is an ancient form of exercise called tai chi (TIE-CHEE). Originally developed in China, tai chi involves slow, gentle, dance-like movements that relax and strengthen muscles and joints. Many people who practice tai chi view it as a form of meditation in motion.

What the research shows

Biofeedback. People with arthritis who underwent biofeedback reported feeling less intense pain when their treatment was combined with cognitive behavioral therapy. Some research shows that biofeedback can be as effective as medication in preventing headaches and that it can help improve headache symptoms.

Studies indicate it may also improve symptoms of asthma, irritable bowel syndrome, chemotherapy-related nausea and vomiting, chronic pain, anxiety, stress, and high blood pressure, among others.

Hypnotherapy. Hypnotherapy may offer relief to those experiencing pain associated with a number of disorders, including cancer, irritable bowel syndrome and fibromyalgia. It may help relieve symptoms of hot flashes associated with menopause. In addition, hypnotherapy has been used with some success in treating insomnia, bed-wetting, smoking, obesity and phobias.

A few studies have evaluated weight-loss hypnotherapy. Most studies show only slight weight loss, with an average loss of about 6 pounds. But the quality of some of these studies has been questioned.

Yoga. Yoga can help you improve your balance, flexibility, range of motion and strength. As with other types of physical activity, yoga can help reduce your risk of chronic diseases, such as heart disease and high blood pressure. It can also help you manage chronic conditions such as depression, pain, anxiety and insomnia.

In one study of overweight adults who were getting little or no physical activity, researchers found that yoga was a "stepping stone" toward regular exercise, helping people stick to a regular physical activity program.

You'll find tai chi classes offered in cities throughout the United States. To locate a class in your community, contact your local YMCA, YWCA, fitness club or senior center.

Research indicates that tai chi can prevent falls in older adults by improving strength and balance. In one large study, those who practiced tai chi reduced their risk of multiple falls by about 47 percent.

Chiropractic treatment

Chiropractic care is based on the idea that your body's structure — nerves, bones, joints and muscles — and its capacity for healthy function are closely intertwined. Most chiropractors use a hands-on type of adjustment called spinal manipulative therapy or spinal manipulation. According to chiropractic theory, misaligned vertebrae can restrict your spine's range of motion and affect nerves that radiate out from your spine. In turn, the organs that depend on those nerves may function improperly or become diseased. Chiropractic adjustments aim to realign your vertebrae, restore range of motion and free up nerve pathways.

People other than chiropractors do spinal manipulation. Many osteopathic doctors and physical therapists are trained in this treatment. The scientific evidence clearly supports chiropractic treatment for musculoskeletal conditions, particularly for neck and back pain. Some chiropractors hold tightly to the theory that spinal manipulation can cure whatever ails you, but no scientific evidence supports this.

Although they can't prescribe drugs or perform surgery, chiropractors use many standard medical procedures. And the services of chiropractors are increasingly covered by medical insurance.

Osteopathic manipulation

Osteopathy is a recognized medical discipline that has much in common with conventional medicine and chiropractic treatment. Like traditional physicians, doctors of osteopathy go through long training in academic and clinical settings. Osteopaths are licensed to perform many of the same therapies and procedures as traditional doctors. They can perform surgery and prescribe medications. Osteopaths may also specialize in various areas of medicine, such as gynecology or cardiology.

Osteopathy does differ from conventional medicine in one area: manipulation to address joint and spinal problems. Similar in this respect to a chiropractor, an osteopath may perform manipulations to release pressure in your joints, align your muscles and joints, and improve the flow of body fluids.

5 tips if you seek chiropractic care

To get the most out of chiropractic care or other treatments that rely on spinal manipulation, here are some tips:
1. Ask your primary doctor to refer you to an appropriate provider. This could be a chiropractor or an osteopath, a doctor specifically trained in manipulation to treat joint and spinal problems.
2. If you seek chiropractic care without a referral, do so carefully. Find someone who's licensed and who completed the training program at a school accredited by the Council on Chiropractic Education.
3. See chiropractors who are willing to send a report to your doctor and give you a written treatment plan.
4. Avoid chiropractors who order frequent X-rays or ask to extend your treatment indefinitely.
5. Avoid chiropractors who view spinal manipulation as a cure for "whatever ails you." There's no evidence to support this idea.

Massage

Massage is often used as part of physical therapy, sports medicine and nursing care. It may be used, for example, to relieve muscle tension or promote relaxation, helping people as they undergo other types of medical treatment. It's also accepted as a simple means for healthy people to relieve stress and just feel good.

Massage is the kneading, stroking and manipulation of your body's soft tissues — your skin, muscles and tendons. Your massage will vary depending on the rhythm, rate, pressure and direction of these movements.

You shouldn't get massage over an open wound, skin infection, phlebitis or areas of weakened bones. If you've been injured, consult your doctor first. Don't rely exclusively on massage to repair damaged tissues.

Generally, a massage should feel good or cause very little discomfort. If this isn't the case, speak up promptly.

Therapeutic touch

Therapeutic touch resembles the religious concept of "laying on of the hands," where healing power is believed to flow from a minister's hands to a person. However, therapeutic touch is not necessarily based on a religious concept. Instead, it comes from the idea that your body is surrounded by a field of energy. Illness results from disturbances in that field.

Some practitioners of therapeutic touch attempt to get rid of these disturbances by moving their hands back and forth across your body. Practitioners believe that by transferring healing energy through their hands to your body, they can reduce pain, stress and anxiety. Many conventional health care providers are skeptical of therapeutic touch, which isn't supported by solid research.

Acupuncture

Acupuncture is a part of Chinese traditional medicine that has been around for at least 2,500 years. According to this Eastern philosophy:

- Health depends on the free circulation of blood and a subtle energy called chi (pronounced "chee" and sometimes written *qi*).
- Chi flows through your body along pathways called meridians.
- Inserting needles into points along the meridians promotes the free flow of chi.

Medical researchers are skeptical about these claims. Even so, acupuncture is one of the most well-researched and accepted practices in integrative medicine. Pain specialists at Mayo Clinic have used acupuncture since 1974 as part of their pain treatment program.

Depending on your reasons for seeking acupuncture, you'll have one or several hair-thin needles inserted under your skin. Some may go in as deep as 3 inches, depending on where they're placed in your body and what the treatment is for. Others will be placed superficially. The needles usually are left in for 15 to 30 minutes. Once inserted, needles are sometimes stimulated with an electrical current.

Expect to have several sessions. If you experience no relief after six to eight sessions, acupuncture probably isn't for you.

To find a qualified practitioner, ask for a referral from your doctor or contact the American Academy of Medical Acupuncture (AAMA). Visit the AAMA website at *www.medicalacupuncture.org*. AAMA's members are all licensed physicians with more than 200 hours of training in acupuncture.

■ Other approaches

Homeopathy

Homeopathy (hoe-me-OP-uh-thee) is a controversial treatment. It's based on two basic beliefs:

- *The law of similars.* When given to a healthy person in large quantities, some plant, animal and mineral substances produce symptoms of disease. But when given to a sick person, much smaller doses of the same substances can (theoretically) relieve the same symptoms.
- *The law of infinitesimals.* Literally, infinitesimal means too small to be measured. According to this belief, substances treat disease most effectively when they are highly diluted, often in distilled water or alcohol.

The law of similars is sometimes stated as "like cures like" — a capsule summary of homeopathy. Vaccination, a conventional practice, is based on a similar idea: Injecting a small dose of a modified infectious agent stimulates the body's immune system to fight diseases caused by that agent.

Homeopathy in general departs widely from conventional medicine. Modern drug therapy primarily uses substances to reverse symptoms, not produce them. In addition, medical doctors find it difficult to accept the law of infinitesimals — especially when many homeopathic treatments are so diluted that no trace of the original substance remains. Although highly diluted substances may not help you, they probably won't harm you either.

People who practice homeopathy (homeopaths) may also recommend changes in diet, exercise and other health-related behaviors. But avoid practitioners who encourage you to use homeopathic remedies instead of the medications that your doctor prescribed.

Many studies of homeopathy examine whether the benefits claimed for this treatment result from a placebo effect — that is, from the belief of people in the treatment rather than the treatment itself. One analysis of 89 controlled studies concluded that homeopathy appeared to have results that went beyond the placebo effect. However, there's little published evidence that homeopathy can effectively treat specific diseases or conditions.

Ayurveda

One of the oldest systems of health care comes from Hindu medicine practiced in India since ancient times. It's called ayurveda (i-YUR-ved-uh), a Sanskrit word that means "the science of life."

Ayurveda begins with the premise that people differ both physically and psychologically. So treatments take these differences into account.

According to ayurvedic practitioners, there are three main types of energy (doshas) that create differences between people and govern health:

- Vata is the energy of movement. People dominated by vata are alert, creative and physically active.
- Pitta is the energy of digestion and metabolism. People with this primary dosha have larger appetites, warmer bodies and more stable temperaments than vata-dominated people.
- Kapha is the energy of lubrication. People dominated by kapha generally have oily skin. They easily gain weight and tend to be less physically active. In addition, kapha types are usually calm, patient and forgiving.

It's believed that one of these energies can go to extremes, creating a lack of balance. For example, kapha types can become lethargic. Treatment in this case might include recommendations to exercise regularly, avoid naps and stay away from fatty, oily foods.

Naturopathy

Based on their belief in the healing power of nature, early naturopaths prescribed hydrotherapy — literally, water treatment — to treat illness. They recommended soaks in hot springs, walking barefoot on grass or through cold streams, and other water-related treatments.

Today, naturopaths employ a combination of therapies, including nutrition, herbs, acupuncture and massage. They also use techniques from homeopathy, ayurveda, Chinese medicine and conventional treatments. The main emphasis of naturopathy is on prevention of illness through a healthy lifestyle, including fresh air, clean water and exercise.

■ 5 steps in considering any treatment

1. Gather information about the treatment

The internet offers a good way to keep up with the latest on integrative treatments. Begin with websites created by national organizations, government agencies, major medical centers or universities. U.S. government websites that provide information on integrative medicine include:

National Center for Complementary and Integrative Health
https://nccih.nih.gov

Office of Dietary Supplements
https://ods.od.nih.gov

National Institutes of Health
www.nih.gov

Department of Health and Human Services
https://healthfinder.gov

For the latest health information from **Mayo Clinic,** visit:
www.MayoClinic.org

Steer clear of misinformation on the internet — Apply the three D's

You can find thousands of websites devoted to health. But, be careful. The material you'll find ranges from solid research to outright quackery.

Remember to look for these three features:

- *Dates.* Search for the most recent information you can find. Reputable websites include a date for each article they post.
- *Documentation.* Check for the source of information and whether articles refer to published medical research. Look for a board of qualified professionals who review content before it's published. Be wary of commercial sites or personal testimonials that push a single point of view or sell miracle cures.
- *Double-checking.* Visit several health sites and compare the information they offer. And before you follow any medical advice, ask your doctor for guidance.

Some websites post a logo from the Health on the Net (HON) Foundation. Sites that display this logo have agreed to abide by the HON Code of Conduct.

---

2. Find and evaluate treatment providers

After gathering information about a treatment, you may decide to find a practitioner who offers it. Choosing a name from a browser search or the classified section of the phone book is risky if you have no other information about the provider. Check your state government listings for agencies that regulate and license health care providers. These agencies may list names of practitioners in your area and offer a way to check credentials.

Talk to people who've received the treatment you're considering and ask about their experience with specific providers. Start by asking friends and family members.

There are risks and side effects with many types of treatment, both conventional and unconventional. With any treatment you consider, find out if the benefits outweigh the risks.

3. Consider treatment cost

Many integrative approaches are not covered by health insurance. Find out exactly how much the treatment will cost you.

4. Check your attitude

When it comes to integrative medicine, steer a middle course between uncritical acceptance and outright rejection. Learn to be both open-minded and skeptical at the same time. Stay open to various treatments but evaluate them carefully. Also remember that the field is changing: What's alternative today may be well-accepted — or discredited — tomorrow.

5. Opt for integrative over alternative medicine

Research indicates that the most popular use of unconventional medical treatments is to *integrate with* rather than *replace* conventional medical care. Ideally, the various forms of treatment should work together.

You can use integrative treatments to maintain good health and to relieve some symptoms. But continue to rely on conventional medicine to diagnose a problem and treat the sources of disease. And tell your medical doctor about all the treatments you get — both conventional and unconventional.

Be sure to seek conventional treatment if you have a sudden, severe or life-threatening health problem. If you break a bone, get injured in a car accident or develop food poisoning, then make the emergency room your first stop.

Also, remember that your lifestyle choices make a difference. Most practitioners — conventional and integrative — will tell you that nutrition, exercise, not smoking, stress management and safety practices are your keys to a longer life and better health.

Too good to be true — Signs of medical fraud

The Food and Drug Administration (FDA) recommends that you watch for the following claims or practices. These are often warning signs of potentially fraudulent herbal products or other "natural" treatments:

- The advertisements or promotional materials include words such as *breakthrough, magical* or *new discovery*. If the product were in fact a cure, it would be widely reported in the media, and your doctor would recommend it.
- Promotional materials include pseudo-medical jargon such as *detoxify, purify* and *energize*. Such claims are difficult to define and to measure.
- The manufacturer claims that the product can treat a wide range of symptoms, or cure or prevent a number of diseases. No single product can do this.
- The product is supposedly backed by scientific studies, but references aren't provided, are limited or are out-of-date.
- The product promotion mentions no negative side effects, only benefits.
- The manufacturer of the product accuses the government or medical profession of suppressing important information about the product's benefits. There is no reason for the government or medical profession to withhold information that could help people.

The healthy traveler

This section suggests ways to deal with common conditions that affect travelers. For most people, especially those with chronic health problems, it's always a good idea to talk with your doctor before you travel internationally.

■ Traveler's diarrhea

Diarrhea affects up to half of the people who travel to developing countries. To reduce your risk:

- Don't drink tap or spring water. Drink only bottled water. Sodas, beer or wine served in their original containers are acceptable. Avoid ice cubes. Beverages from boiled water, such as coffee and tea, are usually safe.
- Use bottled water to brush your teeth. Keep your mouth closed while showering.
- Don't eat food from street vendors.
- Avoid salads, buffet foods, undercooked meats, raw vegetables, grapes, berries, fruits that have been peeled or cut, and unpasteurized milk and dairy products.
- Ask your doctor whether you should take along anti-diarrhea medication.

■ Heat exhaustion

In hot climates, a day of sightseeing can leave you weak, dizzy, nauseated and perspiring faster than you can replenish lost fluids. To prevent heat exhaustion:

- Pace yourself. Go slow the first few days after arriving in a warm climate.
- Plan regular breaks in the shade. Carry water if you're unsure of sources along the way.
- Don't overeat.
- Drink liquids before you feel thirsty. Avoid alcoholic beverages.
- Wear lightweight, light-colored clothing and a broad-brimmed hat.
- At the first sign of heat exhaustion, get out of the sun and rest in the shade or an air-conditioned building.

■ Blisters

Blisters can be an unwelcome reminder to slow down. To avoid them:

- Wear comfortable shoes. Break in new shoes before leaving.
- Wear cotton or wool socks dusted inside with talcum powder.
- Use moleskin as a cushion and to protect areas of friction.

■ Altitude sickness

Decreased oxygen at higher altitudes can cause altitude sickness. Symptoms are usually mild but can be severe enough to require immediate medical help. They include headache, breathlessness, fatigue, nausea and disturbed sleep. To reduce your risk:

- **Start slowly.** Begin at an altitude below 9,000 feet.
- **Allow time to adjust.** Rest a day after arriving to adjust to the altitude.

- **Take it easy.** Slow down if you're out of breath or tired.
- **Limit ascent.** Once you reach 8,000 feet, don't climb more than 1,000 feet a day.
- **Sleep at a lower altitude.** If you're above 11,000 feet during the day, spend your nights at 9,000 feet or lower.
- **Avoid cigarettes, alcohol and too much caffeine.**
- **Consider medication.** Ask your doctor about acetazolamide (Diamox) or other prescription medications that may help prevent or lessen symptoms.
- **Talk with your doctor.** If you've had altitude sickness before, or if you have a chronic lung or heart problem, get your doctor's advice before departing.

■ Motion sickness

Any type of transportation can cause motion sickness. It can progress from a feeling of restlessness to a cold sweat, dizziness, and then vomiting and diarrhea. Motion sickness usually quiets down as soon as the motion stops. You may escape motion sickness by planning ahead.

- If you're traveling by ship, request a cabin in the forward or middle part of the ship, near the waterline. If you're on a plane, ask for a seat over the front edge of a wing. Once aboard, direct the air vent at your face. On a train, take a seat near the front and next to a window, and face forward. In an automobile, drive or sit in the front passenger's seat.
- If you begin to feel sick, focus on the horizon or a stationary object. Don't read. Keep your head still, resting against a seat back. Eat dry crackers or have a carbonated beverage to help settle your stomach. Avoid spicy food and alcohol.
- If you know you'll be sick, take an over-the-counter antihistamine such as meclizine (Bonine) or dimenhydrinate (Dramamine). Talk with your doctor about prescription medications such as scopolamine (Transderm Scop).

■ Traveling abroad

Before traveling overseas, especially if you have a health condition or take medications, review your plans with your doctor. If your plans include travel to a relatively remote location, consider consulting a specialist in travel medicine.

- **Get a head start on immunizations.** Immunizations needed depend on your destination, the length of your visit and your medical history. See your doctor at least four to six weeks — and preferably six months — before you depart to schedule the immunizations. Some require several injections spaced days, weeks or even months apart. Information on immunizations and health precautions for travelers is available from your local health department, your doctor and the Centers for Disease Control and Prevention (see "Travel information sources," page 286).
- **Get medical clearance.** Depending on your circumstances, your doctor may clear you for travel even if you have an unstable health condition. Take your doctor's letter with a list of your diagnoses and medications with you.
- **Take your medical history summary.** Make multiple copies. In case of an emergency, you may need copies for the medical professionals caring for you. If you have a history of heart problems or wear a pacemaker, ask for a copy of a recent electrocardiogram (ECG).
- **Know where medical care will be available.** Take with you a list of the names, addresses and telephone numbers of the recommended English-speaking doctors

and hospitals at your destination. Your doctor, local or state medical society, the International Association for Medical Assistance to Travellers (IAMAT), or the Bureau of Consular Affairs' Overseas Citizens Services (see "Travel information sources," page 286) can help you make your list.

- **Take copies of your prescriptions.** Request typewritten prescriptions (they're easier to read), including prescriptions for syringes and needles if you use these. Take your eyeglasses prescription, too.
- **Pack medication carefully.** Keep your prescription medications in their original containers, with typed labels, in your carry-on luggage. Always fill your prescriptions before you leave home and bring more than you think you'll need. If you're taking a prescription narcotic, obtain a letter of authorization on your physician's letterhead stationery. Know the laws of the countries you'll be in.
- **Double-check your health insurance.** Find out ahead of time how your health insurance plan handles medical care abroad, since many plans, including Medicare, do not cover health care costs overseas.
- **Learn about the countries you plan to visit.** Before you go, read up on the culture, people and history. For up-to-date information, obtain a consular information sheet from the Bureau of Consular Affairs' Overseas Citizens Services. This sheet provides information on health and security conditions.

■ Vaccines for international travel

In addition to making sure you've had your primary vaccine series — measles-mumps-rubella (MMR), chickenpox (varicella), tetanus-diphtheria, pertussis, polio — the Centers for Disease Control and Prevention (*https://wwwnc.cdc.gov/travel*) recommends that you consider these additional vaccines.

Booster vaccines or additional doses
- **Tetanus, diphtheria and whooping cough (pertussis).** Adults and teenagers should receive the tetanus, diphtheria and acellular pertussis booster vaccine (also known as Tdap) in place of one tetanus-diphtheria (Td) injection, and then continue with Td boosters every 10 years thereafter.
- **Polio.** Unless you've had a polio booster as an adult, you may need an additional single dose if you're traveling to parts of Africa, Asia, the Middle East, India and neighboring countries, and most of the former republics of the Soviet Union. For certain countries you may require a polio vaccine within the last year.
- **Measles.** If you were born in 1957 or after, consider a vaccine booster if you've only had one MMR vaccination in your life.
- **Pneumonia.** If you're age 65 or older, you have a chronic health problem (such as lung disease, heart disease or diabetes) or you're a smoker.
- **Influenza.** Recommended once a year for everyone over the age of 6 months and may be needed for destinations in the Southern Hemisphere depending on destination and time of year for travel
- **Shingles.** The shingles vaccine (Zostavax) is advised for people 60 years of age or older, whether or not they had shingles previously, except for those with certain types of immune deficiencies.

Additional vaccines

- **Yellow fever vaccine.** Recommended if you're traveling to certain parts of Africa and South America.
- **Hepatitis B vaccine.** Consider if you'll be staying more than one month in areas with high rates of hepatitis B (Southeast Asia, Africa, the Middle East, islands of the South and Western Pacific, and the Amazon region of South America).
- **Hepatitis A vaccine (or immune globulin).** Recommended for travelers to all areas except Japan, Australia, New Zealand, Northern and Western Europe, Canada and the United States.
- **Typhoid.** Recommended if you'll be staying in areas where food and water precautions are recommended and typhoid commonly occurs, such as many developing countries.
- **Meningococcal vaccine.** Recommended if you'll be traveling to another country for a school semester (and living in a dorm), to sub-Saharan Africa, or to Saudi Arabia for the annual hajj pilgrimage.
- **Japanese encephalitis vaccine.** Consider if you'll be staying longer than four weeks in Asia, including Japan, and particularly in Southeast Asia, where this disease is common.
- **Rabies vaccine.** Recommended if you'll be staying one to two months or longer (or in a rural region) in a developing country.

Air travel hazards

The fastest way to travel — by airplane — is also one of the safest. Yet by placing you thousands of feet in the air, moving at a speed of hundreds of miles per hour, air travel does subject your body to special challenges.

There are issues that only affect a small number of flyers. For example, people who scuba dive should avoid air travel 12 to 24 hours after scuba diving to decrease the risk of decompression sickness (the bends).

However, there are several common problems that you might experience during air travel, and self-care steps you can take to prevent or manage them.

Dehydration

The pressurized cabin of an airplane has extremely low humidity, only 5 to 10 percent. This can cause dehydration. To prevent dehydration, drink liquids such as water and fruit juices during your flight. Limit alcohol and caffeine.

Blood clots and leg swelling

Sitting during a long flight causes fluid to accumulate in the soft tissues in your legs. This increases your risk of a blood clot (deep vein thrombosis). To improve circulation back to your heart:

- Stand up and stretch periodically after the "wear your seat belt" sign is turned off. Take a walk through the cabin once an hour or so.
- Flex your ankles or press your feet against the floor or seat mountings in front of you.
- If you're prone to swollen ankles or have varicose veins, consider wearing support hose or OTC below-knee compression stockings. If you have additional risk factors for blood clots, wearing a prescription compression stocking is advised. In some high-risk situations, a medication for prevention of blood clots also may be needed.

Ear pain

To avoid ear pain during descent, try these strategies to equalize the pressure in your ears. (Also see "Airplane ear," page 68).

- With your lips tightly closed, try to gently blow air as though you were playing a trumpet. Don't blow too hard.
- Pinch your nose and swallow.
- Yawn, move your jaw, chew gum or swallow.
- If you typically have difficulty clearing your ears during air travel, review with your doctor.

Jet lag

If you've traveled by air to a different time zone, you're probably familiar with what it's like to get jet lag — that dragged-out, out-of-sync feeling. Not all jet lag is the same. Flying eastward — and therefore resetting your body clock forward — is often more difficult than flying westward and adding hours to your day. Most peoples' bodies adjust at the rate of about an hour a day. Thus, after a change of four time zones, your body will require about four days to resynchronize its usual rhythms.

- Reset your body's clock. Begin resetting your body's clock several days in advance of your departure by adopting a sleep-wake pattern similar to the day-night cycle at your destination.
- Drink plenty of fluids and eat lightly. Drink extra liquids during your flight to avoid dehydration, but limit beverages with alcohol and caffeine. They increase dehydration and may disrupt your sleep.
- Avoid taking a sleeping pill on the flight over. However, taking an over-the-counter sleep aid for the first three nights after reaching your destination may help you to adjust.

■ Questions and answers

Flying when you have a cold

Question: Can flying make a head cold worse?

Answer: Air travel probably won't make your cold worse. But landing with a cold can cause severe ear pain. The problem is air pressure. At high altitudes, air pressure is low. But as you descend, it increases.

When you have a cold, the tiny tube (eustachian tube) that connects your throat and middle ear is often blocked. Normally, the eustachian tube equalizes air pressure in your middle ear with the increasing outside pressure. Blockage in the tube leaves a vacuum in your middle ear, leading to a buildup of painful pressure on your eardrum. Your body's attempt to fill the vacuum causes fluid and sometimes blood to enter the middle ear.

To prevent ear pain when you fly with a cold, take a decongestant at least an hour before landing. You might also use a decongestant nasal spray before descent. These over-the-counter medicines help keep your eustachian tubes open. Sipping a nonalcoholic drink on takeoff and landing also helps keep these tubes open.

Drink plenty of nonalcoholic fluids when you fly, but especially when you have a cold. Liquids keep your throat and sinus membranes from drying and keep sinus secretions thin and easy to clear.

Melatonin and jet lag

Question: A friend suggested that I take melatonin supplements to prevent jet lag. Do they work?

Answer: Melatonin helps control your body's sleep and wake schedule. Some research suggests that taking a small amount of melatonin may help. You may try taking 1 to 3 milligrams of melatonin at bedtime for several days once you arrive at your destination. However, melatonin's benefits are often exaggerated.

Despite numerous books and articles about melatonin, much remains unknown about this hormone and its effects on the body, particularly when it's used long term or with other medications. If you're considering taking melatonin supplements, check with your doctor first — especially if you have any health conditions. He or she can help you determine the correct dose, which depends on the intended use.

Travel after a heart attack

Question: My husband has had a heart attack. Are there any special precautions we should take when traveling?

Answer: If your husband has heart disease, chest pain (angina) or a history of a heart attack or stroke, he should do the following.

- Be alert to the symptoms of a heart attack or stroke. At the first warning, seek emergency care. Know in advance where this medical care is available.
- Check the expiration date of nitroglycerin tablets. Get a new supply if they're older than 6 months.
- Avoid driving for more than four hours without a rest.
- Stay out of the midday sun if traveling in a hot, humid climate.
- Limit or avoid alcohol. It reduces the heart's pumping action.
- If he wears a pacemaker, have his doctor check the battery before the trip.
- Check with his doctor or cardiologist about the safety of travel with his medical condition. Travel may need to be delayed a few weeks to months.

Traveler's first-aid kit

Accidents and minor injuries can happen away from home. Be prepared to treat yourself and any companions for minor medical mishaps. Include these basic supplies:

Adhesive tape	Hydrocortisone cream (1 percent)
Aloe gel for sunburn	Insect repellent with DEET (20 to 50 percent)
Antacid	Laxative
Antibacterial ointment	Moist towelettes
Antibacterial hand wipes	Moleskin (for blisters)
Anti-diarrheal tablets, over-the-counter	Oral rehydration solution packets
Antihistamine	Pain relievers, over-the-counter
Anti-motion sickness medication	Scissors
Bandages (including elastic type)	Skin cream or moisturizing lotion
Cotton swabs	Sunscreen, sun protection factor (SPF) of at least 30
Cough suppressant	Thermometer, digital
Decongestant	Throat lozenges
Eyedrops, saline	Tweezers
Heartburn medicine, over-the-counter	

Travel information sources

Centers for Disease Control and Prevention (CDC)
Atlanta, Georgia
800-232-4636
https://wwwnc.cdc.gov/travel
The CDC's travel website offers information on specific countries, detailing diseases and how to prevent them, along with immunization recommendations for regions of the world. The site also gives information on useful travel-related mobile apps. The book *CDC Health Information for International Travel* (commonly called the Yellow Book) also is available for purchase.

Bureau of Consular Affairs
Overseas Citizens Services
Washington, D.C.
888-407-4747, if calling from the U.S. or Canada
+1 202-501-4444, if calling from overseas
www.travel.state.gov
The Bureau of Consular Affairs can provide information about overseas travel (such as tips for traveling abroad and how to apply for a passport) and assist with emergencies, if needed.

International Association for Medical Assistance to Travellers (IAMAT)
Niagara Falls, New York
716-754-4883
www.iamat.org
This organization can help you plan a healthy trip and connect you with reputable English-speaking doctors.

International Society of Travel Medicine
Dunwoody, Georgia
404-373-8282
www.istm.org
This organization offers an online global travel clinic directory.

Index

A

abdominal hysterectomy, 152
abdominal pain and discomfort, 56
abdominal thrusts (Heimlich maneuver), 4
abusive behavior, symptoms of, 203
acetaminophen, 163, 257, 258
Achilles tendinitis, 102
acid reflux, 64
acne, 118
acquired immunodeficiency syndrome (AIDS), 184, 185
acupuncture, 275–276
acute bacterial prostatitis, 142
acute pain, 40
acute shoulder pain, 92
addictive behavior
    alcohol use disorders, 188–191
    compulsive gambling, 197
    drug use and dependency, 196–197
    smoking and tobacco use, 192–195
adult immunizations, 226–227
AED. See automated external defibrillator
aerobic activity, 215
age-related hearing loss, 75
aging
    life expectation, 235–236
    maintaining health with age, 236
    physical changes, 235
    positive attitude and, 236
    social connections and, 236
    spirituality and, 236
AIDS. See acquired immuno-deficiency syndrome
airplane ear, 68
air pollution, indoor, 233–234
air travel
    hazards, 283–284
    jet lag, 284–285
    questions and answers, 284–285
    See also travel

alcohol use
    binge drinking, 188
    effects in body, 188
    hangover treatment, 191
    high blood pressure (hypertension) and, 183
    intoxication, 188
    teenage drinking and, 190
    workplace, 241–242
    See also addictive behavior
alcohol use disorders
    defined, 188
    individualized treatment, 190–191
    seeking evaluation, 189
    self-assessment, 189
    warning signs, 189
allergic reactions
    drug, 13
    food, 12–13
allergies, respiratory
    causes of, 158
    colds versus, 159
    hay fever, 114, 159
    immune response and, 158
    inhalers and, 167
    medical help, 159
    restless legs syndrome, 158–159
    self-care, 159
    self-monitoring with peak flow meter, 167
    testing for, 167
allergist, 250
alternative medicine, 268
Alzheimer's disease, 204
anaerobic activity, 215
anaphylaxis, 11
anemia, pregnancy and, 155
anesthesiologist, 250
angina, 111, 177
angioedema, 123
animal bites, 14
ankle and foot pain
    burning feet, 104
    causes of, 102
    flatfeet, 103
    hammertoe, 104
    heel pain, 105–106

    mallet toe, 104
    Morton's neuroma, 105
    self-care, 102
    swelling, 105
anorexia nervosa, 48
antihistamines, 259
anxiety disorders
    generalized anxiety disorder, 198
    obsessive-compulsive disorder (OCD), 198
    panic attacks and panic disorder, 199
    phobias, 199
    post-traumatic stress disorder (PTSD), 199
    social anxiety disorder, 198
appendicitis, 56
arthritis
    chronic pain, 41
    common forms of, 162
    coping at work, 239
    exercise and, 161
    gout, 92, 162
    infectious, 162
    joint protection, 164
    medications, 163
    PAD and, 177
    pain relief methods, 163
    rheumatoid, 162
    warning signs, 161
    See also osteoarthritis
asbestosis, 234
aspirin, 257–258
aspirin therapy, 178
asthma
    activity and, 166
    common triggers, 165
    defined, 165
    illustration, 165
    life-threatening attack, recognizing, 165
    medical help, 167
    self-care, 166
    wheezing and, 110
asymptomatic inflammatory prostatitis, 142
athlete's foot, 122
atopic dermatitis, 121

audiologist, 250
automated external defibrillator (AED), 2–3
automobile safety, 231
ayurveda, 277

B

baby rashes, 125
back
    anatomy, 50
    exercises, 55
    injury prevention, 53
    lifting properly and, 238
    protecting at workplace, 238
backache, pregnancy and, 156
back and neck problems
    back pain, 51–52
    back protection and, 238
    bulging disk, 53
    daily back routine and, 55
    herniated disk, 53
    osteoarthritis, 53
    osteoporosis, 53
    pain issues, 50
    prevention, 54
back pain
    in children, 52
    as job-related disability, 41
    self-care, 51–52
bacteria, in food-borne illness, 27
bad breath, 135
baker's cyst, 101
balance, maintaining, 35
baldness, 131
basal cell cancer, 129
bed-wetting, 45
bee stings, 15–16
belching, 60
binge drinking, 188
binge-eating disorder, 48
biofeedback, 272
birth control, 143, 153
bites and stings
    animal bites, 14
    human bites, 14
    insect bites and stings, 15–16
    snakebites, 15
    spider bites, 16
    tick bites, 16
black cohosh, 262
black eye, 76
bladder cancer, 170

bleeding
    internal, detecting, 10
    between periods, 147
    severe, 10
blepharitis, 79
blisters, 280–281
bloating, 60
blood clot on the brain, 32
blood pressure
    defined, 182
    high, 182–183
    low, 183
    monitoring, 183
    numbers, 182
    reading, 182
BMI. *See* body mass index
BMI calculator, 207
body mass index (BMI)
    chart, 207
    defined, 207
    determining, 206–208
    waist size and, 207–208
body odor, 47
boils, 118–119
bones
    anatomy, 85
    broken, 89
    fusing, 164
    realignment of, 164
boss, relationship with, 244
botulism, 26
brain, blood clot on, 32
breast, lump in, 144
breast cancer, 145–146, 169
breast density, 144
breast pain, 146
breathing
    exercises, 110
    relaxed, 223
bronchitis, 109–110
bronchodilators, 167
bruxism, 45
bulging disk, 53
bulimia nervosa, 48
bunions, 102
bupropion, 194
burning feet, 104
burns
    chemical, 18
    electrical, 19
    emergency treatment, 17–18
    first-degree, 17

    second-degree, 17
    sunburn, 19
    third-degree, 17
bursitis, 90, 101–102

C

caffeine, headaches and, 84
calcium supplements and osteoporosis, 149
calluses, 120
cancer
    breast, 145–146, 169
    cervical, 151
    colorectal, 169–170
    early diagnosis, 168
    endometrial (uterine), 170–171
    Hodgkin's lymphoma, 171
    lung, 169
    non-Hodgkin's lymphoma, 171
    oral, 139
    ovarian, 151, 171
    prostate, 141, 168
    signs, symptoms, and screening, 168
    skin, 129, 171
    statistics, 168
    testicular, 140, 171
    thyroid, 160, 171
canker sores, 136–137
carbon monoxide poisoning, 233
cardiologist, 250
cardiopulmonary resuscitation (CPR)
    defined, 2
    hands-only, 2
    for adults, 2–3
    for children, 3
    for infants, 3
carotenoids, 261
carpal tunnel, 96, 238
carpal tunnel syndrome, 96–97, 238
car safety seats, 231
cataracts, 80
cavities and toothache, 30
cellulitis, 119
cervical cancer, 151
checklist. *See* Ready, Check, Go! checklist
chemical burns, 18

chemical splash, 24
chest pain, 111, 177
chewing tobacco, 195
chickenpox, 125
children
    back pain, 52
    bladder, 170
    car safety, 231
    choking, 4
    ear infections, 71
    eye injuries and, 25
    fever and, 39
    hair loss, 131
    headache, 84
    rashes, 125
    skin cancer and, 129
    sleep disorders, 45
    vaccines schedule for,
        227–228
    weight loss or failure to
        grow, 48
chiropractic treatment, 274–275
chlamydia infections, 184–185
choking, 4
cholesterol
    HDL, 213
    high, causes of, 213
    LDL, 213–214
    lowering, 213–214
    need for, 213
    numbers, 214
chondroitin, 263
chronic bacterial prostatitis, 142
chronic fatigue syndrome, 37
chronic pain
    defined, 40
    forms of, 41
    treatment of, 43
    See also pain
chronic prostatitis/chronic
    pelvic pain syndrome, 142
claudication, 100
clearing objects in eye, 25
cluster headache, 82
coenzyme Q10, 263
cold remedies, 259–260
cold sores (fever blisters),
    137–138
cold-weather problems
    frostbite, 18, 20
    hypothermia, 21
    prevention, 21

colic, 57
colorectal cancer, 169–170
    screening, 170, 225
common cold, 114, 133
complementary and alternative
    medicine (CAM). See integra-
    tive medicine
complementary medicine, 268
compulsive gambling, 197
computer screens and eyestrain,
    245–246
concussion, 32
congestion, nasal, 114
congestive heart failure, 110, 179
conjunctivitis, 78
constipation
    laxatives and, 58
    overview, 58
    pregnancy and, 156
contact dermatitis, 121
contact lenses, 81
corneal abrasion (scratch), 24
corns, 120
coronary artery disease, 177
corticosteroids, 163
cough-cold combinations, 259
coughing, 107–108
co-worker conflict, 243
COX-2 inhibitor, 163
CPR. See cardiopulmonary
    resuscitation
cradle cap, 124
Crohn's disease, 267
croup, 109
cuts and scrapes, 22–23

D
Daily Values (DV), 265–266
dandruff, 120
decongestant nasal sprays, 114
decongestants, 259
deep vein thrombosis, 100
dehydration, 283
dementia, 204
dengue fever, 15
depression
    causes of, 201
    coping with loss and, 201
    major, 200
    minor, 200
    seeking help for, 201
    self-care, 200

suicide signs and, 202
    treatment options, 202
dermatitis, 121
dermatologist, 250
designer/club drugs, 196
DHEA, 263
diabetes
    activity and, 175
    blood sugar monitoring, 174
    complications, 172
    defined, 172
    foot care and, 176
    healthy food selection, 175
    high blood sugar and, 176
    high ketones (diabetic keto-
        acidosis) and, 176
    low blood sugar
        (hypoglycemia) and, 176
    medical emergencies, 176
    medication use, 175
    metabolic syndrome and, 173
    prediabetes, 172, 174
    risk factors, 173
    self-care, 174–175
    testing for, 174
    type 1, 172
    type 2, 172–173
    warning signs, 173
diabetic ketoacidosis, 176
diaper rash, 124
diarrhea, 59
    when traveling, 280
Dietary Reference Intakes
    (DRIs), 265–266
dietary supplements
    antioxidants, 261
    choosing and using, 266–267
    decision to take, 264–265
    defined, 261
    digestive health problems
        and, 267
    fish oil, 262
    herbs, 262–263
    hormones, 263
    how much do you need,
        265–266
    minerals, 265–266
    safety, 267
    storing, 266
    vitamins, 261, 265–266
    whole foods and, 264
    See also healthy consumer

digestive system
    abdominal pain and
      discomfort, 56
    colic, 57
    constipation, 58
    diarrhea, 59
    excessive gas and gas
      pains, 60
    gallstones, 61
    gastritis, 61
    hemorrhoids and rectal
      bleeding, 62
    hernias, 63
    indigestion, 64
    irritable bowel syndrome,
      41, 65
    nausea and vomiting, 66
    peptic ulcers, 67
dislocated elbow, 93
dislocations, 31
dizziness and fainting, 34–35
doctors
    finding, 248–249
    primary care, 248
    specialists, 250
    surgeons, 252
    trusting instincts and, 249
    visiting, 249
    See also health care providers
domestic violence, 203
DRIs. *See* Dietary Reference
  Intakes
drool rash, 124
drooping eyelid, 79
drug allergies, 13
drug use
    common drugs of abuse, 196
    dependency and, 196–197
    teenager, 197
    workplace, 242
dry eyes, 77
dry skin, 121
DV. *See* Daily Values

E
E. coli, 27
ears
    air travel and, 284
    airplane ear, 68
    anatomy, 68
    foreign objects in, 69
    functioning of, 68

hearing loss and, 74–75
infections, 70–71
ringing in, 72
ruptured eardrum, 69
swimmer's ear, 72
wax blockage, 73
ear tubes, 70
earwax blockage, 73
eating disorders, 48
echinacea, 262
eczema (dermatitis), 121
elbow and forearm
    dislocated elbow, 93
    hyperextended elbow, 93
    tennis elbow or golfer's
      elbow, 94
electrical burns, 19
emergencies/urgent care
    allergic reactions, 12–13
    bites and stings, 14–16
    burns, 17–19
    choking, 4
    cold-weather problems,
      20–21
    CPR, 2–3
    cuts, scrapes and wounds,
      22–23
    eye injuries, 24–25
    foodborne illness, 26–27
    heart attack, 5–6
    heat-related problems, 28
    overview, 1
    poisoning, 9
    poisonous plants, 29
    severe bleeding, 10
    shock, 11
    stroke, 7–8
    tooth problems, 30
    trauma: bones and muscles,
      31–32
    trauma: head injuries, 32
emergency medicine specialist,
  250
emergency preparedness
    disaster supply kits, 229–230
    emergency types, 229
    flu epidemic preparation,
      230
    need for action, 229
    workplace, 241
emphysema, 110
endocrinologist, 250

endometrial (uterine) cancer,
  170–171
endometriosis, 152
ephedra (ma-huang), 262
epididymitis, 140
erectile dysfunction (ED), 142–143
essential (primary) hypertension,
  182
excessive gas and gas pains, 60
exercises
    for breathing improvement,
      110
    for heel pain, 106
    interval training, 220
    for office workers, 239–240
    program, 218
    for strengthening leg
      muscles, 98
    for walkers, 219
eye injuries
    chemical splash, 24
    common sense with, 25
    corneal abrasion (scratch), 24
    foreign object, 25
eyelid inflammation, 79
eyelid twitching, 79
eyes and vision
    anatomy, 76
    black eye, 76
    cataracts, 80
    diseases, 80
    drooping eyelid, 79
    dry eyes, 77
    excessive watering, 77
    eye strain, 245–246
    eyelid inflammation, 79
    floaters, 77
    glasses and contact lenses, 81
    glaucoma, 80
    impaired vision,
      transportation and, 80
    macular degeneration, 80
    overview, 76
    pink eye, 78
    sensitivity to glare, 79
    sty, 79
    taking care of, 76
    twitching eyelid, 79

F
fainting, 34–35
falls, preventing, 232

family medical tree, 254
family physician, 250
fatigue
    chronic fatigue syndrome
        and, 37
    common causes, 36
    defined, 36
    self-care, 37
fever
    defined, 38
    kids' care, 39
    self-care, 38
    taking temperatures and, 39
feverfew, 262, 271
fibromyalgia
    defined, 41
    knee pain and, 100
    self-care, 91
    symptoms, 91
fifth disease, 125
first aid
    allergic reactions, 12–13
    bites, 14–16
    bleeding, 10
    breathing problems, 2–4
    burns, 17–19
    choking, 4
    CPR, 2–3
    cuts and scrapes, 22–23
    dislocations, 31
    eye injuries, 24–25
    fractures, 31
    frostbite, 20
    head injury, 32
    heart attack, 5–6
    heat problems, 28
    Heimlich maneuver, 4
    home medical supplies, 260
    hypothermia, 21
    insect stings, 15–16
    object in eye, 25
    poisoning, 9
    poison ivy, oak, sumac, 29
    puncture wounds, 23
    shock, 11
    sprains, 32
    stroke, 7–8
    tooth loss, 30
    trauma, 31–32
    travel supplies, 285
    wounds, 22–23
first-degree burns, 17

fish oil, 262
fitness
    defined, 215
    program, starting, 216
    walking your way to,
        217–218
flatfeet, 103
floaters, 77
flu epidemic, 230
flu pandemic, 229
folic acid, 261
food allergies, 12–13
foodborne illness
    bacteria types and, 27
    defined, 25
    food handling safety and, 26
    self-care, 27
foot care, diabetes and, 176
foot pain. See ankle and
    foot pain
foreign objects
    in ear, 69
    in eye, 24
    in nose, 112
fractures
    ankle and foot pain and, 102
    bone, 31, 89
    skull, 32
frostbite, 20
fungal infections, 122

G
gallstones, 61
gambling, compulsive, 197
ganglion cysts, 95
garlic, 262
gas, passing, 60
gas pains, 60
gastric bypass, 267
gastritis, 61
gastroenteritis, 66
gastroenterologist, 250
gastroparesis, 66, 267
generalized anxiety disorder, 198
geneticist, 250
genital herpes, 184, 185
genital warts, 184, 186
ginger, 262
ginkgo, 262
ginseng, 263
glasses, 81
glaucoma, 80

glucosamine, 263
glue and inhalants, 196
golfer's elbow, 94
gonorrhea, 184, 186
gout, 92, 162
growing pains, 86
gynecologist, 250

H
hair loss, 131
hallucinogens, 196
hammertoe, 104
hand-washing, 234
hay fever, 114, 159
headache
    caffeine and, 84
    in children, 84
    cluster, 83
    defined, 82
    migraine, 41, 83
    self-care, 83
    tension-type, 41, 82
    triggers, avoiding, 84
    types of, 82
head injuries, 32
health
    age and, 235–236
    workplace and, 237–246
health care providers
    finding, 248–249
    nurses, 251
    occupational therapists, 251
    pharmacists, 251
    physical therapists, 251
    physician assistants, 251
    primary care, 248
    specialists, 250
    surgeons, 252
    trusting instincts and, 249
    visiting, 249
healthy consumer
    dietary supplements,
        261–267
    family medical tree, 254
    health care provider and,
        248–252
    home medical testing kits,
        253
    integrative medicine,
        268–279
    medications, 255–260
healthy cooking, 212

healthy eating
  aging and, 236
  cooking and, 212
  high blood pressure
    (hypertension) and, 183
  Mayo Clinic Healthy Weight
    Pyramid and, 211
  mix-and-match salads and,
    212
  plant foods, 210
  self-care, 210
  serving recommendations,
    211
  weight loss and, 208–209
  whole foods, 264
healthy traveler, 280
healthy weight
  body mass index (BMI) and,
    206–208
  determination, 206–208
  high blood pressure
    (hypertension) and, 183
  Mayo Clinic Healthy Weight
    Pyramid and, 211
  See also weight loss
hearing
  age-related hearing loss, 75
  earwax blockage and, 73
  noise-related hearing loss, 74
  See also ears
hearing aids, 75
heart attack
  coronary artery disease and,
    177
  getting help fast, 5
  medications, 6
  prevention, 6
  signs and symptoms, 5, 177
  surgical and other
    procedures, 6
  travel after, 285
  while waiting for help, 6
heartburn
  chest pain and, 111
  defined, 64
  pregnancy and, 156
  self-care, 64
heart disease
  aspirin therapy and, 178
  coronary artery disease, 177
  medical help, 179
  risk factors, 178

self-care, 179
signs and symptoms, 177
heart failure, 100, 179
heart rate, checking pulse to get,
  218
heat exhaustion, 28
heat problems, 28
heat rash, 124
heatstroke, 28
heel pain, 105–106
Heimlich maneuver, 4
hematologist, 250
hemorrhagic strokes, 7
hemorrhoids
  formation of, 62
  pregnancy and, 156
  self-care, 62
hepatitis
  defined, 180
  hepatitis A, 180
  hepatitis B, 180–181, 184, 186
  hepatitis C, 181
  virus spreading prevention
    of, 181
hepatitis A vaccine, 283
hepatitis B vaccine, 283
herbs
  dangerous, avoiding, 271
  dietary supplements, 262–263
  drug interactions, 271
  limited FDA regulation, 270
  research, 271
  safe use of, 270–271
hernias, 63
herniated disk, 53
hiatal hernia, 63
high blood cholesterol, 213
high blood pressure
  (hypertension)
  defined, 182
  medications, 183
  readings, 182
  self-care, 183
  terminology, 182
high-intensity interval training
  (HIIT), 220
hip pain, 97
HIV. See human immuno-
  deficiency virus)
hives, 123
hoarseness or loss of voice,
  135–136

Hodgkin's lymphoma, 171
home medical supplies, 260
home medical testing kits, 253
homeopathy, 276–277
hormones, 263
hostility, workplace, 244
human bites, 14
human immunodeficiency virus
  (HIV), 184
human papillomavirus (HPV),
  151
humidifiers, 108
hyperextended elbow, 93
hypertension, 182–183
hyperthyroidism, 160
hypnosis, 272–273
hypoglycemia, 176
hypotension, 183
hypothermia, 21
hypothyroidism, 160
hysterectomy, 152

I
ibuprofen, 258
illness, stress and, 222
immunizations
  adult, 226–227
    well-child schedule, 227–228
immunologist, 250
impetigo, 123
indigestion, 64
indoor air pollution, 233–234
infants
  colic, 57
  CPR for, 3
infectious arthritis, 162
infectious disease specialist, 250
influenza
  cold versus, 115
  sore throat and, 133
  vaccine, 282
ingrown toenails, 132
inguinal hernia, 63
insect bites and stings, 15–16
integrative medicine
  ayurveda, 277
  claims of treatment success,
    269
  complementary and alterna-
    tive medicine versus, 279
  defined, 268
  homeopathy, 276–277

medical fraud and, 279
mind-body medicine, 272–276
misinformation on the internet, 278
most commonly used, 269
natural products, 270–272
naturopathy, 277
promise and peril of new treatment options, 268
research, 269
steps in considering treatment, 278–279
strategies, 268
international travel
  doctor consultation before, 281
  tips for, 281
  vaccines for, 282–283
  See also travel
internet
  misinformation on, 278
  ordering medications on, 256
internist, 250
interval training, 220
intestinal pseudo-obstruction, 267
irregular periods, 147
irritable bowel syndrome
  defined, 41
  self-care, 65
  signs and symptoms, 65
ischemic strokes, 7

J
jammed finger, 95
Japanese encephalitis vaccine, 283
jet lag, 284, 285
job-noise exposure levels, 74
jock itch, 122
joint replacement, 164
joints
  anatomy, 85
  arthritis and protection of, 164
  ball-and-socket, 86
  hinge, 86
  R.I.C.E. for injury, 87

K
kava, 263
knee pain, 100–101
knee supports and braces, 101

L
lactose intolerance, 60
laryngitis, 135–136
LASIK eye surgery, 81
laxative use, 58
lead poisoning, 232
leg pain
  defined, 98
  muscle cramps, 98–99
  pulled hamstring muscle, 98
  shin splints, 99
  swollen legs, 99–100
leg swelling, 99–100
leukoplakia, 138
lice, 126
life expectancy, 235
lifting properly, 54
ligaments, sprains, 88
lightheadedness and fainting, 34
limbs, muscles, bones and joints
  ankle and foot pain, 102–106
  bones, 85
  bursitis, 90
  elbow and forearm pain, 93–94
  fibromyalgia, 91
  fractures, 89
  gout, 92, 162
  hip pain, 97
  joints, 86
  knee pain, 100–101
  leg pain, 98–100
  muscles and tendons, 85
  nerves, 86
  shoulder pain, 92–93
  sprains, 88
  strains, 87
  tendinitis, 90–91
  wrist, hand, and finger pain, 95–97
long-term memory, 204
loss, coping with, 201
low blood pressure (hypotension), 183
lung cancer
  checkups and screening, 169
  risk factors, 169
  warning signs, 169
  wheezing and, 110
lungs, chest and breathing
  bronchitis, 109
  chest pain, 111
  coughing, 107–108
  croup, 109
  palpitations, 111
  shortness of breath, 110
  wheezing, 110
Lyme disease, 16
lymphedema, 100

M
macular degeneration, 80
male birth control, 143
mallet toe, 104
mammograms, 145
marijuana and hashish, 196
massage, 275
Mayo Clinic, about, vi
Mayo Clinic Healthy Weight Pyramid, 208, 210–211
measles, 125
measles vaccine, 282
medical fraud, 279
medical history, 254
medical supplies, home, 260
medications
  cold remedies, 259–260
  home medical supplies, 260
  ordering on the internet, 256
  pain relievers, 257–258
  rules when taking, 255
melanoma, 129
melatonin
  defined, 263
  jet lag and, 285
memory, improving, 204
memory loss, 204
meningococcal vaccine, 283
menopause, 149
men's health
  age-specific tests, 225–226
  enlarged prostate, 141
  erectile dysfunction (ED), 142–143
  male birth control, 143
  prostatitis, 142
  testicular pain, 140
menstrual cramps, 146
metabolic syndrome, 173
middle ear infection, 70
migraine
  characteristics of, 82
  as chronic pain, 41
  theory, 82

mind-body medicine
    acupuncture, 275–276
    biofeedback, 272
    chiropractic treatment, 274, 275
    hypnosis, 272–273
    massage, 275
    osteopathic manipulation, 274–275
    tai chi, 273–274
    therapeutic touch, 275
    yoga, 273
    See also integrative medicine
moles, 127
mononucleosis, 133
mood, xvii
morning sickness, 155
mosquito bites, 15
motion sickness, 281
mouth sores, 136–138
muscle cramps, 98–99
muscles
    anatomy, 85
    R.I.C.E. for injury, 87
    strains, 87

N

nail fungal infections, 132
naproxen sodium, 258
natural products, 270–272
naturopathy, 277
nausea and vomiting, 66
neonatologist, 250
nephrologist, 250
nerves, 85
neurodermatitis, 121
neurologist, 250
neuropathic pain, 41
nicotine
    as addictive substance, 192
    gum, 193
    inhalers, 193–194
    lozenges, 193
    nasal spray, 193
    patches, 193
    replacement therapy, 193–194
    teenage, 195
    withdrawal, coping with, 194
    See also smoking
nightmares, 45
night terrors, 45
noise-related hearing loss, 74

noises, sound levels of, 74
nonallergic rhinitis, 114
non-Hodgkin's lymphoma, 171
nonsteroidal anti-inflammatory drugs (NSAIDs), 163, 257
noroviruses, 27
nose and sinuses
    cold versus flu and, 115
    foreign objects in nose, 112
    loss of sense of smell, 112
    nosebleeds, 113
    runny nose, 114
    sinusitis, 115
    stuffy nose, 114
nosebleeds, 113
NSAIDs. *See* nonsteroidal anti-inflammatory drugs
nurses, 251
nutrition, xvi

O

obesity, 207
obsessive-compulsive disorder (OCD), 198
obstetrician, 250
occupational therapists, 251
oncologist, 250
oophorectomy, 152
ophthalmologist, 250
opioids, 196
oral cancer, 139
oral thrush, 138
orchitis, 140
organization, this book, v
orthopedist, 250
osteoarthritis
    as back and neck problem, 53
    cause and frequency, 162
    defined, 41
    joint protection, 164
    key symptoms, 162
    knee pain and, 101
    medications, 163
    methods to relieve pain, 163
    surgery for, 164
    See also arthritis
osteopathic manipulation, 274–275
osteoporosis
    defined, 53, 149
    menopause and, 149
otorhinolaryngologist, 250

ovarian cancer, 151, 171
over-the-counter medications
    cold remedies, 259
    oral pain relievers, 258

P

PAD. *See* peripheral artery disease
pain
    abdominal, 56
    acute, 40
    after shingles, 128
    ankle and foot, 102–106
    back, 41, 50–52
    in breast, 146
    chest, 111
    chronic, 41–43
    ear, 284
    elbow and forearm, 93–94
    functioning of, 40
    gas, 60
    heel, 105–106
    hip, 97
    knee, 100–101
    leg, 98–100
    medication use, 43
    natural painkillers and, 42
    role of emotions and behavior in, 41
    self-care, 42
    shoulder, 92–93
    testicular, 140
    wrist, hand, and finger, 95–96
painkillers, natural, 42
pain relievers
    matching the pill to the pain, 257
    over-the-counter, 258
    self-care, 258
    separating help from hype, 257
pain-relieving medications, 43
palpitations, 111
pancreatitis, 267
panic attacks, 199
panic disorder, 199
Pap test, 151
pathologist, 250
pediatrician, 250
peptic ulcers, 67
Percent Daily Values (%DV), 266

periods
    bleeding between, 147
    irregular, 147
peripheral artery disease (PAD), 177
peripheral neuropathy, 41
pharmacists, 251
phlebitis, 100
phobias, 199
physiatrist, 250
physical activity
    aerobic activity, 215
    aging and, 236
    anaerobic activity, 215
    benefits of, 215
    calories burned by, 216
    checklist and, xviii
    defined, 220
    heart rate and, 218
    high blood pressure
        (hypertension) and, 183
    walking, 217–218
    weight loss and, 209
    See also exercises; fitness
physical therapists, 251
physician assistants, 251
pink eye, 78
plant foods, 210
plants, poisonous, 29
PMS. See premenstrual
    syndrome
pneumonia
    vaccine, 282
    wheezing and, 110
poisoning
    carbon monoxide, 233
    emergencies, 9
    lead, 232
poisonous plants, 29
polio vaccine, 282
postherpetic neuralgia, 128
post-traumatic stress disorder
    (PTSD), 199
postural hypotension, 183
precordial catch, 111
prediabetes, 172, 174
pregnancy
    common problems during,
        155–156
    home tests, 154
    self-care, 154
prehypertension, 182

premenstrual syndrome (PMS),
    147–148
presbyopia, 81
preventive care, xvii
preventive medicine specialist,
    250
primary biliary cirrhosis, 267
progressive muscle relaxation, 223
prostate cancer, 141, 168
prostate gland enlargement, 141
prostatitis, 142
protection
    carbon monoxide poisoning,
        233
    emergency preparedness,
        229–230
    fall prevention, 232
    flu epidemic, 230
    hand-washing, 234–235
    indoor air pollution, 233–234
    lead exposure, 232
    risk at home, 231
    risk on the road, 231
psoriasis, 127
psychiatrist, 250
psychologist, 250
PTSD. See post-traumatic stress
    disorder
pulled hamstring muscle, 98
pulmonologist, 250
puncture wounds, 23

R
rabies, risk of, 14
rabies vaccine, 283
radiologist, 250
radon, 233
rashes
    baby, 124
    childhood, 125
Ready, Check, Go! checklist
    getting started, xiv
    mood, xvii
    nutrition, xvi
    overview, xiii
    physical activity, xviii
    preventive care, xvii
    safety, xix
    tobacco use, xiv
    weight, xv
rectal bleeding, 62
relaxation techniques, 223

restless legs syndrome, 45
rheumatoid arthritis, 41, 162
rheumatologist, 250
R.I.C.E., 87
ringing in the ear, 72
ringworm, 122
roseola, 125
rotator cuff disorder, 92
runny nose, 114
ruptured eardrum, 69

S
safety
    carbon monoxide poisoning,
        233
    checklist and, xix
    dietary supplements, 267
    emergency preparedness,
        229–230
    fall prevention, 232
    hand-washing, 234–235
    herbal treatments, 270–271
    at home, 231
    indoor air pollution, 233–234
    lead exposure, 232
    on the road, 231
    workplace, 241
salads, mix-and-match, 212
salmonella, 27
SAMe, 264
saw palmetto, 263, 271
scabies, 126
scarring, 23
screening
    age-specific tests for men,
        225–226
    age-specific tests for
        women, 225
    cancer, 140, 151, 168, 169
    men's health, 140, 225–226
    recommendations, 226
    women's health, 151, 225
seborrheic dermatitis, 121
secondary hypertension, 182
second-degree burns, 17
secondhand smoke, 195
selenium, 263
sensitivity to glare, 79
sensory memory, 204
serving recommendations,
    healthy eating, 211
severe bleeding, 10

sexually transmitted infections (STIs)
 AIDS, 184, 185
 chlamydia infections, 184, 185
 genital herpes, 184, 185
 genital warts, 184, 186
 gonorrhea, 184, 186
 hepatitis B, 184, 186
 risky behaviors and, 184
 syphilis, 184, 186
 types of, 184
 use of condoms and, 184
shift workers, sleep tips for, 241–242
shingles
 defined, 128
 self-care, 128
 vaccine, 282
shin splints, 99
shock, 11
shoes, proper fitting, 104
shortness of breath, 110
short-term memory, 204
shoulder pain, 92–93
simple wounds, 22
sinusitis, 115
skin, hair and nails
 acne, 118
 baby rashes, 124
 boils, 118–119
 cellulitis, 119
 corns and calluses, 119
 dandruff, 120
 dry skin, 121
 eczema (dermatitis), 121
 fungal infections, 122
 hair loss, 131
 hives, 123
 impetigo, 123
 ingrown toenails, 132
 itching and rashes, 124
 lice, 126
 moles, 127
 MRSA infection, 119
 nail fungal infections, 132
 proper skin care and, 117
 psoriasis, 127
 scabies, 126
 signs of skin cancer and, 129
 warts, 130
 wrinkled skin, 130
skin cancer, 129, 171

skin care, 117
skull fracture, 32
sleep
 back and neck problems and, 54
 disorders, 44–45
 pregnancy and, 156
 for shift workers, 241–242
sleep apnea, 45
sleepiness, excessive, 45
sleepwalking, 45
smell, loss of sense of, 112
smoking
 aging and, 236
 checklist and, xiv
 chewing tobacco and, 195
 deaths related to, 192
 high blood pressure (hypertension) and, 183
 as indoor air pollution, 233
 nicotine and, 192
 nicotine replacement therapy and, 193–194
 secondhand smoke and, 195
 suggestions for stopping, 192
snakebites, 15
social anxiety disorder, 198
social connections, aging and, 236
sore throat, 133–134
specialists, health care, 250
spider bites, 16
spirituality, aging and, 236
sports injuries, 88
sprains, 32, 88, 100, 102
squamous cell cancer, 129
St. John's wort, 263, 271
stasis dermatitis, 121
STIs. See sexually transmitted infections
stimulants, 196
stings, 15–16
strains, 87, 100, 102
strangulated hernia, 63
strep throat, 133
stress
 causes of, 221
 heart and blood vessel disease and, 221
 illnesses and, 222
 immune system suppression and, 221
 signs and symptoms of, 222

stress management
 defined, 221
 high blood pressure (hypertension) and, 183
 importance of, 221
 progressive muscle relaxation, 223
 relaxed breathing, 223
 self-care, 224
 visual imagery, 223
 workplace, 243–244
stroke
 prevention, 8
 risk factors beyond control, 8
 TIAs and, 7–8
 treatment, 8
 types of, 7
 warning signs, 7
stuffy nose, 114
sty, 79
suicide warning signs, 202
sunburn, 19
supplements. See dietary supplements
surgeons, 250, 252
surgery, questions to ask before, 252
sweating, 46
swelling (edema), 155
swimmer's ear, 72
swollen feet, 105
syphilis, 184, 186

T
tai chi, 273–274
technology, coping with, 245–246
teenagers
 alcohol use, 190
 drug use, 197
 smoking, 195
temperatures, taking, 39
tendinitis, 90–91, 100, 102
tennis elbow, 94
tension-type headache, 41, 82
testicular cancer, 140, 171
testicular pain, 140
testicular torsion, 140
tetanus, diphtheria and whooping cough vaccine, 282
tetanus infection, 23
tetanus vaccine, 23
therapeutic touch, 275

third-degree burns, 17
throat and mouth
  bad breath, 135
  cold sores (fever blisters), 137–138
  hoarseness or loss of voice, 135–136
  leukoplakia, 138
  mouth sores, 136–137
  oral cancer, 139
  oral thrush, 138
  sore throat, 133–134
thumb pain, 97
thyroid cancer, 160, 171
thyroid disorders, 160
TIA (transient ischemic attack), 7–8
tick bites, 16
time management, 244
tinnitus, 72
toenail, ingrown, 132
toenail fungal infections, 132
toe problems
  bunions, 102
  gout, 92, 162
  hammertoe, 104
  mallet toe, 104
toothache, 30
tooth loss, 30
toxic shock syndrome, 148
transient ischemic attack (TIA), 7–8
trauma
  bones and muscles, 31–32
  head injuries, 32
travel
  air travel hazards, 283–284
  blisters and, 280
  first-aid kit, 285
  after heart attack, 285
  information sources, 286
  international, 281–283
  motion sickness, 281
  questions and answers, 284–285
  tips for traveling abroad, 281–282
  traveler's diarrhea and, 280
  vaccines for, 282–283
traveler's diarrhea, 280–281
trigger finger, 95
typhoid vaccine, 283

U
ulcers, stomach, 67
urgent care. See emergencies/ urgent care
urinary incontinence, 150
urinary tract infections (UTIs), 150
urination problems
  in men, 141, 142
  in women, 150
urologists, 250
uterine fibroids, 152
uterine polyps, 152
UTIs. See urinary tract infections

V
vaccines
  adult, 226–227
  for international travel, 282–283
  schedule for children, 227–228
vaginal bleeding, 147
vaginal discharge, 150
vaginal hysterectomy, 152
vaginal yeast infections, 150
vaginitis, 150
varenicline, 194
varicose veins, 155
venous insufficiency, 100
vertigo, 34
vision problems. See eyes and vision
visual imagery, 223
vitamins, 261
voice, loss of, 135–136
vomiting, 66

W
waist size, 207–208
walking
  benefits of, 217
  calories burned by, 216, 218
  exercises for walkers and, 219
  frequency and duration, 218
  intensity, 217–218
  planning your program, 217–219
  tips, 217
  warm-up/cool-down, 218
  See also fitness; physical activity
warts, 130
watery eyes, 77
weight
  checklist and, xv
  gain, 47
  unexpected changes, 47–48
  See also healthy weight
weight loss
  body mass index (BMI) and, 206–208
  eating behaviors and, 209
  getting started, 208
  healthy eating and, 208–209
  as healthy goal, 206
  physical activity and, 209
  tips on, 208–209
  unexplained, 47–48
  See also healthy weight
well-child immunization schedule, 227–228
West Nile virus, 15
wheezing, 110
whole foods, 264
whooping cough (pertussis) vaccine, 226, 227, 228
women's health
  age-specific tests, 225
  birth control methods, 153
  bleeding between periods, 147
  breast cancer, 145–146
  cancer screening, 151
  endometriosis, 152
  hysterectomy, 152
  irregular periods, 147
  lump in your breast, 144
  mammograms and, 145
  menopause, 149
  menstrual cramps, 146
  osteoporosis, 149
  pain in your breast, 146
  pregnancy, 154–156
  premenstrual syndrome (PMS), 147–148
  toxic shock syndrome, 148
  urinary problems, 150
  uterine fibroids, 152
  uterine polyps, 151
  vaginal discharge, 150
  vaginal dryness, 149

workplace
  alcohol use, 241, 242
  arthritis at, 239
  back protection, 238
  burnout, 243
  computer screens and
    eyestrain and, 245–246
  co-worker conflict, 243
  drugs and, 242
  emergency preparedness,
    241
  exercise for office workers,
    239–240
  hand and wrist care, 238
  health and, 237–246
  hostility and, 244
  medication and alcohol use,
    241
  relationship with boss, 244
  sleeping tips for shift
    workers, 241–242
  stress relievers, 243–244
  technology, 245–246
  time management, 244
  workstation, 245–246
workstation, 245–246
wounds
  puncture, 23
  scarring and, 23
  simple, 22–23
wrinkled skin, 130
wrist, hand and finger pain
  carpal tunnel syndrome,
    96–97
  ganglion cysts, 95
  jammed finger, 95
  overview, 95
  self-care, 95
  thumb pain, 97
  trigger finger, 96

Y
yellow fever vaccine, 283
yoga, 273

Z
Zika virus, 15